Hot Stone MASSAGE

A Three-Dimensional Approach

Hot Stone MASSAGE

A Three-Dimensional Approach

LESLIE BRUDER
Founder of the Institute for Phenomenal Touch Massage
Eldorado Springs, Colorado

LEARNING RESOURCES CENTRE
Havering College of Further and Higher education
HAVERING COLLEGE

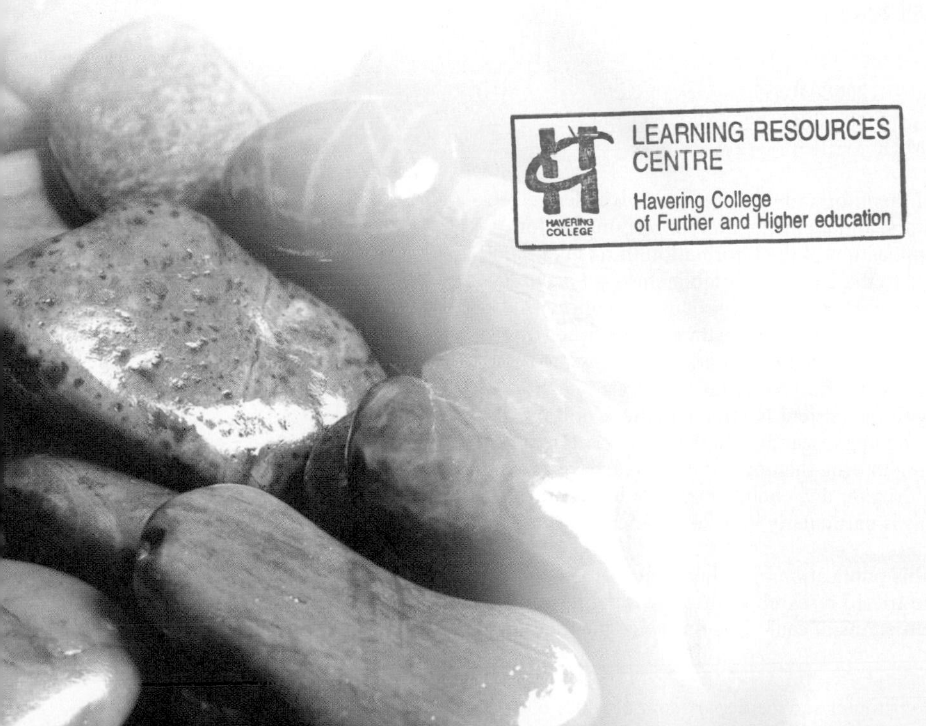

Wolters Kluwer | Lippincott Williams & Wilkins
Philadelphia • Baltimore • New York • London
Buenos Aires • Hong Kong • Sydney • Tokyo

615.822 AG.
170829

Acquisitions Editor: John Goucher
Managing Editor: Jennifer Walsh, Rachelle Detweiler
Marketing Manager: Zhan Caplan
Designer: Doug Smock
Production Editor: Julie Montalbano
Compositor: Aptara, Inc.

Copyright © 2010 Lippincott Williams & Wilkins, a Wolters Kluwer business.

351 West Camden Street
Baltimore, MD 21201

530 Walnut Street
Philadelphia, PA 19106

Printed in China.

Phenomenal Touch is a registered trademark.

All rights reserved. This book is protected by copyright. No part of this book may be reproduced or transmitted in any form or by any means, including as photocopies or scanned-in or other electronic copies, or utilized by any information storage and retrieval system without written permission from the copyright owner, except for brief quotations embodied in critical articles and reviews. Materials appearing in this book prepared by individuals as part of their official duties as U.S. government employees are not covered by the above-mentioned copyright. To request permission, please contact Lippincott Williams & Wilkins at 530 Walnut Street, Philadelphia, PA 19106, via email at permissions@lww.com, or via website at lww.com (products and services).

9 8 7 6 5 4 3 2 1

Library of Congress Cataloging-in-Publication Data

Bruder, Leslie.
Hot stone massage : a three-dimensional approach / Leslie Bruder.
p. ; cm.
Includes bibliographical references and index.
ISBN 978-0-7817-6327-1 (alk. paper)
1. Hydrostone therapy. I. Title.
[DNLM: 1. Massage—methods. WB 537 B888h 2010]
RM723.H93B78 2010
615.8'22—dc22

2008040335

DISCLAIMER

Care has been taken to confirm the accuracy of the information present and to describe generally accepted practices. However, the authors, editors, and publisher are not responsible for errors or omissions or for any consequences from application of the information in this book and make no warranty, expressed or implied, with respect to the currency, completeness, or accuracy of the contents of the publication. Application of this information in a particular situation remains the professional responsibility of the practitioner; the clinical treatments described and recommended may not be considered absolute and universal recommendations.

The authors, editors, and publisher have exerted every effort to ensure that drug selection and dosage set forth in this text are in accordance with the current recommendations and practice at the time of publication. However, in view of ongoing research, changes in government regulations, and the constant flow of information relating to drug therapy and drug reactions, the reader is urged to check the package insert for each drug for any change in indications and dosage and for added warnings and precautions. This is particularly important when the recommended agent is a new or infrequently employed drug.

Some drugs and medical devices presented in this publication have Food and Drug Administration (FDA) clearance for limited use in restricted research settings. It is the responsibility of the health care provider to ascertain the FDA status of each drug or device planned for use in their clinical practice.

To purchase additional copies of this book, call our customer service department at **(800) 638-3030** or fax orders to **(301) 223-2320**. International customers should call **(301) 223-2300**.

Visit Lippincott Williams & Wilkins on the Internet: http://www.lww.com. Lippincott Williams & Wilkins customer service representatives are available from 8:30 am to 6:00 pm, EST.

RRS0811

This book is dedicated to:

My darling dogs Chicalita, Monkey, Chilkoot, and Jelly who patiently forfeited many hikes for the sake of this book.

My beloved wise father, Bert Bruder, who taught me the meaning of love, kindness, and adventure.

My precious, loving brother-in-law Mark Moore, who forever listened deeply to my heart . . .

All of who have passed to the spirit world before I could finish this book. May you read it from heaven and smile.

Preface

CONTENT AND STRUCTURE OF BOOK

Hot Stone Massage: A Three-Dimensional Approach guides the professional massage therapist in how to give a safe, effective, and all-encompassing hot stone massage. This book is an easy to follow manual to this ancient, exquisite art. It covers every aspect required to administer a flowing hot stone massage including: the purpose and benefits of using hot and cold stones; precautions and safety guidelines; the necessary equipment and varieties of stones required; the arrangement of the tools, stones, and accessories, including a description of the environmental set-up; a guide to obtaining the proper stone temperatures; static and flowing stone placement; a system of stone management for optimal flow; guidelines and techniques for using the stones; three-dimensional massage principles and strokes; tips on draping and body mechanics; and a guided step-by-step example of a three-dimensional hot stone massage.

This book also includes information on the history of hot stone use, the physiological effects of heat and cold on the body, the impact of integrating hot stones into your practice, special applications for stone use and an appendix with supplemental information on hot stone massage trainings, suggested readings and videos, and a brief list of where to acquire hot stone kits. *Hot Stone Massage: A Three-Dimensional Approach* leaves no stone unturned, revealing secrets not covered by other sources.

It is important to note, however, that while this book describes everything needed to perform a safe and effective hot stone massage, the written word is not a sufficient "tool" for learning three-dimensional hot stone massage on its own. This book is not intended to replace "live" training, but rather to serve as an adjunct to accompany in-person instruction given by a certified trainer of three-dimensional hot stone massage. This book is a perfect accompaniment to these courses. A list of certified trainers can be found in Appendix C.

It is imperative that classes taught on this modality are done so **only** by instructors that have been certified through the 3-Dimensional Hot Stone Training Program, given at the Institute for Phenomenal Touch Massage, or the information passed on may be inaccurate and potentially dangerous.

The chapters of this book are organized progressively, beginning with the basics of a hot stone massage and then moving on to more advanced techniques. Each chapter includes an outline of its contents and gives a bulleted list of objectives, an introduction, and a list of key terms with definitions. Special tip and caution boxes appear throughout each chapter offering reminders and easy access to important information. At the end of each chapter, there is a summary and a list of review questions to make sure you have effectively digested the material. All techniques and descriptions are supported with photographs. This helpful format further demonstrates the user-friendly nature of the book.

Why Learn Hot Stone Massage?

As a massage therapist interested in broadening your horizons, you will benefit greatly from the incorporation of hot stones into your massage. Not only will learning hot stone massage increase your clientele, but it will also extend the lifetime of your career by saving your hands from overuse. The stones do much of the work for you. And yet, simply rubbing the stones against a body without any training is neither safe nor recommended. This book, along with hands-on training in three-dimensional hot stone massage, provides vital information you will need to perform miracles with stones.

In the 20 years I have taught and practiced massage, hot stone massage has generated more interest and excitement that any other modality I have experienced. Just within the last few years, hundreds of spas, schools, distributors, and conferences across the nation have included and promoted hot stone massage as part of their programs. It is becoming extraordinarily popular and for a good reason. Hot stones deepen the effect of a massage and make conventional touch seem magical. One does not have to cultivate a taste for hot stones. Once the heated stones make contact with the skin, massage alone becomes obsolete. The hot stones, gliding along the oiled skin, melt the muscles and feel like warm water being poured down your bones. There is no sensation comparable.

Since the onset of hot stone massage, the number of classes I teach has tripled. Despite all this interest, there have been few viable in-depth guidebooks about hot stone massage. This book meets that need.

UNIQUE QUALITIES OF THIS BOOK

In my efforts to become completely knowledgeable, I continuously research the field to experience all existing versions of hot stone massage. I have critiqued various teaching styles, compared different stone kits on the market, learned every technique and method being offered, and assessed most articles and videos available. This book is a culmination of the extensive knowledge I have amassed. It eliminates ineffective methods and includes important aspects so often overlooked by many who teach hot stone massage.

This book contains information not covered in other hot stone massage books or trainings. It teaches a unique system for managing the flow and temperature of your stones. It also contains a novel three-dimensional approach and demonstrates how to move the body in space to allow the use of stones on both sides of the client's body at once. This original approach enables the therapist to remove the stones from underneath the body without having to engage the client. The experience of having both sides of the body massaged with stones at the same time is like none other. It will allow your hot stone massage to stand out from all others.

My focus on creating a seamless flow with the stones will enable you to break the myth that hot stone massage has to be completely interruptive. The emphasis on smooth entrance and holding the stone in such a way that the hand and the stone become one, will convince your clients that stones do not have to be invasive. Stones are not substitutes, but extensions of the hands. This seamless approach creates a much more satisfying, fluid experience of hot stone massage. With this three-dimensional style, you will learn to truly dance with the stones.

Stones are a natural and sacred gift given to us from the earth. May their power combined with your newly honed ability to navigate them along the body in a three-dimensional, fluid fashion bring deep relaxation, peace, and pleasure to all of those who will be fortunate enough to receive a hot stone massage from you. Enjoy.

Leslie Bruder

Additional Resources

Hot Stone Massage: A Three-Dimensional Approach includes additional resources for both instructors and students that are available on the book's companion Web site at http://thePoint.lww.com/Bruder.

Instructors

Approved 3-D hot stone massage instructors will be given access to the following additional resources:

- Image bank containing figures from the book and additional images
- Syllabi for courses of various hours

Students

Students who have purchased *Hot Stone Massage: A Three-Dimensional Approach* have access to the following additional resource:

- Image bank containing figures from the book and additional images

In addition, purchasers of the text can access the searchable full text online by going to the *Hot Stone Massage: A Three-Dimensional Approach* Web site at http://thePoint.lww.com/Bruder. See the inside front cover of this text for more details, including the pass code you will need to gain access to the Web site.

Acknowledgments

This book would not have been written if not for the following people who blessed and paved the way . . . my beloved mother and father, Tama and Bert Bruder, who taught me to love stones from the get-go and who always encouraged and believed in my ability to create, write and teach. Their love and zest for life contributed greatly to the creation of this unique approach to massage; my beloved step-father Don Pasternak, who lovingly and painstakingly transformed my first submissions from poetic verbiage into clear, precise, and accurate sentences; Andrea Van de Loop for exposing me to my very first hot stone massage; Gary White and Elyn Aviva for teaching me how to write a book proposal; Doug Richards for editing my proposal to the bone and for managing the house while I wrote; Helen Cartwright, my first dedicated secretary, who dared to proofread my attempts at chapters and held the office together like a tight ship; Sally Hacking for believing in me enough to connect me with Lippincott; Peter Darcy for accepting my book proposal; David Payne for getting me through the first draft; John Goucher for approving the photographs in color; Jennifer Walsh for getting me through the second draft; Laura Bonazolli for patiently and fervently editing my writing to its next level of clarity and organization; Rachelle Detweiler for elegantly stepping in to complete the editorial phase; Julie Montalbano and production crew for their artistry with design; Mary Axelrod for her kind help with research; Chelsea Ogelsby for her comprehensive formatting of references; Ric Breese and Omer Raup for their detailed geological explanations; Edye Rose, my noble office manager, for staying the late hours slaving over references and for lovingly attempting to manage my complex life; my loyal clients who so patiently waited during my absence while writing this book; my generous friends that posed as models and camera people for the first and second photo shoot: Anya Worshan, Mario Sauceda, Sherry Rosamond, Michael Romano, Jessica Baker, Nancy Lawrence, Kurt Smith, Michelle Moore, Cary Ambraziunas, Colleen Vistara, Tyrone Pearson, Edye Rose, and Selina Borquez; Rick Giasi for his patient artistry that created these gorgeous photographs; Prana for the generous donation of the clothing worn; my extraordinary students at the Institute for Phenomenal Touch Massage whose hunger has given me the reason to write this book; Michelle Moore, whose steadfast, calm and loving presence both as a teacher and a friend helped to keep me and the school on track; Cary Ambraziunas, whose loyal commitment to both me and to this work pushed himself past his own limits for the sake of a greater success; Elena Klaver, whose plentiful organic food full of love kept me alive; Cygalle Dias, whose love and support of this work brought it to her organic healing spa; Jo Brewer, the wise laughing sage who kept me grounded, sane, and laughing throughout the most intense times of the writing; Nancy Lawrence, whose love, dedication and vehement belief in me and my stone skills inspired and encouraged me to teach my first hot stone class; Dana Hutson, whose angelic smile, voice, heart, and eternal belief in mankind refueled my tank; Zetta Alderman, whose enthusiastic love and dedication to the work and support of my heart has helped to create a balance between my emotions and the task at hand; Michelle Helms, whose deep heart, loyalty, and hysterical British accent kept me going even when the steam was running out; my dear friend Cedar, whose love, support, and loyal dedication to both this work and to me held me afloat and shined a light into my darkest overwhelming moments; and the rest of my treasured friends and family who have been so patient with my absence since I started writing this book, namely: Debbie Panish; Suzanne Blanch; Vicki Catalina; Sherry Rosamond; Anya Worshan; Mario Sauceda; Michele Merhib; Karen Zupko; Carlos Steybe; Kevin Cowan; Jan and Karin Delany "the Eldorado crew"; Sarah Townes; Randy Compton;

Mark (Wolfsburg!) Cervelli; Terri Kirwin; David Sawyor; Suzanne Marie; Evan Hodkins; Heart and Jeffrey Weisberg; Puja, Gayan, Pamela, Jan and J.D., David and Tamara, Hosen and the rest of the Jemez caravan; Dan Taslitz; Tirzah Firestone; Emily Hodkins; Saffire; Kathy Curless; Neysa Griffith; Ehren Miller; Dawn Burke; Donna McLean; Pamela Rojas; Jerome Phillips; Helaine and Mike Bernstein; my loyal and beloved sister Ellen Bruder-Moore; my cool nephew Erik Bruder-Moore; my devoted brother Jay Bruder; my loving sister-in-law Jodi Mraz; my hip niece and nephew Kristen and Joey; my extended Bruder/Busch/ Frankel aunts, uncles, and heartfelt cousins who helped to shape me with love as I grew up; my great new loving, open, and fantastic Pasternak family; and finally all of my devoted past and present doggy children Monkey, Girlie Whirlie, Chilkoot, Cedar, Bruno, Tellis, Caico, Gus, Pecas, Brownie, Morena, Alien, and Happy, whose love never wavers. I thank you all from the bottom of my heart for both contributing to the creation of and being the foundation beneath this book.

Contents

Hot Stone MASSAGE

A Three-Dimensional Approach

CHAPTER 1

Introduction to Hot Stone Massage

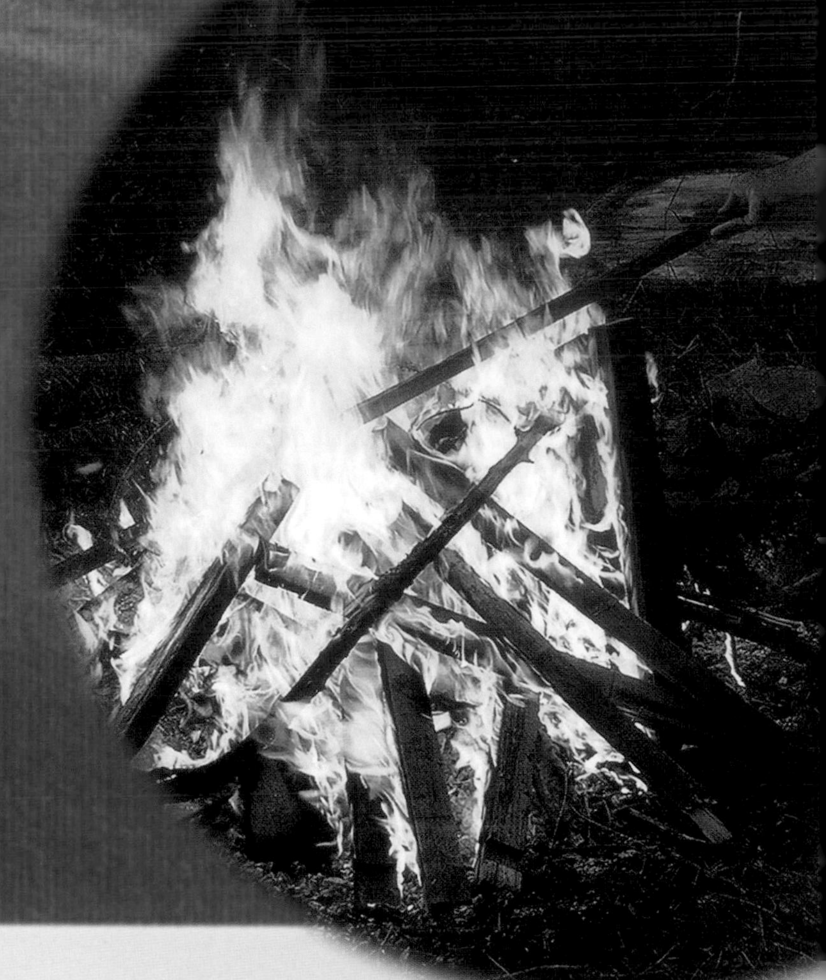

Outline

Healing with Hot Stones: A Brief History
- Ancient Uses of Healing Stones
- Development of Hot Stone Massage

What Is a Hot Stone Massage?
- Fundamental Elements of Hot Stone Massage
- The Benefits of Hot Stone Massage
  - *Benefits for Clients*
  - *Benefits for Therapists*
- Three-Dimensional Approach to Hot Stone Massage

Incorporating Hot Stones into Your Healing Practice
- Potential Impact on Existing Massage Practice
  - *Rewards*
  - *Challenges*
  - *Possible Concerns*
- Incorporating Hot Stones into Other Healing Modalities
  - *Cranial Sacral, Reiki, and Other Energy Work*
  - *Rolfing and Deep Tissue Work*
  - *Facials, Pedicures, and Manicures*
  - *Acupuncture, Chiropractic, and Physical Therapy*
  - *Other Uses for Hot Stones*

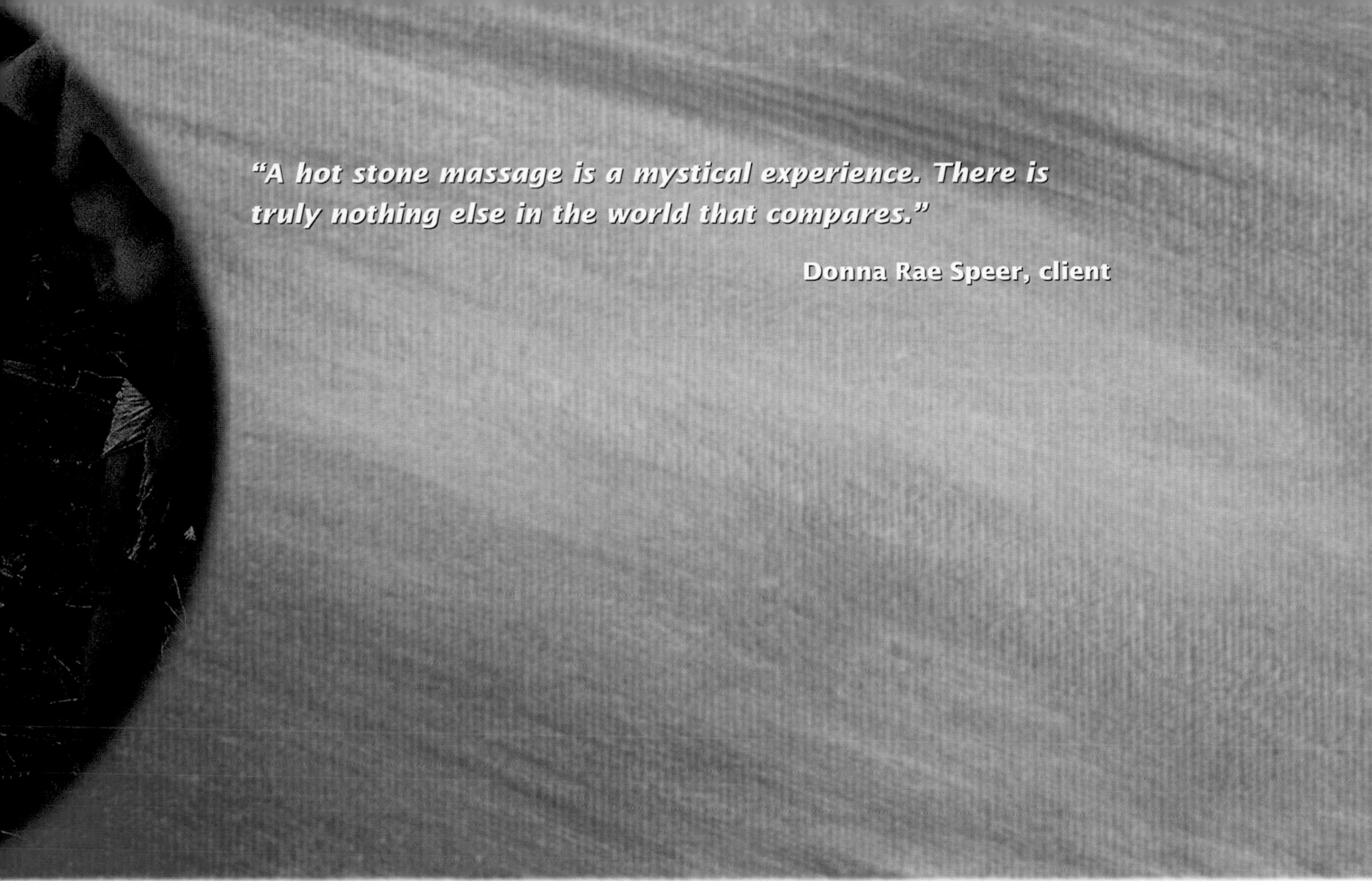

"A hot stone massage is a mystical experience. There is truly nothing else in the world that compares."

Donna Rae Speer, client

Objectives

After reading this chapter, you should be able to:

- Describe the use of stones in the healing practices of several cultural groups.
- Identify the key elements that distinguish hot stone massage from traditional massage therapy.
- Discuss the therapeutic benefits of a hot stone massage.
- Explain how the three-dimensional approach to hot stone massage benefits both the client and the therapist.
- Discuss the rewards and challenges of integrating hot stone massage into a massage therapy practice.
- Explain how hot stones can be incorporated into other healing modalities.

Key Terms

Ayurveda: A 2,000-year-old system of medicine practiced in India that is based on a holistic approach that focuses on establishing and maintaining balance of the life energies within us, rather than on individual symptoms. The Sanskrit definition of *ayu* is life, while *veda* means knowledge.

Chi: A form of energy that the ancient Chinese believed flowed through the body via channels called "meridians." Traditional Chinese medicine explains that the blockage of chi causes both mental and physical diseases.

Geo-thermotherapy: Another term for hot stone massage.

Hot stone massage: The incorporation of heated (and cooled) stones into a session of traditional massage or other bodywork.

Three-dimensional hot stone massage: An approach to hot stone massage in which the therapist effortlessly moves the client's body in space in order to massage both sides simultaneously with stones.

Hot stone massage, technically known as **geothermotherapy,** is the incorporation of heated (and cooled) stones into a session of traditional massage for the purpose of treating an injury or other disorder, relieving pain, and increasing a client's general state of well-being. The use of stones enables the therapist to offer clients the well-known therapeutic benefits of heat and cold, as well as to create movement, friction, pressure, and vibration with the stones. Adding the benefits of stone use to the many acknowledged benefits of a traditional hands-on massage increases the healing potential of your work with clients.

This chapter provides an introduction to hot stone massage. Where did the technique originate? How did it develop? And what are the benefits of using hot and cold stones in a massage, not only for your clients, but also for you? The chapter also describes my own unique approach, which I call **three-dimensional hot stone massage,** and explains how it differs from other hot stone massage approaches. The chapter concludes with a brief overview of the rewards, challenges, and possible concerns relating to the incorporation of hot stones into an existing massage practice and other healing modalities in which hot stones can be used. In short, reading this chapter should give you all of the background information you need to begin your journey of discovery into the world of hot stones.

HEALING WITH HOT STONES: A BRIEF HISTORY

A client experiencing hot stone massage for the first time may think of it as the latest "new" technique, but the use of stones as a healing modality is as old as the stones themselves. Hot stones have been used for centuries in different cultures worldwide as a means of healing.

Ancient Uses of Healing Stones

Let's step back in time. . . . Over the years, stones have been used in saunas, steam baths, and sweat lodges; for healing disease or relieving pain; for assisting childbirth; for smoothing skin; and as a source of heat. Warmed stones have been used to comfort the elderly and children, calm the nervous system, assist the dying process, aid digestion, and improve the function of internal organs.

Records from ancient Japan and China describe using pointed stones, rather than needles, to stimulate meridians and acupuncture points (otherwise known as *tsubo*). The heated stones act to penetrate blockages and stimulate the flow of **chi.** The technique is not unlike *moxabustion*, a traditional Chinese heat therapy in which a compacted stick of mugwort (an herb) is burned over an area of the skin to simulate chi and blood flow. Heated stones were used in this way when the mugwort was not available.

Stones also play an important role in Native American healing rituals. Mario Sauceda, an ordained medicine man descended from the Yaqui Indian tribe, explains:

TESTIMONIAL

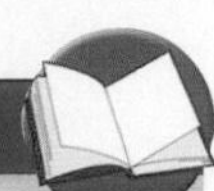

In sweat lodges we refer to the rocks as stone people. The creator gave stones to us as tools for healing. My ancestors put stones from the fire into a bladder bag of water to cool them enough to be held. They would then pass the stones around from person to person to hold or rub them on specific parts of their body for healing. They would also use stones to heat and steep herbs for healing illnesses. When making medicine wheels, my ancestors taught me to place the stones according to their different properties. They believed in the power of stones to give us visions. Crazy Horse did his vision quest on a bed of stones. Native Americans have been using stones for healing for thousands of years and yet make no claims for having discovered their healing properties. They simply accept and respect them as a gift from Wankantonka, the great mystery.

The Moqui Indians, who lived in an area now within the state of Utah, used a rare stone with a metal outer shell for healing and ceremonial rituals. These mysterious stones called *Moqui marbles* or *shaman stones* are thought to have been used by shamans in a variety of rituals; for example, they were rolled along the body with varying pressure to induce healing. The Indians would also hold them in their pockets and hands for their "grounding" energy. After they were used for healing, the stones would be set outside in lightning and thunder or smudged with sage in order to recharge their energy.

In warm regions, such as Costa Rica and Hawaii, black lava stones heated by the sun are used during childbirth. Women in labor lie on the warm, dry lava stones for pain relief and midwives hold stones on their lower backs to help stimulate childbirth. Pools lined with lava stones and heated by solar energy provide warm baths for birthing. The warm water, heated by the black sun-drenched stones, provides a gentle transition for the newborn to move from the temperate amniotic fluid to the outside world. Similarly, Roman, Greek, Egyptian, Japanese, and Turkish steam baths utilized heated stones to help warm the waters.

Every hot stone class I teach invariably calls forth stories from students telling how their ancestors used heated stones. Students of European descent talk about their grandparents using hot stones to prewarm their feather beds on cold nights before the advent of central heating. They claimed the warmth of the stones helped them fall asleep and stave off illness. Students of Scandinavian origin describe how stones are used for the operation of their culture's ubiquitous saunas. Stones are taken from the river beds and dried overnight to prevent them from exploding during the next morning's rapid heating process. They are then heated by fire and placed in the corner of a small wooden room lined with benches on which people sit. By inducing sweating, the sauna is thought to help the body eliminate toxins. Russian students tell stories of the *banyas* that their grandparents made. Banyas are similar to saunas; however, water and essential oils are doused over the stones and large oak-leaf fans are used to beat the body and stimulate perspiration. Stories are also told of cowboys from the American West who placed heated stones in their pockets, mittens, socks, or sleeping sack to keep their hands, feet, or internal organs warm in the cold weather.

Every culture has probably been touched by the healing power of stones. And yet, even though stones have been used for thousands of years to comfort and promote healing, it was not until the early 1990s that the integration of hot stones into massage became popular and was formalized into what is now commonly known as hot stone massage.

Development of Hot Stone Massage

Although there are no clear records and thus no way of determining who was first to introduce heated and chilled stones into a massage session, Mary Nelson is the woman who deserves credit for making hot stone massage both a formal and popular healing art. As Jane Scrivner explains in her book *LaStone Therapy*, Mary Nelson introduced LaStone therapy, a form of hot and cold stone massage, in 1993. Mary was a massage therapist who was looking for a way to work the muscles deeply without causing damage to her own joints and muscles. She states that she was led by her Native American spirit guide to use stones in the massage. LaStone has become popular around the country and has influenced many practitioners and spas to integrate stones into the massages they offer. However, LaStone therapy is only one method of performing a hot stone massage.

Since the popularization of hot stone massage, many other versions and variations of this art have developed. Sonia Alexandra, author of *The Art of Stone Healing*, focuses more on crystal healing and balancing the chakras in method. Both Karyn Chabot of the Sacred Stone Center and Carollanne Crichton of the Stone Temple Institute use an **ayurvedic** approach to their stone massage. These are just a few of the people who have developed their own methodology of hot stone massage.

I came to discover hot stone massage on my own in 1995. I did not study stone massage with a teacher; it came from inside of me.

As a child, I collected stones with my mom on the Jersey shores and beaches of Rhode Island, Maine, and New Hampshire. I relished helping my mom find the smoothest and roundest stones for her to paint. We collected so many stones my dad would tease us about the old station wagon not being able to make it home with the weight of the stones. My mom had stones piled in all the spare rooms and on shelves in the garage. And while she painted many of them, there were still plenty of plain stones left in their natural state for my own growing collection. Little did I know that these stones would eventually become my tools.

Years later, I became a river guide and began collecting smooth river-beaten stones from the many river banks of the West. Eventually, I began frequenting the beaches of Big Sur, California, and Mexico and collected stones from their shores as well. My home became a sanctuary of magnificent stones, as full as my mother's house once was. However, I had nothing to do with them except admire them. My massage room was filled with beautiful stones. I would gaze at them, thank them for their beauty, turn them in my hands, and instinctively rub them against my skin. After contact with my stones, I always felt better; somehow my heart felt warmed by the natural energy given off from the stones. I always knew they were in my life to serve a higher purpose, but I was never quite clear what that purpose would be.

Then one winter day, I was massaging in my wood-heated studio on the river in Eldorado Springs, Colorado. It was a particularly cold day, and my client expressed being slightly chilled even though the fire was going. I looked over at a large, flat stone that I'd had for years and thought, "Why not heat that up on the stove and place it on my client's belly to warm her up?" I did, and that was the beginning of my own integration of stones into my practice.

Little by little, I kept adding more stones from around my room to the top of the wood-burning stove, until there was no more space. I then started placing stones on my oil radiator. I experimented with these stones for years—first simply placing them on top of or beneath the client's body, then actually massaging with them.

Meanwhile, my 20 precious stones kept falling off the edge of the oil radiator and stove, clanking loudly on their way down. I finally decided that a skillet would be a much more efficient and quiet way of heating the stones! And I began keeping a bowl of ice water nearby for quickly cooling the stones. Step by step, stone by stone, I came up with new and innovative ways to use and manage my stones. I had no idea what I was doing, but my clients loved it. Eventually, I received a hot stone massage from a friend, Andrea Van de Loop, who had also come to hot stone massage on her own. Her use of stones inspired me to become adept at this ancient art.

Over a 10-year period, I developed the three-dimensional approach: the system of stone management, guidelines, principles, techniques, and embracing strokes that are taught in this book. During this time, a dear friend, Nancy Lawrence, as well as many massage therapists who came to me for hot stone massages, encouraged me to teach my approach. My experience of teaching informs every page of this book. Before I say more about the three-dimensional approach, let's look at the fundamental elements that make up a basic hot stone massage.

WHAT IS A HOT STONE MASSAGE?

A hot stone massage is similar to a traditional massage, but in addition to his or her hands, the therapist also uses hot stones. The gliding of the heated, oiled stones along the body creates a relaxing sensation while simultaneously warming the client's joints and tissues, increasing the client's circulation, and promoting release of toxins. Hot stones may also be placed on and/or beneath particular body regions to enhance these effects.

Even though most hot stone massages predominately use heated stones, cold stones can also be used to stimulate body tissues, reduce inflammation, aid in pain relief, or enhance alertness. An in-depth discussion on the physiological effects of both heat and cold will be included in Chapter 2.

Fundamental Elements of Hot Stone Massage

When first hearing about hot stone massage, many people think that the stones are simply placed on the body and that there is very little contact with the therapist's hands. This is a misunderstanding. While static placement of heated stones is an important element, a professional hot stone massage also includes traditional massage strokes, with the therapist holding smooth, hot, oiled stones while he or she works. The client receiving the massage experiences the contact of the therapist's hands simultaneously with the heat of the stone. You'll know a hot stone massage is going well if the client exclaims, "I can't tell the difference between your hands and the stone!" This indicates that you have woven the use of stones into the massage so seamlessly that the client experiences stone and hands as one.

In addition, when giving a hot stone massage, the therapist also works without stones. Hands have a sensitivity that stones do not, and a great deal of feedback passes to and from the client via the therapist's hands. Thus, it is the combination of stone and hands precisely balanced that creates the unique experience of a hot stone massage.

Students of hot stone massage often assume that the modality is more physically taxing than traditional massage. This is another misconception. Once the therapist has become accustomed to using the stones, it is actually easier on his or her body to perform a hot stone massage than a traditional massage. This is because the stones provide weight and heat that help to soften the muscles, making them more pliable. In short, the stones do some of the work for you, relaxing the tissue more rapidly and with less stress on the wrists and hands.

A hot stone massage can be simple or complex. If you are a novice massage therapist, you might begin by experimenting with the simplest techniques for sliding the stones along the client's skin. If you are a seasoned massage therapist, you might feel comfortable employing the advanced techniques for using the stones and creating an optimal flow. These are all described in the later chapters of this book.

The Benefits of Hot Stone Massage

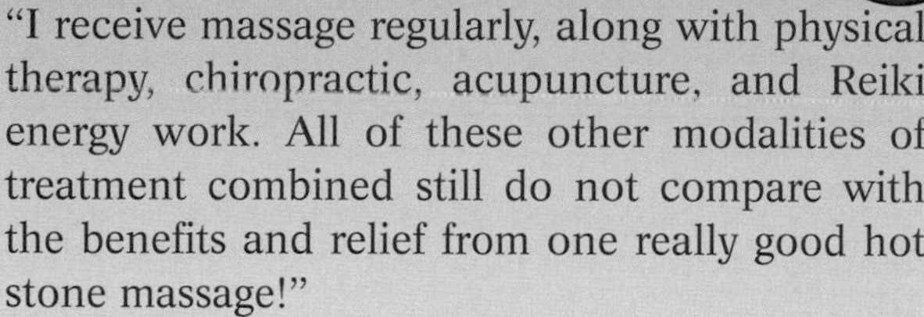

TESTIMONIAL

"I receive massage regularly, along with physical therapy, chiropractic, acupuncture, and Reiki energy work. All of these other modalities of treatment combined still do not compare with the benefits and relief from one really good hot stone massage!"

Mary Axelrod, client

The feeling that hot stones induce is reason enough to use them. The sensation has been described as warm water being poured down the bones, floating in the ocean, lying on hot sand, or making a transcendent journey. However, there are a great many other benefits to using them.

The following is a thorough list of the benefits of hot stone massage for the client as well as the therapist. Because a hot stone massage incorporates the use of cold stones, this list includes the benefits of using chilled as well as heated stones. Much of this information is a compilation of my many years of study and practice in the field. In time, you may come to discover other benefits that are not included in this list.

Benefits for Clients

A hot stone massage:

- **Nurtures**: Hot stones have a very nurturing quality. Recipients report that they feel safe, as if they are in the arms of a loving mother. Some clients cry when they first experience the nurturing property of the stones. This nurturing quality is wonderful for elderly people, for people who have not been touched in a long time, and for people who are hospitalized.
- **Centers**: The earth element of the stones helps to ground clients, calming them down and inviting them back into their body. Hot stones are settling and help clients become present; their warmth brings the attention to each part of the body the stones are touching, taking clients out of the future and into the now.
- **Induces relaxation**: The penetrating heat of the stones elicits deep relaxation immediately, melting away stress and soothing the nervous system. It is like a warm bath for the nerves, aiding in sleep at the end of the day.
- **Moves tissue with heat**: Hot stones allow clients to actually be *massaged* with the heat, rather than just have the heat placed upon them. Therapists can heat their hands or the oil they use, but this heat lasts only a few seconds. An electric heating pad, a hot grain bag, a hot gel pad, or a heating balm can be used to heat up an area of the body, but none of these items can be used as devices to perform massage.
- **Penetrates and lasts**: Within a minute or two of use on the body, the heat within a stone is dissipated. Where did that heat go? It penetrated the muscles. This process is repeated with each stone so that by the end of a hot stone massage, the muscles of the body have taken in enough heat to help the tissue remain supple and warm for hours after the massage. This is particularly appreciated on a cold day. After a hot stone massage, a client can walk out into the snowy weather and still feel warm. This helps to prevent injuries hours after the massage has ended.
- **Reduces residual pain**: It is very common, after receiving a traditional deep-tissue massage, for the recipient to report feeling sore the next day. Using the heated stones protects the tissue from damage or injury during a deep massage, and it reduces the amount of soreness felt the next day. Many of my clients have reported feeling absolutely no soreness the day after receiving a deep hot stone massage. Hot stones also help athletes recover more quickly and feel less pain the day after athletic exertion.
- **Opens meridians and chakras**: The combination of the energy from the stones and the heat within them helps to open energy channels and energy centers, thus increasing the flow of vital energy or chi in both meridians and chakras. Some practitioners place particular gem stones on energy centers of the body to increase the energy experienced in that area.
- **Softens muscular armor**: The heat of the stone helps to soften the armor of tight muscles. This can help clients to access and release emotional issues that may have been hiding beneath the protective shield of their gripped muscles. A muscle that has softened as a result of the release of a withheld emotion, versus being kneaded from the outside, tends to stay released much longer.
- **Acts as a boundary**: The stones can serve as boundaries to help clients feel safe if they have issues about being touched in certain parts of their

bodies. For instance, it is common for clients who have been sexually abused to tighten up or pull away when they are touched in the areas around their pelvis or on their bellies, inner thighs, or buttocks. A stone placed between the client's body and the therapist's hand acts as a protective shield and makes it much easier for clients to relax and be touched in those sensitive areas, perhaps for the first time since the traumatic event.

- **Feels like extra hands**: When hot stones are statically placed on the body, their warmth penetrates and feels like a hand rather than a stone. This means that clients experiencing hot stone massage often feel as if there are several hands on their body at one time. Even when the therapist moves to the skillet for more hot stones, clients feel that his or her hands are still on them because of the hot stones that remain upon their body. Many clients have commented that it feels as if two people are massaging them at once because of the stones.
- **Decreases tissue swelling**: Cold stones help to reduce swelling following an acute injury or an inflammatory response, limiting fluid infiltration into an injured area. Cold stones on the eyes help to reduce puffiness. They are wonderful to integrate into a facial.
- **Acts as an analgesic**: Massage with cold stones eases the sensation of pain and increases the pain threshold. This is helpful when attempting to "break up" trigger points. It can also increase range of motion in an injured joint; however, you must use cold stones with caution because their analgesic effect can mask the necessary limits of an injury.
- **Invigorates**: Cold stones stimulate the body, creating a sensation of vitality. For clients who are suffering from depression, this "shock" of cold can be therapeutic, energizing the mind–body system. Cold stones can also help a tired client to feel refreshed.
- **Increases brain function**: Cold stones used around the face and temples of the head aid a client in increasing his or her brain function. If a client must take an exam or work diligently on a project, cold stones can help clear the head.
- **Restores lucidity**: Cold stones help to bring a client back to the present moment at the end of a massage. It is important to use cold stones toward the completion of a massage if the client is foggy and must go immediately back to work or drive for any significant distance.

Benefits for Therapists

In comparison to a traditional hands-only massage, a hot stone massage:

- **Increases tissue pliability**: Massaging the tissue with heat allows the muscles to open up, relax, and become supple and pliable significantly faster than with hands alone. An area of the body that would normally take 15 to 20 minutes of regular massage to release takes only 2 to 3 minutes with the aid of hot stones. This saves and makes your job much easier.
- **Relieves therapist's hands**: Because the heat of the stones dissolves so much of the muscle tightness, massage is much easier on your hands. The heat does much of the work the hands previously had to do. The stones can also be used as tools to give pressure, acting as a substitute for thumbs or fingers. Most massage tools feel very hard on the body because they are not hot. The heat of the stone removes any sensation of hardness, and this allows stones to become friendly tools.
- **Extends career longevity**: Many practitioners discover that they can continue performing massage for more years than they might have been able to without the use of stones.
- **Increases revenue**: You can charge more for a hot stone massage than you can for a regular massage, and you can take more clients in a day because it is easier on your body. Offering hot stone massage will also attract more clients than before and keep those who might have become bored with your regular massage. Thus, hot stone massage increases your revenue.
- **Quiets hyper clients**: Many therapists struggle with how to massage clients who won't stop talking or helping throughout the massage. The heat from the stones really helps to calm and quiet this type of client, making the work easier for you.
- **Energizes**: Many massage therapists have shared with me that they often feel more energized after administering a hot stone massage than they do after giving a regular hands-only massage. Whether it is the stones, the heat, or the simple act of working with the stones, giving a hot stone massage does seem to have an energizing effect on many therapists.
- **Warms joints**: Working with hot stones warms the muscles in your fingers, palms, wrists, and forearms as you work. This helps to prevent injury and

chronic pain from overuse of the joints even as the joints are working.

- **Relaxes therapist**: The stones and the heat seem to have a grounding effect not only for clients, but also for you. In addition, during the massage, you can relax your own muscles by placing hot stones strategically on your own body in such a way that they will remain in place while you work (e.g., in pockets or inside tight-fitting clothes). Sitting on a warm stone helps to ground you as well.
- **Advances competency**: For therapists who are just starting out in their massage career and are not yet proficient at the massage strokes, the use of hot stones can increase their clients' satisfaction with the massage. Because the sensation of the heated stones gliding along the body is so satisfying in and of itself, it can take the place of fancy strokes. This affords new therapists more opportunities to develop and increase their level of competency as they develop in their practice.

As mentioned earlier, these are just some of the benefits of using hot and cold stones in a massage. Once you gain experience, you'll come to observe many others.

Three-Dimensional Approach to Hot Stone Massage

Three-dimensional hot stone massage differs from the common method of using stones in that the therapist effortlessly moves the client's body in space in order to massage both sides simultaneously. This approach to touch acknowledges the three-dimensional nature of the body: When a body part is cradled and embraced, no portion of that part is left out of the experience. Instead, the entire area feels acknowledged and complete.

Working three dimensionally also enables you to take advantage of the force of gravity and the weight of the client's body to create pressure against the stone. This means that the therapist does not have to exert effort to press the stone into the tissue. When the weight of the client's body is allowed to drape over the hand or stone, the muscle softens and opens much more easily than it does when the therapist pushes in from above with strength. This gives three-dimensional massage a fluid quality that is often missing from traditional manual therapy.

Many therapists currently providing hot stone massage require their clients to sit up, lie down, and roll to one side during the massage so that they can place or remove the stones from beneath the body. With the three-dimensional approach, you will learn how to place and remove the hot stones without ever having to require your clients to do anything but enjoy. You'll discover how to incorporate the stones into the massage sequence in such a flowing fashion that clients will be unaware of the process that is taking place.

Three-dimensional hot stone massage also embodies many of the same holistic principles that underlie all forms of successful body therapy. Some of these include paying close attention to the way in which the hands make contact with the body, overlapping the strokes, entering the muscles in their shortened position, revisiting parts of the body as appropriate, preventing client pain and injury, and ensuring client comfort. A more comprehensive discussion of the principles and techniques of a three-dimensional hot stone massage are given in Chapters 8 through 10.

TESTIMONIAL

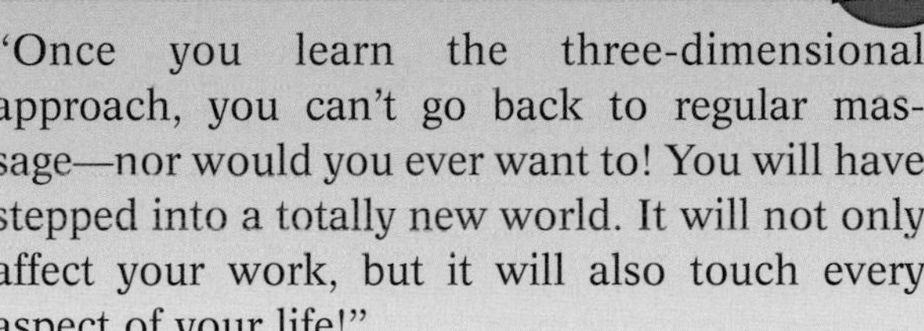

"Once you learn the three-dimensional approach, you can't go back to regular massage—nor would you ever want to! You will have stepped into a totally new world. It will not only affect your work, but it will also touch every aspect of your life!"

Anya Worshom, massage therapist

INCORPORATING HOT STONES INTO YOUR HEALING PRACTICE

Before deciding to incorporate three-dimensional hot stone massage into your practice, you should be aware of several considerations that are particular to this modality. Because hot stone massage is a specialized service, it can create a larger and more satisfied clientele, but it also involves a greater amount of forethought, not only in terms of managing supplies, but also in the very way in which you approach massage. We touch on these topics briefly here, and they are explored in detail in later chapters of this book.

Potential Impact on Existing Massage Practice

As with most things in life, there are both rewards and challenges to adding hot stone massage into your regular massage practice. The following overview will help you gain a sense of what hot stone massage involves.

Rewards

Adding hot stone massage to your practice will enable you to compete in a highly specialized niche market. This, in turn, will expand your potential clientele by attracting new clients, generating a higher return rate from pre-existing clients, and increasing the number of referrals you receive. Adding a new modality may also enable you to motivate inactive clients.

Because hot stone massage is much easier on your hands, you will also be able to increase the number of clients you can see in your practice without injuring or exhausting yourself. Clients will also pay more for hot stone massage. Thus, by adding hot stone massage to your repertoire, your revenue will increase from an expanded clientele and from pre-existing clients whenever they choose your new specialty.

Sometimes, after years of doing the same thing, massage work can become stale. Adding hot stone massage to your traditional practice can increase the enjoyment you get from your work. In addition, because hot stones are so effective in releasing tension and reducing stiffness and pain, your clients will likely report increased satisfaction with your massage. This will enhance your excitement about and commitment to your work as well as increase your feelings of accomplishment.

In addition to simply adding hot stones to your massage, you will also be integrating the three-dimensional approach. This will not only set your hot stone practice apart from others, but will also influence your regular massage practice as well. That's because many of the three-dimensional principles taught in this book are applicable to massage without stones. The reward for your efforts will not only include a new modality to offer to clients, but a more satisfying traditional massage as well.

Challenges

Although adding hot stone massage to your practice should increase your revenues, some start-up costs are involved. You will need to make some minor adjustments to your treatment area and purchase supplies (see Chapters 3 and 4). Also, if you are not using this book as part of a training program, you will need to enroll in a specialized course or workshop to ensure that you can work with hot stones safely and effectively. Again, this book is not intended to replace training, but rather to serve as a reference before, during, and after training—and throughout your career.

One of the most significant differences between a traditional massage and a hot stone massage is the extra time and planning that is required. For instance, you'll need to allow extra time before a session to heat up and lay out a placement of the stones. You'll also need extra time after each session for clean-up. Planning is also required throughout the hot stone massage, as you create stone piles, keep track of stone temperatures, manage the placement of stones, reheat the used stones, and pay attention to timing. Although such planning becomes second nature with time, you need patience and practice to get over that hurdle. Planning is probably the biggest adjustment therapists must undertake when beginning to incorporate hot stone massage into their healing practice.

A word of comfort, however . . . What seems like a great deal of thinking and a fair amount of interruption to you may go entirely unnoticed by a client who is immersed in the pleasure of the stones. This is illustrated by the following story:

TESTIMONIAL

A new client of mine who was trying to decide between receiving a regular and a hot stone massage asked me, what the advantages were of one over the other. I explained that a hot stone massage involves some interruption, because I have to leave the body to go and fetch the stones from time to time throughout the massage. I gave assurances, however, that the benefits far outweigh the interruptions, and then I let the client choose. After pondering the choice, the client decided to try using hot stones. In order to fully appreciate my story, you should know that my office is located on the edge of a small river.

About 45 minutes into the massage, the client remarked, "I thought you were going to have to leave me to go get the stones from time to time." This comment surprised me, and I replied, "I have been leaving you to get the stones throughout the massage." The client asked, "When did this happen?" and I replied, "Every time I go to the skillet, I get you new stones." The client laughed and said that he had been expecting me to leave the room and trek to the river for new stones! Now it was my turn to laugh. It amazed me that a client had been willing to try a hot stone massage, even though he thought I would have to leave the office to go down to the river several times during the massage. Meanwhile, I had been worried about the short moments I left the client's side to get stones from the skillet, but the client was never even aware of those short interruptions.

Possible Concerns

The following questions are indicative of some of the concerns that both students and new clients have asked me over the years. Perhaps some of yours or your clients' questions will be answered here.

Therapists sometimes wonder:

1. **Question**: What's wrong with just using my hands? Why do I need to use stones? Will my clients like stones as much as my hands?

   Answer: There is nothing wrong with your hands. They are an integral part of giving a hot stone massage. In a three-dimensional hot stone massage, you always use your hands without stones before you introduce stones to each part of the body. Stones are an addition to your hands rather than a substitute for your hands. Stones offer you the ability to massage with heat and cold. This deepens the good work you are already doing with your hands.
2. **Question**: What if my clients prefer the stones to my hands?

   Answer: That won't happen. They might prefer to have you use hot stones in addition to your hands rather than go back to a hands-only massage, but they will rarely want you to use only stones. Your hands are an integral part of a hot stone massage, and they will not enjoy the experience nearly as much without contact with your hands alone as well. The stones will never replace the power of your human touch. They will just enhance it.
3. **Question**: Won't I burn my hands using stones?

   Answer: There is no reason to burn yourself if you are careful and abide by the safety precautions taught in this book. At first, the stones may feel hot to your hands, but over time your skin becomes desensitized to the heat and you will be able to hold hotter stones without the stones feeling too hot. However, regardless of how sensitive you are to heat, following the safety guidelines will prevent you from ever burning yourself.
4. **Question**: What if I burn my client? Will my client have an adverse reaction to the heat or cold? Do I risk getting sued?

   Answer: There is no reason to burn your client or cause an adverse reaction if you take care to follow the safety precautions and contraindications explained in this book. I have given thousands of hot stone massages without burning or causing an adverse reaction in a client. In theory, adding the element of heated stones to your massage could increase your risk of being sued; however, I have never heard of it happening. Liability insurance covers both hot stone as well as regular massage. It is a good idea to be covered no matter what kind of massage you perform.
5. **Question**: Will I overheat while giving a hot stone massage? Will I get ill from my hands being hot for so long?

   Answer: Given that hot stone massage does slightly increase the temperature of the room and of your own body, it is important to have ventilation available (either a window, door, or fan) and to dress lightly when using hot stones. Because you periodically dip the hot stones in cold water to cool them, and because a good portion of the massage is done with stoneless hands, you do not have to worry about your hands being hot for an extended period of time. However, I have also never heard of anyone getting sick from having his or her hands warm for prolonged periods of time.
6. **Question**: Can I learn hot stone massage entirely from a book or a video? If not, will the extra cost for hot stone training pay off for me?

   Answer: I do not recommend relying solely on a book or video to learn hot stone massage. The beauty of doing hands-on training is that you can watch the instructor manage the stones, demonstrate the guidelines, and perform the techniques and strokes in person. You will then practice the strokes and be assisted in improving your performance. Classes help prevent you from learning something incorrectly that could displease or injure a client. Although this book reviews all of the most important information about performing hot stone massage, it cannot show movement. The extra cost of training will pay off because you will become more competent at using hot stones more quickly and thus have a richer practice.

7. **Question**: How will I ever learn how to manage a full set of stones?

   Answer: Managing an entire set of stones takes time and practice. It's best to begin with a small number, say 10 stones, then add a few more stones at a time until you work your way up. It's important not to overwhelm yourself with too many stones at first. This could turn you away prematurely from learning how to manage what later will seem natural and easy. Take your time and make sure it feels good to you each step of the way.

8. **Question**: How can I afford the additional cost of stones and supplies along with the cost of training?

   Answer: You can collect your own set of stones, or purchase them very inexpensively at a stone yard. There is no need to spend an enormous amount of money on stones. As just noted, start small. As far as the rest of the equipment, avoid purchasing it from a hot stone massage retailer, as they charge more than it will cost you to find it on your own. You can purchase all equipment needed very inexpensively or even find it used at a garage sale.

9. **Question**: Do I need to have my stones and skillet by the time I take the class?

   Answer: In order to retain what you learn in class, it is important to either have or have access to a set of stones and the rest of the equipment needed. If you cannot find a way to get a set of stones and equipment by the time of the class, see if you can borrow from a friend. It is best to wait to learn hot stone massage until you have (or have access to) a set of stones and a skillet.

10. **Question**: So many people do hot stone massage these days; how can my hot stone massage stand out from the others? How will I compare to my competition?

    Answer: If you learn the unique approach offered in this book, your hot stone massage will stand out from others offered. Many clients have shared their disappointment with other hot stone modalities. Once they experienced the three-dimensional approach, they were sold.

Clients may ask you or be simply wondering the following:

1. **Question**: Is this just another gimmick, or is it truly going to help me?

   Answer: It would be understandable for you to think of a massage given with stones as a gimmick; however, the best way of deciding for yourself is to experience it. The benefits of getting massaged with both heated and cooled stones are numerous and can help you in ways a hands-alone massage does not.

2. **Question**: Will I still get deep, specific work if you use the stones?

   Answer: Absolutely. The hot stones make it possible to work deeply with much less discomfort than you would feel without the heat. The pointed tool stones allow the work to be very specific. In addition, hands are used as well as the stones throughout the massage, so nothing will be lost from what you are used to receiving in the past.

3. **Question**: Can I get hot stone massage with my particular disease or illness?

   Answer: The answer to that will be based on what your condition is, how long you have had it, how acute or chronic it is, and how it is affected by heat or cold. I will also have you check with your doctor. Once I have the information I need, I will be able to determine if it is safe and advisable to give you a hot stone massage.

4. **Question**: Won't I get burned with the stones?

   Answer: If I can hold the stone comfortably in my hands, you will not get burned. I will take all precautions and check in with you regularly to make sure that no stone feels too hot for you at any time. You are also invited to communicate with me at all times to let me know if a stone temperature is uncomfortable for you. I will make sure to glide the stones at the proper speed so no heat is left too long in one spot. Thus, burning will not be possible. I would not be able to perform hot stone massage on my clients if burning were a common and regular occurrence!

5. **Question**: What if a stone gets dropped on me?

   Answer: I make sure I never carry stones across your face so that one can never drop on you there. Stones rarely drop on my clients and if they do, it is never from very high above your body and always on a place of your body that won't be damaged by the stone dropping on it. That being said, if you are ever feeling unsafe as far as a stone dropping on you, tell me and I will slow down my massage so that you can feel safe. But truly, dropping a stone on a client is a very rare occurrence with minimal repercussions.

6. **Question**: Why do I have to pay more for a hot stone massage?

   Answer: In order to perform a safe, fluid, and soothing hot stone massage, I need to spend additional time planning and setting up the massage, as well as cleaning up the area and clearing the stones afterward. In addition, I invested in a training and proper equipment in order that I could give an effective hot stone massage.

7. **Question**: Won't the massage be interrupted constantly while you get the stones?

   Answer: The approach of hot stone massage that I use involves a system of stone management that cuts back greatly on the amount of interruption involved in the massage, so the massage will be interrupted only occasionally. You need to weigh the benefits of being massaged with heated stones over the drawback of these sporadic interruptions. If you are not sure what you want to do, we can start the massage using stones and you can tell me whether or not you want to continue with them.

Now that you know the rewards and challenges of incorporating hot stone massage into your practice and have answers to some of the most common concerns of students and clients, you're in a better position to decide whether adding hot stone massage to your practice is the right step for you. In addition, hands-on training in hot stones will give you a feeling of what it's like to work with hot stones. But perhaps the best way to decide whether to add hot stone massage to your practice is to experience it for yourself. Once you do, you will probably be determined to do whatever it takes to offer this powerful ancient healing modality to your clients.

Incorporating Hot Stones into Other Healing Modalities

Hot stone massage does not always need to be done as an exclusive full-on stone massage. Stones can be incorporated into many other healing modalities and serve to enhance and deepen the effects of each modality. If hot stones are going to be used as an adjunct therapy, these practitioners do not need to focus on special techniques and the organization of stones for optimal flow, but they do need to be trained in the basics of stone use, entrance, placement, and temperature.

Cranial Sacral, Reiki, and Other Energy Work

Cranial sacral, Reiki, and other energy work can create a very deep state of relaxation; however, when the body contains a fair amount of tension and pain, or the mind is very active, it can be challenging to stay present with the movement or absorb the movement of the subtler energies. Hot stones can be used with energy work in two different ways. The hot stones can be massaged on a part of the body that is tense or in pain before the energy work begins, and/or they can be placed strategically on the body and left in place during the energy work. The heat and grounding effect of the stones will help the client to shift their focus within and allow the energy to move.

Rolfing and Deep Tissue Work

Rolfing and deep tissue work both attempt to penetrate the tissue at a much deeper level than ordinary massage. This can cause intense pain as a result of the stripping of adhered fascia that is involved in such work. Using hot stones to massage the tissue before entering with depth can cause a softening to occur, making it possible to penetrate with less pain. Placing hot stones on the body, in the hands, or on the feet can help to relax clients and allow them to receive the deep penetration more easily. Massaging with hot stones after the body has received Rolfing or deep tissue work will lessen residual pain and calm the nervous system.

Facials, Pedicures, and Manicures

Facials can be extremely relaxing, but the focus is primarily on the face. When stones are added to the treatment, they lift facials to another dimension. The warmth of the stones spreads throughout the entire body and deepens the relaxation effect. Hot stones can be placed on the client's abdomen, beneath their lower back, under their shoulders, in their hands, on their feet, between their toes, and beneath their knees. Both hot and cold stones can be used to massage the face adding another element to the facial itself. This is an easy, inexpensive way to enhance a well-known treatment and set it apart from the others.

Pedicures and manicures can also benefit from the incorporation of hot stones. They can be used to massage the client's feet or hands, be set in the client's lap, or placed in the client's hand(s). You can also deepen the relaxation effects of a manicure or pedicure by having the client sit upon a large, flat warm stone.

Acupuncture, Chiropractic, and Physical Therapy

The effects of acupuncture, chiropractic, and physical therapy can all be heightened by the integration of hot stones. Acupuncture needles penetrate the body much more easily after it has been massaged briefly with hot stones or has had hot stones placed on it. Chiropractic adjustments move much more freely and painlessly when the area to be adjusted has been massaged briefly beforehand with hot stones. Physical therapy already utilizes massage and moist heat applications in the treatment of injuries. Hot stones provide the opportunity to join these separate modalities together, enhancing their individual effects.

Other Uses for Hot Stones

Hot stones can also be incorporated into a multitude of other modalities and life situations:

- Psychotherapists can calm clients by giving them warm stones to hold or sit on.
- Veterinarians can warm and soothe post-surgical animals by gently running warm stones along their fur or placing a few warm stones against their body.
- Nurses can use hot stones to massage their bedridden patients or comfort them with the placement of warm stones in their beds.
- Hair stylists can include a hot stone shoulder massage with their hair treatment.
- Parents can help their children get to sleep at night or calm their anxieties with a few simple strokes of the hot stones.
- People who work outside in the cold can place hot stones in their pockets to warm their hands.

Using the tools gained from this book, you'll be able to take hot stone massage beyond the workplace, touching as many people as possible with the power of hot stones.

"You are not alone. The stones speak to you. They have their own language. Listen to them and they will guide you."

Denise Christiana, client

SUMMARY

For centuries, people from around the world have used stones for healing purposes. Although rooted in ancient traditions, hot stone massage, which is the incorporation of heated (and cooled) stones into a bodywork session, developed as a unique massage modality in the United States in the early 1990s. Since that time, hot stone massage has become increasingly popular among both therapists and clients.

The unique element of hot stone massage is its use of oiled, heated stones both for static placement and for active massage. Cooled stones may also be used. Like traditional massage, hot stone massage also requires the therapist to use his or her hands without stones. Thus, hot stones do not replace but rather enhance traditional massage methods.

The benefits of hot stone massage are numerous for both the client and the therapist and extend beyond the obvious feel-good aspect to attributes such as muscle softening, pain reduction, relief of the therapist's hands, and many more.

The three-dimensional approach to hot stone massage is unique. Other forms of hot stone massage use the stones primarily on one side of the client's body at a time. Using three-dimensional techniques to move the client's body in space enables the therapist to massage an area from above and beneath simultaneously, as well as to remove stones without engaging the client. This provides a richer experience for clients and places less physical stress on the therapist. This approach also includes a seamless incorporation of the heated stones into the massage, further enhancing the relaxation experience.

Incorporating hot stone massage into a practice requires purchasing supplies, slightly altering the layout of your treatment area, allowing for more time per session, and learning to plan for the seamless integration of the stones into the massage experience. The benefits to be derived are substantial and include the expansion of clientele, increased revenues, less stress on your body, more satisfied clients, and greater personal gratification.

REVIEW QUESTIONS

TRUE/FALSE

1. Hot stones were commonly used by ancient peoples living in cold climates, but there is little evidence that hot stones were used by peoples living in warmer regions.

   Circle: True False

2. A hot stone massage uses stones instead of hands to massage the body.

   Circle: True False

3. A hot stone massage includes the movement of oiled stones along the client's body along with the static placement of stones.

   Circle: True False

4. The experience of giving a hot stone massage is somewhat more physically stressful on the therapist's body than the experience of giving a traditional massage.

   Circle: True False

5. In three-dimensional massage, the therapist uses both hands on the same side of the client's body at once.

   Circle: True False

MULTIPLE CHOICE

6. A three-dimensional hot stone massage differs from a traditional hot stone massage in which way?
   a. It uses stones on both sides of the body at once.
   b. It allows therapists to remove stones from beneath clients without having to involve them.
   c. It creates a fluid, seamless experience for both the client and therapist.
   d. It utilizes gravity and the weight of the client, rather than strength, to penetrate the tissue.
   e. All of the above

7. A reason clients give for seeking a hot stone massage is:
   a. Relief of joint pain
   b. Increased circulation
   c. Sensual pleasure
   d. Detoxification
   e. All of the above

8. Hot stones can be incorporated into:
   a. Energy work
   b. Animal care
   c. Physical therapy
   d. Facials
   e. All of the above

9. A client may experience the following benefit from receiving massage with hot stones:
   a. Cure of cancer
   b. Weight loss
   c. Deep penetration in the muscle without pain
   d. Feeling of being "shocked" with energy
   e. None of the above

10. A possible challenge for integrating stones into an existing massage practice is:
    a. Slight alterations to layout of treatment area
    b. Increase in clientele and revenue
    c. Creation of a niche market
    d. Having to strategize when managing stones
    e. Both a and d

SHORT ANSWER

11. The ancient Japanese used hot stones as an alternative to a treatment called ______________ in which heat stimulates the flow of chi.

12. Scandinavians use heated stones in structures called ________________________ to stimulate sweating.

13. Instead of their fingers or thumbs, therapists can use ________________________ stones to achieve deep penetration of tissues.

14. Parents can use hot stones to ________________ ________________________.

15. People who work outdoors in the winter can use hot stones to ________________.

Answers to Review Questions can be found in Appendix D.

CHAPTER 2

Physiologic Effects of Hot Stone Massage

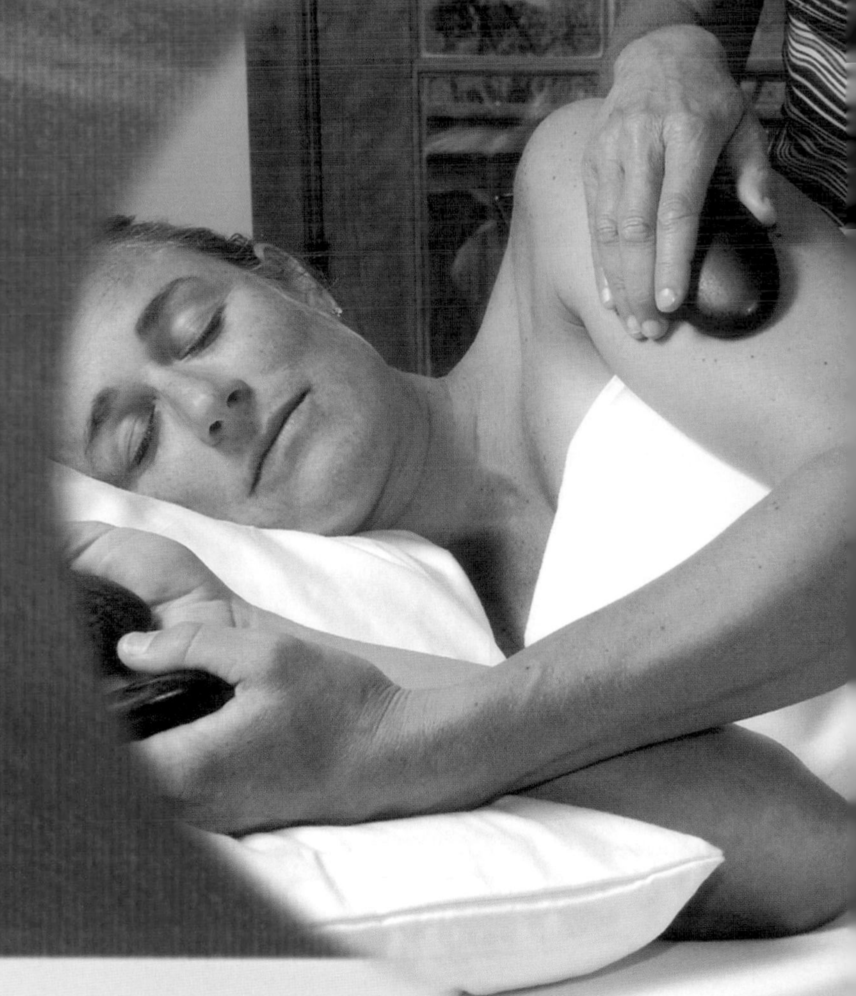

Outline

Objectives

- Compare and contrast the effects of heat and cold on the human body.
- Discuss the appropriate use of thermotherapy and cryotherapy.
- Explain the effect of heat on balms and essential oils.
- Describe the effects on the body and therapeutic use of thermo-cryotherapy.
- Identify disease conditions in which hot and/or cold stone use is contraindicated and explain why.
- Identify disease conditions for which special care is required in order to provide hot stone massage safely.

Key Terms

Active hyperemia: Physiologic response in which blood rushes to an area recovering from an application of cold.

Acute: Having a sudden onset and involving intense pain and other symptoms that typically resolve promptly with appropriate medical intervention. Contrast *Chronic.*

Aromatherapy: The use of essential oils to promote health and well-being. The fragrances and oils can be applied to the body or introduced into the air through a variety of heating methods.

Balm: An ointment, cream, or other skin product that relieves muscular pain and inflammation through dissemination of heat.

Chronic: Having a gradual onset and characterized by signs and symptoms that are difficult to interpret, persist for a long time, and generally cannot be prevented by medical interventions. Contrast *Acute.*

(Continued)

Key Terms (Continued)

Counterirritant: Substance applied topically to produce a slight irritation or inflammation in order to relieve pain or deeper inflammation.

Cryotherapy: Clinical application of cold to treat an ailment, relieve pain, and/or improve the client's general state of well-being.

Derivation: Physiologic process by which heat draws blood to the surface of the body.

Nerve conduction velocity: The speed of conduction of impulses through a nerve.

Occlusion: Clinically induced, temporary blockage of blood supply, trapping toxins next to the skin.

Reactive hyperemia: Physiologic response to the removal of an occlusion in which blood rushes to the site.

Retrostasis: Physiologic process by which cold draws blood away from the surface and to the interior of the body.

Thermo-cryotherapy: Clinical application of alternating heat and cold to treat an ailment, relieve pain, and/or improve the client's general state of well-being.

Thermotherapy: Clinical application of heat to treat an ailment, relieve pain, and/or improve the client's general state of well-being.

Tonify: To enhance or restore balance and to strengthen various parts of the body, including blood and all organs.

Trigger point: A small, isolated tight spot in the muscle tissue that is tender to touch and causes referred pain to another area distant from itself.

Vascular gymnastics (also *vascular whip* or *circulatory whip*)**:** Physiologic response to the rapid and constant alternation of applications of heat and cold in which vessels repeatedly dilate and constrict.

Heat and cold not only add a different type of sensory stimulation to traditional massage, but also have physiologic effects that can be healing. This chapter identifies the effects of heat and cold on the body, both in general and during a hot stone massage. An understanding of these effects will enable you to safely include both temperatures in a massage. This chapter will also help you determine which temperature to use for different clients and how long to use an application. It will also enable you to explain to your clients how hot stone massage is likely to affect them.

Despite the numerous benefits of massage with hot and cold stones, you should be aware of situations that warrant caution, consultation with a physician, or strict avoidance. These situations and disorders are discussed in the final section of this chapter.

EFFECTS OF HEAT AND COLD ON THE BODY

Two opposing physiological processes are prompted by the application of heat and cold to the body. Heat draws blood to the surface, or periphery, of the body through the physiological process known as **derivation**. Cold drives blood to the interior of the body through the physiological process known as **retrostasis**. These are the primary, initial effects of heat and cold; however, secondary effects also occur with long-term applications. The secondary effect of long-term cold is to draw blood once again to the body surface, thus warming the surface tissues. This process is known as *secondary derivation*. The secondary effect of long-term heat, although not quite as dramatic as cold's reverse effect, is to increase blood flow back to the interior over time.

In extremes of environmental temperature, the body uses these processes of derivation and retrostasis in an attempt to maintain homeostasis (1).

The autonomic nervous system also utilizes the processes of derivation and retrostasis as part of the sympathetic and parasympathetic responses. For instance, with sympathetic nervous system arousal (known as the "fight or flight" response), blood rushes away from the skin and digestive organs towards the brain, heart, and lungs, promoting quick, clear thinking and increasing heart rate and breath. These effects prepare the body to take actions necessary for survival. When the parasympathetic nervous system is activated, blood rushes towards the skin and digestive organs, lowering the blood pressure and respiratory rate. This "resting and digesting" response helps the body to calm down, relax, and regenerate (2).

When a client's body is appropriately warmed, activation of the parasympathetic nervous system reduces blood pressure and prompts relaxation. Conversely, when cold is applied to the body, the sympathetic nervous system is stimulated, blood rushes away from the periphery towards the heart to preserve core temperature, and the client typically feels invigorated.

These effects differ somewhat according to whether the heat or cold is applied locally (over a specific area of the body) or globally (over a large area). When heat or cold are applied locally, with a heat or ice pack or an individual stone placement, the effect on the blood flow is limited to that specific area. When heat or cold is applied in a global way, such as by gliding hot or cold stones over the body, the effect in blood flow is experienced over more of the body.

As a massage therapist interested in working with heat and cold, you need to understand that exposure to *extreme* heat or cold is dangerous. If you apply excessive heat, you will stimulate the client's sympathetic nervous system and possibly shock or burn the body part. In contrast, applying extreme cold for an excessive amount of time will eventually activate the parasympathetic nervous system and have a sedating effect, as in the later stages of hypothermia.

It is also important to note that although hot and cold applications usually have the effects discussed in this chapter, this is not always the case for every client. For example, you may have a client who responds to heat the way most people respond to cold. If you pay close attention to your clients, you will notice these differences. The following discussions of the effects of both heat and cold identify the most common primary effects rather than the delayed or unusual.

Thermotherapy

Thermotherapy involves the application of heat to the body for the purpose of treating an injury or other disorder, relieving pain, or increasing the client's general state of well-being.

Effects of Heat on the Body

Widely known for its relaxing and sedating effects, heat has been used for ages to offer relief from sore, stiff muscles as well as from stress. Application of heat to the body also produces the following effects:

- Vasodilatation (widening of blood vessels) in the treated area
- Increased flow of blood and lymph to the area of application
- Increased peripheral blood flow
- Decreased blood pressure
- Increased gastrointestinal functioning
- Increased cellular metabolism
- Increased detoxification of the body's tissues
- Heightened immune response
- Decreased muscle pain and tension
- Decreased muscle spasms
- Increased muscle flexibility
- Softened muscle tissue
- Increased range of motion
- Increased extensibility of collagen
- Decreased viscosity of synovial fluid
- Decreased cardiac activity
- Decreased breathing rate
- Decreased flow of blood to the brain
- Increased sedative effect on the nerves
- Activation of the parasympathetic nervous system

The following is a basic explanation of what happens when heat is applied to the body and why it has these effects. As stated previously, heat causes the blood vessels to dilate (widen), thus promoting an increase in blood flow to the area where the heat is applied. Increased blood flow brings fresh oxygen, nutrients, and lymph to distressed tissues and cleanses the body through the increased removal of toxins. In this way, heat helps to restore tissue strength and health. Heating the surface of the skin also increases the ability of the immune cells to destroy germs.

In addition, heating a part of the body that harbors an active infection hastens the speed at which leukocytes (white blood cells) move into that area to fight the infection. Furthermore, anaerobic bacteria cannot reproduce in a high-oxygen environment, and because increased blood flow means increased oxygenation of tissues, this type of bacteria will die out. Other microbes cannot tolerate high temperatures and, therefore, perish in heated body tissues. Finally, heat increases cellular metabolism. This is tolerated well by healthy tissues, but is detrimental to bacteria already challenged by high temperatures, oxygen, and white blood cells. Thus, heat application heightens the body's defense mechanisms and increases the microbial death rate (3). It can, however, cause a temporary exacerbation of the symptoms of infection while the healing is occurring.

When heat is applied to muscles, it increases spindle activity, promoting greater flexibility and range of motion. Heat also increases the extensibility of collagen, creating elasticity, softening the muscles, and reducing stiffness and muscle spasms. All of these effects allow deeper and easier penetration into a muscle during a massage. In addition, heat reduces the viscosity of synovial fluid, creating more freedom and less pain in joints.

Heat has a calming effect on the nervous system and prompts blood pressure, heart rate, and breathing to slow down. This contributes to the feeling of relaxation and the dulling of brain activity that heat brings to the body.

Because of its derivative nature, strategic placement of heat on the body will help to draw the blood away from an area of congestion. For instance, congestion in the head can be reduced by applying heat on the feet or legs. If there is congestion in the lungs, heat can be placed on the lower torso, hands, and on the chest to draw the congestion towards the body periphery and the surface of the skin. For congestion in the middle ear, heat can be placed on the sides of the head.

As you can see, the effects of massaging with heat are vast. And although the majority of them are quite positive, certain conditions and disorders do require special care. Contraindications to the use of heat and special precautions that must be taken into account before applying heat to the body will be covered later in this chapter.

CAUTION

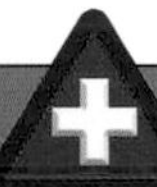

Both you and your client need to drink extra water after a hot stone massage because the heat against the skin can have a cumulative dehydrating effect.

Appropriate Use of Thermotherapy

Heat is best used for chronic rather than acute injuries. An **acute** injury is the result of sudden trauma and usually involves severe symptoms such as sharp pain, heat, bruising and/or bleeding, and inflammation. A **chronic** injury is one that appears gradually, can be intermittent, and may cause dull pain or soreness. It is often the result of overuse but can also develop or intensify over time, particularly when an acute injury is not properly treated. Heat should be applied to a chronic injury just before exercise or when resting.

Generally, heat should be applied to the body for periods ranging from 5 to 20 minutes. Prolonged applications of over 30 minutes may have adverse results. The overheating of a body part can cause burns as well as less obvious problems such as pooling, stagnation, and congestion of blood in an area. This can actually reverse the positive effects of the heat and cause inflammation or slight bruising to an area. So, while heat is predominantly a safe and healing modality, care must be taken with the length of its application (4).

Effects of Heat on Balms and Essential Oils

Balms (or *liniments*) are topical analgesics designed to relieve pain and heal muscle injuries. Different balms may have heating, anti-inflammatory, and/or counterirritant effects. The heat that is created on the skin by the herbs in a balm stimulates an increase in blood flow. Lavender, rosemary, and camphor are examples of herbs that draw blood to the skin and thereby create heat. Balms containing calendula, ginger, and chamomile have anti-inflammatory effects. Balms made with eucalyptus and wintergreen irritate and stimulate the muscles, causing toxins to be flushed out. Otherwise known as **counterirritants,** this last group of remedies serves to distract the brain from the source of original pain, offering temporary relief by creating an opposing nerve pathway for pain. This technique is similar to that of pinching an arm to counteract the pain of a toothache. Adding an external source of heat to any of these balms will help to increase their anti-inflammatory, detoxifying, counterirritant, and analgesic effects (5).

Essential oils are concentrated extracts derived from plants, roots, and flowers. They have many therapeutic qualities, including heating, oxygenating, and irritating a local area of the skin. Essential oils can also be added to the hot water in the skillet to create **aromatherapy.** Adding heat to essential oils magnifies their healing potential. Both static heat and the heat from stones gliding along the body increase the diffusion of the oil's fragrance and help to drive it more deeply into the client's tissues.

Be sure your clients have no physical conditions that could result in an adverse reaction from the application or inhalation of balms or essential oils. You should always double check with your clients before applying balms or essential oils, and even more so during a hot stone massage, as the effects are magnified. This magnification is generally a good thing, but in the case of a negative reaction, it can result in a serious rash, allergic reaction, or other problem.

Cryotherapy

Cryotherapy involves the application of cold to the body for the purpose of treating an injury or other disorder, relieving pain, or increasing the client's general state of well-being.

Effects of Cold on the Body

Applying cold to the body is generally known to induce feelings of being awakened, stimulated, and vitalized. Application of cold to the body also produces the following effects. Notice that some are surprisingly similar to the effects of heat.

- Vasoconstriction (narrowing of blood vessels) in area of application
- Increased blood pressure
- Decreased blood and lymph flow to area of application, limiting hemorrhaging
- Decreased peripheral blood flow
- Lowered inflammatory response
- Decreased edema and swelling by limiting fluid infiltration
- Reduction in pain by lowered **nerve conduction velocity** (acts as an analgesic)
- Raised pain threshold
- Decreased gastrointestinal functioning
- Decreased cellular metabolism
- Increased amount of favorable hormones in blood serum
- Increased detoxification of body
- Heightened immune response
- Lowered muscle contractility
- Decreased muscle spasms
- Increased muscle flexibility
- Increased range of motion
- Increased muscle tone
- Increased viscosity of synovial fluid
- Increased cardiac activity
- Increased breathing rate
- Increased flow of blood to brain
- Stimulation of the sympathetic nervous system

The application of cold is one of the simplest, safest, fastest, and most effective techniques for caring for acute injuries, pain, and chronic discomfort of muscles and joints. Because cold causes the blood vessels to constrict, blood flow is decreased to an injured area. This in turn limits fluid infiltration and internal bleeding that would normally cause additional edema or swelling. This decrease in the inflammatory response helps to prevent further inflammation of an already injured tissue.

Cold combined with compression can produce even more dramatic results in reducing tissue swelling. Cold constricts the walls of blood vessels while the compression restricts the amount of blood that can reach an injured area. Draining a cooled area by means of elevation further eliminates inflammation from the damaged area.

Cooling a muscle reduces its ability to maintain a contraction (contractility). This lessens muscle spasms and induces relaxation. The inability of muscles to maintain contraction when cooled also allows for greater mobility.

By means of retrostasis, cold tends to drive blood to the interior of the body and away from the locus of application. Thus, when extra blood is needed to improve the function of the internal organs, such as the heart, lungs, or brain, cold can be applied to the extremities, forcing blood inward. Because blood tends to move away from cold, it is effective for treating headaches, migraines, and sinus congestion. Application of cold to the head or face draws away excess heat or congestion and can relieve pressure. When blood eventually rushes back to an area that has been cooled, as its secondary response, it flushes the area with freshly oxygenated blood, cleansing the body and aiding in detoxification.

Cold has a stimulating effect on the brain as well as the entire nervous system. Because of the constriction of blood flow to the area of application, there will be more blood available to supply the brain. Thus, cold contributes to mental alertness and higher levels of energy. It can even elevate mood in someone who is depressed. Cold's anti-inflammatory effect reduces puffiness beneath eyes and edema in tissue and thus contributes to a youthful appearance of the skin on the face. Because cold stimulates the sympathetic nervous system, increasing the heart rate, breathing, and blood pressure, it strengthens the entire body.

Cold lowers the conduction velocity of nerves, thus acting as an analgesic and decreasing the sensation of pain while increasing the pain threshold. Although cold has a valuable capacity to break the cycle of pain, it can also mask the extent of an injury. Thus, injured clients need to be careful that they don't prematurely resume rigorous activities after cold therapies have relieved their pain. Doing so may cause further trauma.

The combination of cold's capacity to decrease inflammation and muscle spasms, increase range of motion, and decrease pain all make it possible for an injury to heal more quickly with the application of cold.

Appropriate Use of Cryotherapy

For the treatment of acute injuries, it is best to apply cold immediately after the onset and then every few hours for the first 48 hours. It is also useful to apply cold to a chronic injury immediately after it has been used for exercise (6).

CAUTION

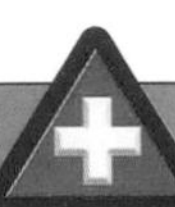

Applications of cold should be done gradually and gently, warming the area first before applying the cold. The shock of the sudden cold can have a detrimental effect, causing clients to tighten their muscles and hold their breath.

Cold applications should be limited to approximately 10 to 20 minutes at a time. As with heat, the positive effects of cold can be reversed if the application is prolonged. Exposure to cold lasting over 30 minutes can cause permanent numbing of tissues as well as an increase in inflammation because of the secondary response to derivation (reactive vasodilatation). Contraindications to and precautions in the application of cold are discussed later in this chapter.

Thermo-Cryotherapy

Thermo-cryotherapy (also called *contrast therapy*) involves the clinical application of alternating heat and cold to the body for the purpose of treating an injury or other disorder, relieving pain, or increasing the client's general state of well-being. The contrast application of alternating heat and cold can be more comfortable than cold by itself and is a very powerful treatment, integrating the primary effects of both exposures.

Effects of Contrasting Temperatures on the Body

Alternating derivation and retrostasis provides the optimal effects of both hot and cold applications, increasing the local blood flow by up to 100%. The heat brings freshly oxygenated blood to an area to begin healing and to carry away toxins, while the cold limits pain and inflammation and slows down the metabolism that causes the buildup of waste products. Applying heat (which is a vasodilator) to an area that has just had an application of cold (which is a vasoconstrictor) brings more blood than would be drawn following heat alone. The constant alternating of blood flow and blood deprivation to an area of application is referred to as **vascular gymnastics** (or *vascular whip or circulatory whip*). The result is a reddening of the area called **active hyperemia**, hyper- meaning above normal, and *-emia* meaning blood. This is a normal and desirable response and should not be confused with a rash, allergic reaction, or other complication.

A similar flushing of an area of the body can be produced without the aid of hot or cold, but instead by temporarily holding a stone firmly in place on a **trigger point**, thereby preventing blood flow to the constricted area. When the stone is released, the pooled blood rushes into the recently occluded area and cleans it in the same way that alternations of hot and cold do. This process is known as **reactive hyperemia** because the blood flow increases in reaction to the therapist's induced **occlusion** of the area.

The combination of active hyperemia from the alternate application of heat and cold with reactive hyperemia from induced occlusion creates a strong cleansing experience for the body (7). Thermo-cryotherapy, along with trigger point work, is the fastest and most powerful way to boost the immune system, detoxify the body, **tonify** the muscles, promote a deep state of relaxation, and return the body back to balance.

Appropriate Use of Thermo-Cryotherapy

When alternating temperatures, use each for a shorter duration of time than you would when using either temperature alone; ideally, from about 2 to 5 minutes each. Short periods of time between contrasting temperatures induces optimal flushing of the blood. A full contrast therapy treatment should last no less than 10 minutes with at least four different alternations of temperatures. In addition, contrast therapy can be done over a longer period than either cold or heat can be applied alone—you can safely make alternating applications for up to 30 minutes without causing any damage to the body.

CONTRAINDICATIONS TO HOT STONE MASSAGE

Given the effects of heat and cold on human physiology, it is essential that you determine in the initial interview whether or not it is safe to perform hot stone massage on clients with illness or injury. If the medical literature does not recommend massage for the client's condition, then obviously hot stone massage also would be contraindicated. Less obviously, some conditions benefit from massage, but the added element of heat or cold would be detrimental. Thus, upon discussing the health condition with the client, if you have any doubt, request a consult with the client's primary care practitioner before proceeding.

In general, avoid massage with hot or cold stones for any client who has a health condition for which other types of heat or cold therapy are contraindicated. Western medicine discourages the use of heat with disorders that involve inflammation, acute injury, edema, skin rash, open wounds, malignant tumors, compromised circulation, impaired sensation, and heart disease. Cold is discouraged with disorders that involve high blood pressure, heart disease, circulatory problems, impaired sensation, nerve damage, and frostbite. However, individual cases may dictate exceptions to these general guidelines.

Figure 2.1 is an intake form that you may photocopy and use with your clients. It identifies several health conditions, discussed next, that should alert you to proceed with caution or avoid hot stone massage altogether. A detailed description of the etiology and pathophysiology of these disorders is beyond the scope of this text; for more information, see *A Massage Therapist's Guide to Pathology* by Ruth Werner, published by Lippincott Williams & Wilkins. When combined with the subsequent text, this excellent reference will provide you with comprehensive information about these conditions and will increase your confidence when making decisions about the appropriateness of hot stone massage with your clients. The conditions discussed here are summarized in Table 2-1.

Abdominal Distress

Abdominal distress is an experience of discomfort, pain, bloating, gas, cramping, constipation, and/or diarrhea. It may accompany any of a variety of conditions, from transient menstrual cramps, irritable bowel syndrome, or a mild infection to severe gastrointestinal tract disorders such as Crohn's disease, colitis, celiac disease, or cancer.

For all cases of abdominal distress, the use of cold stones is contraindicated, as cold will exacerbate the symptoms. Warm stones applied gently in a clockwise circular fashion over the abdomen mimics the movement of bowel contents and may help reduce the client's symptoms. Moving stones in a counter-clockwise direction could increase constipation and should be avoided, unless diarrhea is present.

Acquired Immunodeficiency Syndrome

Acquired immune deficiency syndrome (AIDS) is a cluster of signs and symptoms that can typically develop several years after infection with the human immunodeficiency virus (HIV). The virus invades and destroys immune cells called T-lymphocytes, leaving the body immuno-compromised; that is, susceptible to opportunistic infections and certain types of cancer (8).

Research has shown that HIV is heat sensitive and will become increasingly inactive as the body temperature is progressively raised above normal (9). Because of this, hot stone massage can be beneficial to HIV-positive clients. And because research has also proven that AIDS is not spread through sweat or tears, it would be safe to perform hot stone massage on clients who suffer from this disorder (10). However, accompanying symptoms may make the use of hot stones detrimental to the client. For example, clients with fever, unexplained sweats, or skin rashes should not receive hot stone therapy. Because the symptoms of AIDS are constantly changing, it is important to check with these clients prior to each session to determine whether or not any presenting symptoms would preclude the use of hot or cold stones. If a decision is made to use hot stones, the treatment regimen, including the duration, intensity, and temperature of the stones, needs to be individualized. Since HIV becomes increasingly inactive when heated, there is the chance that it could become increasingly active when cooled. Since this is unclear, it is safest to avoid the use of cold stones.

Allergic Reactions

Some people are heat or cold sensitive and thus can react to extended applications of hot or cold stones with allergic symptoms. Reactions can range from asthma attacks to red and white blotches, hives, welts,

Hot Stone Massage Intake Form

Name________________________ Phone #________________ Age _______

Have you ever received a hot stone massage before? Yes______ No______

If yes, and there were any negative effects or outcomes, please explain below:

____

____

____

Do you have any of the following health conditions? Please circle all that apply.

Abdominal Distress	Insect Bites
AIDS	Irregular Blood Pressure
Allergic Reactions	Kidney Disease
Arteriosclerosis	Medications (please specify below):
Arthritis	Migraines
Asthma	Multiple Sclerosis
Blood Clots	Muscle Injuries and Sciatica
Bursitis	Neuropraxia
Cancer	Parkinson's Disease
Cleansing Fast	Pregnancy
Cold	Previous Threatening Conditions
Diabetes	Raynaud's Disease
Edema	Scleroderma
Fibromyalgia	Skin Irritations
Gout	Tendonitis
Hepatitis	Varicose Veins
Infection	Vertigo

Other____

To help me to understand your particular condition, please state whether or not you are in the care of a doctor, as well as any treatments you are receiving, including self-care.

____

____

____

List any reasons, including medications that you are taking, that might make it uncomfortable or unsafe for you to receive heat or cold in your massage. (Use back of sheet if necessary.)

____

____

____

Figure 2-1 Intake Form. Ask each client to fill out this intake form and review the information with the client before agreeing to provide a hot stone massage.

or problems with breathing. If a client tends to have an allergic reaction to either heat or cold, moderate your use of hot or cold stones or in extreme cases avoid all use of either temperature. This is important to determine before attempting a hot stone massage.

If a client is already experiencing an allergic reaction not related to temperature, such as in response to pollen, food, or an insect bite, the use of heat should be avoided as it will exacerbate the allergy symptoms by increasing production of histamine. However, in these cases, cold may be useful. Clients should be consulted before using cold when a preexisting allergic reaction is present in case they are sensitive to cold.

Table 2-1 Appropriateness of Heat and Cold Therapies with Various Health Conditions

The use of hot or cold stones is contraindicated with several of the following health conditions. Others require that you proceed with caution or moderate the duration or temperature of the treatment. There may be exceptions to these temperature indicators based on the state of the individual condition. There may also be additional conditions unmentioned here for which heat and cold should be avoided.

Condition	Brief Definition	Heat	Cold
Abdominal Distress	Abdominal discomfort due to IBS, constipation, cramps, etc.	Moderate	No
AIDS	Immune deficiency following HIV infection	Caution	No
Allergic Reactions	Overproduction of histamine due to systemic reaction	No	Yes
Arteriosclerosis	Cardiovascular disease causing hardening of the arteries	No	No
Arthritis	A rheumatic disease causing inflammation and pain to joints	Contrast	Contrast
Asthma	Inflammatory respiratory illness that constricts the airways	Caution	Caution
Blood Clots	Occlusion of blood vessel by mass of clotted blood tissue	No/Caution	Moderate
Bursitis	Inflammation of a bursa	No	Yes
Cancer	Disease involving uncontrolled growth of abnormal cells	Caution	Caution
Cleansing Fast	Temporary elimination of food for purpose of cleansing body	Moderate	Moderate
Diabetes	Insufficient/defective production or uptake of insulin	Moderate	Caution
Edema	Soft tissue swelling due to expansion of interstitial fluid	No	Caution
Fibromyalgia	Inflammatory condition resulting in muscle pain and stiffness	Contrast	Contrast
Gout	Rheumatic disease marked by uric acid deposits in tissues	Moderate	Yes
Hepatitis	Inflammation of liver	Caution	No
Infection or Cold	State resulting from invasion by pathogenic microorganisms	Caution	Caution
Insect Bites	A sting or bite from an insect that causes an allergic reaction	No	Yes
Irreg. Blood Pressure	Blood pressure above or below the normal 120/70	Moderate	Caution
Kidney Disease	Impaired ability of kidneys to filter blood and regulate fluids	No	No
Medications	Medications that would cause adverse reaction to heat or cold	Caution	Caution
Migraine	A headache accompanied by nausea/dizziness/light sensitivity	No	Yes
Multiple Sclerosis	CNS disease marked by destruction of myelin	Moderate	Moderate
Muscle Injury/Sciatica	Injury to muscle that causes inflammation, spasm, and pain	Caution	Caution
Neuropraxia	Nerve insult that impairs transmission of electrical impulses	Moderate	Moderate
Parkinson's Disease	Involves death of brain cells that control muscle movement	Moderate	Moderate
Pregnancy	Period from conception to birth	Caution	Moderate
Previous Conditions	Previous life-threatening conditions that preclude heat/cold	Caution	Caution
Raynaud's Disease	Peripheral vascular disease marked by decreased circulation to extremities	Moderate	No/Contrast
Scleroderma	An overproduction of collagen leading to hardening of skin	Moderate	No/Contrast
Skin Irritations	Rashes, abrasions, fungal infections, acne, burns, hives, etc.	No	Caution
Tendonitis	Painful inflammation of a tendon	Contrast	Yes
Vertigo	Dizziness	Caution	No

Arteriosclerosis

Cardiovascular disease is a general term that denotes disorders of the heart and blood vessels. Of the numerous distinct disorders that fall into this category, arteriosclerosis is one of the more common. The term refers to the thickening and hardening ("sclerosis") of artery walls as a result of a build-up of plaque deposits. The sclerosis narrows the arteries and interferes with the normal flow of blood through the vessels. This makes the heart work harder, which, in turn, can cause high blood pressure, a heart attack, or a stroke (occlusion of a blood vessel in the brain).

When arteries leading to the limbs are affected, circulation problems may develop in the arms and legs. Signs and symptoms in the lower extremities include: Coldness or paleness in the legs and feet; blue/red discoloration of the feet or toes; dry, fragile, or shiny-looking skin; numbness, tingling, or pain in the legs, feet, or toes; and sores that do not heal (11). Because poor arterial circulation blunts sensations to heat or cold, there is a greater susceptibility to damage from both burns and freezing (12).

Use of cold should be avoided with clients who have arteriosclerosis, especially if they have high blood pressure, a common symptom of the disease. Cold causes blood pressure to increase, and it also shocks the heart, placing an additional strain on an already compromised organ, thus further risking the possibility of a heart attack. Cold can also cause injury to an extremity that has impaired sensation.

Heat should also be avoided or used very cautiously. Heat increases circulation, which can overload already constricted arteries, forcing too much blood into a narrowed passage too quickly. In addition, the decreased sensation in the extremities increases the client's risk of a burn injury when heat is applied. Thus, the risk of using hot stones outweighs any possible benefit. If a client with arteriosclerosis requests a hot stone massage, it is strongly recommended that you consult with the client's physician before complying.

Arthritis

Arthritis is a joint disorder characterized by inflammation, heat, redness, and limited range of motion. It is frequently accompanied by joint pain or tenderness, referred to as arthralgia. There are more than 100 forms of arthritis, ranging from those related to wear and tear of cartilage (osteoarthritis) to those associated with inflammation resulting from an overactive immune system (rheumatoid arthritis) (13).

As we have stated, heat therapy is discouraged with disorders that involve inflammation, and yet much of the research recommends the use of heat for relieving symptoms of arthritis. The decision to use heat or cold is an individual one and should be determined by the level of pain, redness, heat, and inflammation present in an affected area (14).

If the swelling is accompanied by a high degree of pain, heat can be useful for relaxing the muscles and lessening the pain and stiffness in a particular area, but care must be taken not to use too much heat, as it can exacerbate the symptoms. Cold stones can be helpful in relieving heat, pain, and swelling, thereby increasing range of motion, but paradoxically they can also increase stiffness.

Because much of the research calls for heat applications to an arthritic joint, it would be wise to alternate use of hot and cold stones. Contrasting hot with cold stones addresses the issue of stiffness and pain as well as the inflammation and heat in the arthritic joints. The results of this alternation of temperatures should be assessed individually, both during and after the treatment to decide what is best for each client.

Asthma

Asthma is an inflammatory respiratory illness that causes mild to severe difficulty in breathing as a result of constriction and swelling of the airways. There is also an increase in secretions of mucus, which congest the smaller airways. As a result, air moves into and out of the lungs with difficulty. Wheezing is a characteristic squealing sound produced as a consequence of the air moving through the narrowed and inflamed air passages (15).

Cold stones used on the chest may help with the inflammation; however, because cold, dry air is a common trigger of asthma, cold stones should be applied gradually, one at a time. Too much weight on the chest could increase breathing difficulties and should be avoided. The moisture and warmth of hot stones can be relaxing to the airways, and yet too much humidity and heat in the air can also trigger asthma symptoms (16). Check with clients before and during the session to regulate temperatures for their immediate comfort.

Blood Clots

Blood clots are jelly-like masses of blood tissue formed by clotting factors in the blood. Blood clotting is a natural and necessary process in which blood cells and fibrin strands clump together to stop bleeding after a blood vessel has been injured. Sometimes, however, blood clots form within an artery or vein, even when a person has not been injured, and these can cause problems. Blood clots can form during prolonged inactivity, or as a side effect of a medicine or a more serious illness. Although many blood clots tend to dissolve on their own, they become dangerous when they block blood flow through an artery or vein, especially in the heart or brain. In such cases, a heart attack or stroke may occur (17).

Thrombophlebitis occurs when a blood clot causes inflammation in one or more veins, typically in the legs and occasionally the arms. The affected vein may be near the surface of the skin (superficial thrombophlebitis) or deep within a muscle (deep vein thrombosis). Heat is helpful for dissolving a blood clot in a superficial vein. However, if varicose veins are present, heat would not be advisable because it can cause more varicose veins to develop or worsen existing ones. Massage either with or without hot stones over an area with deep vein thrombosis can prove risky, as both the heat and the act of massaging with the stones can dislodge the blood clots and cause more serious problems. Additionally, it is not advisable to use hot stones over a limb that is swollen. Even if there are no signs or symptoms of deep vein thrombosis, caution should still be taken.

If a client is being treated for heart disease, is taking thrombolytics to dissolve a present blood clot, or using anticoagulants for the prevention of blood clots, avoid heat and deep massage. Cold stones will not help to dissolve a superficial blood clot, but they may be able to aid in reducing the swelling of thrombophlebitis. If cold stones are used for inflammation, simply place the stones lightly on the area, but do not massage in order to avoid dislodging a blood clot.

Bursitis

Bursitis is the inflammation of a bursa, a tiny fluid-filled sac that reduces friction by acting as a gliding surface. The body contains 160 bursae, with the major ones located adjacent to the tendons near the large joints such as the shoulders, elbows, hips, and knees. A bursa can become inflamed from injury, infection, or an underlying rheumatic condition. Heat tends to exacerbate the inflammation and should be avoided. Cold is the treatment of choice with bursitis.

Cancer

Cancer is a group of diseases characterized by uncontrolled growth and spread of abnormal cells. Because both massage and heat increase the flow and circulation of blood and lymph, they can also serve to aid in the spread of cancer present in the body. Therefore, both traditional massage and hot stone massage are contraindicated during the very early stages of cancer treatment.

For women with breast cancer, following mastectomy, hot stone massage is very helpful in regaining the lost range of motion in the arms. Hot stones can also add a much-needed nurturing quality to the medical treatment of cancer. Therapists should avoid use of hot stones, however, if lymph edema is present. Cold stones can be helpful in reducing lymph edema (see section on edema).

Research indicates that gradually raising the temperature of cancer-riddled tissue to anywhere from 105°F to 113°F, otherwise known as hyperthermia, can enhance the effect of chemotherapy and radiation treatment (18). When cells in the body are subjected to higher-than-normal temperatures, changes take place within the cells that make them more likely to be affected by these medical therapies. Very high temperatures can kill cancer cells directly (19). Thus, using very hot stones in areas of cancer may enhance the effectiveness of chemotherapy. Hot stones can also be used during the radiation phase of treatment, but not directly on the skin because it can become thin and slightly burned during radiation. Cold stones are soothing for skin that has undergone radiation treatment.

Ask your clients to check with their doctors to determine whether or not massage with hot or cold stones is suitable for them. Even if both the client and the doctor opt for hot stones, you still need to feel comfortable with the decision. If you don't, then you need to ask the client to seek a different massage therapist.

TESTIMONIAL

I have personally worked with many cancer clients who swore that the hot stones were the only things that helped them to feel good throughout the healing process.

Cleansing Fast

A cleansing fast is a treatment in which a person avoids eating solid food for a period of time in order to cleanse the body of toxins or allergens. Usually juice, broth, or water is ingested during a cleansing fast, along with vitamins, herbs, and intestinal tract cleansers, such as bentonite clay and ground psyllium husks. If a client is on a cleansing fast, it would be wise to either avoid the use of hot and cold stones, or use them with moderate temperatures, as fasting can cause lightheadedness and weakness, which may be increased by the heat or challenged by the cold.

Diabetes

Diabetes is a chronic disorder characterized by insufficient or defective production or uptake of the hormone insulin. Without insulin, glucose (the sugar produced from the breakdown of carbohydrates) cannot be transported into the body's cells. Instead, it remains in the bloodstream, causing a condition commonly known as high blood sugar and depriving cells of the energy they need to maintain their functions.

There are two types of diabetes. Type I is inherited and is usually diagnosed during childhood. It involves such a severe lack of insulin that it must be supplied by injection or a continuous infusion pump every day. Type II was once called *adult-onset diabetes*, but is now being seen in children as young as school-age. It is characterized by insulin resistance, and can often be managed with a nutritious diet, weight loss, exercise, and oral medication rather than injections of insulin (20).

Although the use of hot and cold stones for clients with diabetes is not completely contraindicated, special care must be taken. Heat and massage speed up the breakdown of glucose and fatty acids and can affect insulin absorption rates (21). Thus, it is important to avoid insulin injection sites (22). In addition, clients should monitor their blood glucose levels after, and sometimes while, receiving a hot stone massage.

One of the later-stage symptoms of diabetes is *peripheral neuropathy*, nerve damage (usually affecting the feet and legs) that causes pain, numbness, or a tingling feeling. Clients suffering from peripheral neuropathy may be unable to perceive variations in temperature in affected areas; thus, it is imperative that you use great caution with both heat and cold, especially on the client's legs and feet, as you could burn client or cause further nerve damage.

Edema

Edema is defined as soft-tissue swelling due to expansion of the interstitial fluid volume. Edema can be limited to a specific part of the body such as the feet and ankles (localized) or occur throughout the body (generalized). Edema is a sign of an underlying problem, rather than a disease itself. Some of its many causes are: Prolonged sitting, excess of sodium, antihistamine reactions, sunburns, pregnancy, medications, altitude, significant protein deficiency, heart or kidney failure, and cancer (23).

In all cases of edema, use of heat should be avoided, as warm temperatures cause the blood vessels to expand, making it easier for fluid to cross into surrounding tissues. Deep tissue massage has an effect that is similar to heat because it increases circulation and fluids into the tissues. Thus, using hot stones is not appropriate with any form of edema. Cold stones used with light pressure would be helpful for treating all forms of edema, as they restrict the flow of fluids into surrounding areas.

Lymph drainage is a type of massage that uses very light strokes in a specific direction to stimulate the lymph vessels just below the surface of the skin without increasing blood circulation or reaching a depth in the muscle tissue. This type of gentle massage would be recommended to do with cold stones for helping lymph edema.

Fibromyalgia

Although fibromyalgia is a relatively new term, it is used to describe an age-old problem: Muscle and joint pain that persists for no discernible reason. The primary symptoms include stiff, aching muscles and burning or throbbing pain, especially at specific points on the body. It is believed to be an inflammatory condition akin to rheumatism and may be related to a malfunction of the immune system (24).

As both heat and cold are forms of pain relief and immune boosters, and cold assists in relieving inflammation, hot and cold stone massage can be very useful in reducing symptoms of fibromyalgia. It is important to note, however, that heat and cold can sometimes initiate pain for some clients with fibromyalgia. Consult with clients on an individual basis as the symptoms and reactions to temperatures vary.

Avoid massaging deeply with hot stones, as their relaxing effect can mask the depth of the massage and cause exacerbations of symptoms the following day. Although cold is not very pleasurable for people with fibromyalgia, if they are able and willing to endure it, they will usually experience excellent results, including significantly decreased inflammation the next day. Thermo-cryotherapy is also useful: Hot stones offer relief from muscular tension, while cold stones reduce hidden swelling within the muscle fibers. Both hot and cold stones can offer pain relief if used with moderate temperatures and pressure.

Gout

Gout is one of the most painful rheumatic diseases. It results from deposits of needle-like crystals made of uric acid in connective tissue, in the joint space between two bones, or in both. These deposits lead to inflammatory arthritis, which causes swelling, redness, heat, pain, and stiffness in the joints.

As with other forms of arthritis, many of the resources on gout suggest using heat for pain relief. And yet my personal experience and testimonies from people with gout suggest that cold is more effective. Certainly you should discuss the matter with clients before thrusting heat upon an already heated and inflamed area. I recommend gliding cold stones gently on the affected area. But if the client states that warmth seems to help them, use gently warmed stones.

Hepatitis

Hepatitis is an umbrella term for inflammation of the liver, which could over time lead to extensive scarring of the liver tissue. There are many types of hepatitis, some caused by a virus, which can be spread either through infected food or blood exchange, and others caused by autoimmune disorders, which are not contagious. The liver is the gatekeeper and regulator of nutritional health and acts as a purifying system, cleansing toxins from the body. Because the liver plays a significant role in the circulation and composition of blood, its vitality affects all systems of the body (25).

Heat applied directly over the liver can be detrimental to a client with hepatitis as it could increase inflammation. However, hot stones that are glided globally over the entire body can serve to increase blood circulation to the liver, aiding it in its job of detoxification. Prolonged applications of cold can slow down the circulation and increase the levels of toxicity in the body. Many clients who are experiencing hepatitis prefer heat as it encourages perspiration and thus aids the body in ridding itself of toxins. Because neither heat nor cold are life-threatening to clients with hepatitis, it is best to ask the clients what works best for them. If you do use hot or cold during the massage, ask clients to pay attention and report to you the results of either therapy.

Infections and Colds

Heat can increase the level of leukocytes to help fight infection and raise the body temperature, making it less hospitable to microbes. However, it can temporarily exacerbate the symptoms of an infection or a cold in the process. If an infected area of the body is warm and red, cool stones will offer temporary soothing relief but may slightly deter the healing process. Cold stones will increase the symptoms of a cold and should be avoided.

Consult with clients who have an infection or cold before providing a hot stone massage. Let them know of the advantages and disadvantages to using either hot or cool stones so that they can be informed and make the choice for themselves.

Insect Bites

Insect bites that are accompanied by an allergic reaction of histamine production will usually have symptoms of swelling, heat, edema, itching, and pain. All of these symptoms will be exacerbated with the application of heat. Heat can also serve to spread the venom of the bite. Thus, it is important to avoid using hot stones on or near the area of an insect bite, even if no symptoms exist, as heat can elicit a symptom that would have otherwise remained dormant. If the allergic reaction to the bite is localized, hot stones can be used on other areas of the body. But if the reaction is systemic, with a red rash or itching on most of the body, it is imperative to avoid use of hot stones altogether. Once the reaction is under control, cold stones glided along the affected areas of the body will aid greatly in slowing down the spread of the venom and removing the itch, inflammation, heat, and irritation from the reaction to the bite (26).

Irregular Blood Pressure

When a client normally has low blood pressure, hot stones can further reduce blood pressure to a point that can cause lightheadedness. In clients with high blood pressure, the reduction of blood pressure produced by hot stones can be stressful to the body. Thus, both low and high blood pressure call for using hot stones in moderation. Hot stones can be used when these conditions exist, but it is prudent to integrate them slowly with slightly less heat.

The use of cold stones is also discouraged for clients with high blood pressure as the cold will constrict the blood vessels and increase blood pressure. Cold stones will be useful with clients who have low blood pressure, especially at the end of the massage to help bring their blood pressure back up into its normal range, rather than leaving the client lightheaded.

Kidney Disease

Kidney disease is an impairment of the kidneys' ability to filter blood and regulate fluids in the body. It can be caused by any condition that affects the blood vessels, including diabetes, high blood pressure, arteriosclerosis, heart surgery, severe dehydration, severe infection, and more than 100 others (27). When a person has kidney disease, there is also the chance that they may develop blood clots. As kidney disease can result from or involve a multitude of conditions where hot or cold temperatures are contraindicated, it is safest to simply avoid using both hot and cold stones on such clients.

Medications

Ask clients what medications, if any, they are taking, and also ask about their possible side effects. For example, skin hypersensitivity can be caused by antibiotics, seizure medications, and AIDS medications, and many medications affect blood pressure. Make sure you consider all client medications, including over-the-counter drugs and herbal remedies, before deciding to use hot or cold stones in the massage.

Migraines

Hot stones are effective in preventing migraine headaches from occurring by relaxing the muscles around the head, jaw, and neck. But once a migraine headache has developed, heat used on the head or neck can aggravate the condition because it dilates the blood vessels and stimulates the flow of blood to the head. When migraine headaches occur, the application of cold stones to the face, scalp, eyes, and wrists, is indicated (28). Heat would be helpful on the feet to draw blood away from the head.

Multiple Sclerosis

Multiple sclerosis (MS) is a progressive disease of the central nervous system in which areas of the myelin sheath covering nerve cells in the brain and spinal cord are destroyed by inflammation and scarring. As more and more of the sheath is stripped away, a process called *demyelination*, electrical impulses proceed more and more slowly down the fiber. This leads to various neurological defects such as impaired vision, unsteadiness of the limbs, and loss of feeling or tingling of various parts of the body (29). The symptoms may unpredictably occur and then disappear, and they range from moderate to severe.

One common feature of multiple sclerosis is that many symptoms worsen when the patient is exposed to heat. This is because elevated temperatures further slow the conduction of electrical impulses in nerve fibers. Too much heat can cause the muscles to spasm or become flaccid. Mild heat, however, can help to improve circulation and decrease spasticity of the muscles. Because extreme heat can make the symptoms worse, use only moderate temperatures.

Conversely, cryotherapy can sometimes temporarily relieve symptoms or reduce some of the fatigue multiple sclerosis patients often feel. Thermo-cryotherapy with moderate temperatures for warm and cool stones can help reduce spasticity, maintain flexibility, and relieve muscle pain. Discuss all therapy options with clients first, as they may be able to provide important information about whether or not even warm and cool stones are appropriate to use. Err on the conservative side if there is any uncertainty (30).

Muscle Injury and Sciatica Pain

Treatment of muscle injury varies according to whether the injury is acute, subacute, or chronic. Heat should never be used during the acute stage of an injury, which is the first 48 to 72 hours after its onset, or with acute inflammation. Heat will increase circulation to the area, increasing the swelling and microscopic bleeding, causing the injury to worsen and the pain to increase. Cold is very important to use with an acute injury, reducing inflammation, pain, and spasticity. Occasionally, a muscle is under such severe tension that heat is the only therapy that can immediately relieve the pain. In these situations, ice can be applied afterwards. Heat does not need to be ruled out entirely if the acute injury does not involve substantial inflammation.

After 2 to 3 days, the injury is considered subacute. If the injury persists over a week, the body's healing process enters the chronic stage, which persists as long as the injury is present. In the subacute and chronic stages of healing, both cold and heat can be beneficial. Cold may continue to be of more benefit when swelling remains in the area. Cold can also be very useful when muscle spasms are present. Heat can decrease pain, promote healing by increasing circulation, help tight muscles or muscle spasms to relax, and prepare stiff joints for movement. The effects of heat do not last as long as cold, but can give temporary relief for up to 1 hour or more. Alternating hot and cold stones is often the best treatment for a subacute and chronic injury (31).

Be careful when using cold stones over an injured area, as their analgesic effect can mask the pain that would have normally been felt by the stones without the cold's numbing effect. This can lead to residual pain or injury that is only noticed after the analgesic effect has worn off.

For clients suffering from sciatica (pain along the sciatic nerve), thermo-cryotherapy is the treatment of choice. Using just heat or cold on an inflamed or impinged sciatic nerve can be damaging. The heated stones alone can increase the inflammation, whereas cold stones alone can cause the muscles to constrict around the nerve causing more pressure on it. The combination of the two temperatures helps to relax the tense muscles that are pinching the nerve while eliminating inflammation.

Neuropraxia

Neuropraxia is a reversible form of nerve damage. It results in abnormal conduction of nerve impulses at the specific site of the injury, with normal conduction both proximal and distal to the injured site. Whether mild or severe, neuropraxia can result from a variety of causes such as a crush injury, compression, repetitive use, stretch injury, surgical procedures, radiation therapy, burns, and cold (32).

As with any condition that involves nerve impairment, both hot and cold stones should be used cautiously over the injured area. Because of primary and secondary derivation, both hot and cold temperatures will help to increase the blood circulation to the injured areas. But because the clients have diminished feeling in the injured area, they will not be able to know if a temperature is too hot or too cold. In addition, the impaired area will be more affected by heat and cold than the areas peripheral to it. Moderate degrees of temperature are called for with this disorder.

Parkinson's Disease

Parkinson's disease (PD) is a chronic, progressive disorder of the nervous system that affects a person's muscular coordination. Symptoms of PD include tremors (shaking), rigidity in some muscles, slow movements, and problems maintaining normal posture. The disease is caused by the death of certain brain cells that release a neurotransmitter called dopamine, which is needed to transmit messages from one brain cell to another. Without sufficient amounts of dopamine, the instructions that brain cells need to move muscles do not reach their targets (33).

Parkinson's disease is yet another condition that calls for the use of moderate temperatures of stones. High heat can exacerbate the symptoms of PD and must be avoided (34). In addition, some medications used for the treatment of PD inhibit perspiration, so exposure to high temperatures should be avoided (35). Both warm and cool stones are helpful in relieving some of the muscular tension and spasms. Alternating both temperatures yields the best results. Begin and end the alternations of warm and cool with a warm temperature to achieve the highest level of relaxation for clients.

Pregnancy

During the first trimester, massage with hot stones should be entirely avoided. After the first trimester, hot stones can be used on all parts of the body except the belly, as too much direct heat can cause injuries to the fetus (36).

When massaging with hot stones, be careful to regulate the amount of heat used and make sure to allow for appropriate heat dissipation in order to prevent raising the mother's body temperature too high. Augment heat dissipation by keeping the client's hands and feet out from under the top sheet. Use moderate stone temperatures and fewer stones. Ventilating the room will also help to keep pregnant women from overheating from the warm stones. Weave in the use of cold stones, especially on extremities, to further aid in the dissipation of the heat.

TESTIMONIAL

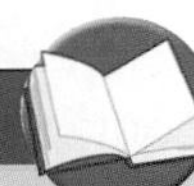

I have massaged pregnant women with warm to hot stones after their first trimester up to the time of birth and all of them have reported a much easier birth that they attribute to increased muscular relaxation over time from the stones.

Previous Life-Threatening Conditions

If clients have had a heart attack, stroke, aneurism, embolism, congestive heart failure, or heart surgery that resulted in the installment of a pacemaker, it is prudent to avoid using hot or cold stones during the massage, or use only a few with moderate temperatures, checking with the client both before and during the session to ensure that the temperatures being used are entirely comfortable. A prior consult with the client's physician is advisable.

Raynaud's Disease

Raynaud's disease is a peripheral arterial disease in which the fingers, hands, toes, and/or feet suddenly experience decreased circulation due to spasms of the arteries supplying them. Episodes most often result from exposure to cold (37). The duration of the attacks can be variable and can sometimes last for hours. Numbness and pain can be severe, particularly in the rewarming phase. Because of the restriction in circulation and nerve impingement, Raynaud's disease makes the body more vulnerable to frostbite. Very cold temperatures can cause a sharp drop in circulation to the fingers and toes and sometimes even the nose and ears (38).

Cold stones should not be used alone over areas that are affected by Raynaud's disease or that have been previously frostbitten. During the rewarming phase, heated stones can be introduced slowly, with moderate warmth, working up to higher temperatures with caution. To minimize the symptoms of

Raynaud's disease, hands and feet should be kept warm. Receiving hot stone massage regularly will help the body to maintain a higher level of warmth in its digits and be a preventative measure for cold days. Alternating hot with cold stones can help acclimatize sensitive areas when clients are not experiencing symptoms (39).

Scleroderma

Scleroderma means "hard skin" and is a rare, noncontagious, progressive disease that leads to hardening and tightening of the skin and connective tissues due to an overproduction and accumulation of collagen in body tissues. It usually begins with a few dry patches of skin on the hands or face that begin getting thicker and harder. These patches then spread to other areas of the skin. In some cases, scleroderma also affects the blood vessels and internal organs. Some of the accompanying symptoms of scleroderma are numbness, pain, or color changes in the fingers, toes, nose, and ears (Raynaud's disease); stiffness or pain of the joints; and puffy hands and feet (40).

Because scleroderma can include the symptoms of Raynaud's disease, use of cold stones should be avoided when there is numbness or lack of color in the extremities. Hot stones can be used, but only with moderation, as the lack of sensation will impair the client's ability to determine if the temperature is too hot. If no signs of numbness are present, alternating warm and cold stones can ease the stiffness, pain, and inflammation.

Skin Irritations

Eczema, psoriasis, and other skin rashes can become more irritated by heated stones, and it is possible for these skin irritations to propagate as a result of their use. Also avoid using hot stones on areas where there are skin eruptions from poison ivy or fungal infections such as athlete's foot and ringworm, as the heat can spread and exacerbate symptoms. Cold stones can be used to help with inflammation, itch, and pain, but need to be kept away from other parts of the body in order to avoid spreading the rash. Avoid using hot stones on abrasions and open wounds, as they can create or further enhance an infection. Clients with acne rosacea are not good candidates for either hot or cold stones because either temperature may worsen the condition (41).

Both hot and cold stones should be used with caution on areas of transplanted (grafted) skin or scar tissue due to burns, as there is usually no sensation in these areas. Make sure clients have not had a recent microdermabrasion, an acid peel, or a face-lift before using hot or cold stones on their faces (42).

Avoid the use of hot stones on sunburned skin; however, cold stones can be used to offer relief from the pain and inflammation of such burns. Do not use hot stones on clients that have applied a niacin-based sun tanning lotion to their skin.

Hot stones can be used on the parts of the body that are not affected by the skin irritations unless the rash is due to a systemic problem such as hives, heat rash, an allergic reaction, a virus, detoxification, shingles, or scabies. All skin irritations involving a systemic reaction absolutely preclude the use of hot stones. However, cold stones can be very helpful and comforting with systemic skin reactions, especially for relieving the itch and heat that often accompanies these rashes.

Tendonitis

Tendonitis is the painful inflammation of a tendon, which attaches the muscle to the bone. It often results from the stress of repetitive movements. Acute tendonitis may become chronic if it is not treated. Symptoms include minor swelling, tenderness in affected limb, pain that worsens with movement, warmth, and redness (43).

Do not use hot stones by themselves because their heat can aggravate tendonitis by adding more swelling to the joint. Hot stones can only be used for tendonitis if they are alternated with cold stones, which are very helpful in relieving the pain and inflammation of tendonitis. The contrast of the two temperatures speeds up the circulation to the area and encourages healing. However, if the addition of hot stones to the cold ones makes the tendon feel worse, then eliminate the hot stones altogether and use only cold stones for treatment.

Vertigo

Vertigo is a feeling of dizziness that occurs when the sense of balance is disrupted. This can be a temporary sensation from turning around too quickly or a more serious condition that can last for periods of a month or even up to a year. The most common known cause of vertigo is a disturbance or infection of the inner ear. However, research has shown that tight muscles in the jaw and around the teeth, such as from temporomandibular joint syndrome (TMJ), can also cause vertigo (44).

If the vertigo is connected with pain in the inner ear, consult the client's physician before attempting to treat. However, if the vertigo symptoms are being caused by tight jaw muscles, teeth grinding, or clenching, using hot stones to massage the tempomandibular joint would be excellent for relaxing the muscles in that area and thus reducing or removing the symptoms of vertigo. If hot stones make the vertigo worse, stop immediately and advise the client to see a doctor. Cold stones may exacerbate the symptoms and thus, should be avoided.

SUMMARY

The application of heat and cold to the body has very specific effects on the circulatory, lymphatic, and nervous systems. Heat increases blood and lymph flow while reducing blood pressure. Cold decreases blood and lymph flow while increasing blood pressure. Heat creates a calming affect on the nervous system and brain, whereas cold stimulates and tones the body, increasing alertness. Generally, heat brings the blood to the periphery of the body, while cold brings blood flow to the interior.

Both heat and cold lessen the contractility of a muscle, aiding in reducing muscle spasms. Both heat and cold also offer pain relief. Heat softens a muscle, thus relieving tension, whereas cold numbs a muscle, thereby acting as an analgesic. Alternating heat and cold offers the highest form of detoxification for the body, flushing it with freshly oxygenated blood and enhancing the immune system response.

Giving a safe hot stone massage requires that you become knowledgeable about the various conditions that may either preclude hot stone massage or require special care with the temperature of the stones.

In general, avoid the use of heat with disorders that involve inflammation, acute injury, edema, skin rash, open wounds, infection, malignant tumors, compromised circulation, impaired sensation, and heart disease. Cold is discouraged with disorders that involve high blood pressure, heart disease, circulatory problems, impaired sensation, nerve damage, and frostbite.

There is always the risk that a client has a condition of which he or she is not yet aware; thus, there is no way to be certain that giving a hot stone massage will never have an adverse affect upon a client. But you cannot take responsibility for conditions not known to you. The best protection for you and your clients is to become knowledgeable of their health history by using an intake form like the one that is included in this chapter.

REVIEW QUESTIONS

TRUE/FALSE

1. Thermotherapy is the application of heat to the body for purposes of healing.

   Circle: True False

2. A chronic injury is treated by icing it before exercise and heating it immediately afterward.

   Circle: True False

3. Occlusion is a temporary arterial blockage that can be used therapeutically.

   Circle: True False

4. Sometimes clients can have an allergic reaction to cold.

   Circle: True False

5. After the first trimester, hot stones can be used everywhere on a pregnant body.

   Circle: True False

MULTIPLE CHOICE

6. The physiological process that draws blood to the surface or periphery of the body by means of heat is known as:
   a. Retrostasis
   b. Homeostasis
   c. Derivation
   d. Hyperemia
   e. Geo-thermotherapy
7. Heat causes the viscosity of synovial fluids in the joints to:
   a. Thicken
   b. Thin
   c. Stiffen
   d. Break down
   e. Become granular
8. Cold's analgesic effect is caused by:
   a. Reduced nerve conduction
   b. Damage to cells
   c. Increased blood flow
   d. Decreased metabolism
   e. Increased respiration

9. Asthma attacks can be brought on by:
   a. Too much heat
   b. Cold, dry air
   c. Cold, moist air
   d. Too much weight on client's chest
   e. Any of these
10. Which of the following statements about treatment of clients with arthritis is true?
   a. Cold should never be used on arthritic joints.
   b. Heat should never be used on arthritic joints.
   c. Heat and cold treatments should be alternated over arthritic joints.
   d. Both thermotherapy and cryotherapy are contraindicated for clients with arthritis.
   e. None of the above statements are true.

SHORT ANSWER

11. A good way for therapists to be certain they have a full health report on their clients is to use the ______________________________.
12. What might a client with a head cold experience following the use of hot stones? ____________________
13. It is best to avoid the use of ____________ stones when a client is experiencing a migraine.
14. It is best to use ____________ stones on an insect bite that has an allergic reaction.
15. It is safest to use ________________ temperatures with clients who have either high or low blood pressure.

MATCHING

a. Heat   c. Rosemary   e. Counterirritant
b. Tonify   d. Ginger

16. Distracts the brain from the original source of pain. _____
17. A root with anti-inflammatory effects that is sometimes used in balms. _____
18. To enhance and restore balance in various parts of the body. _____
19. An ingredient in healing balms that creates heat by drawing blood to the skin. _____
20. Helpful in lowering a client's blood pressure. _____

Answers to Review Questions can be found in Appendix D.

CHAPTER 3

Equipment and Set-Up

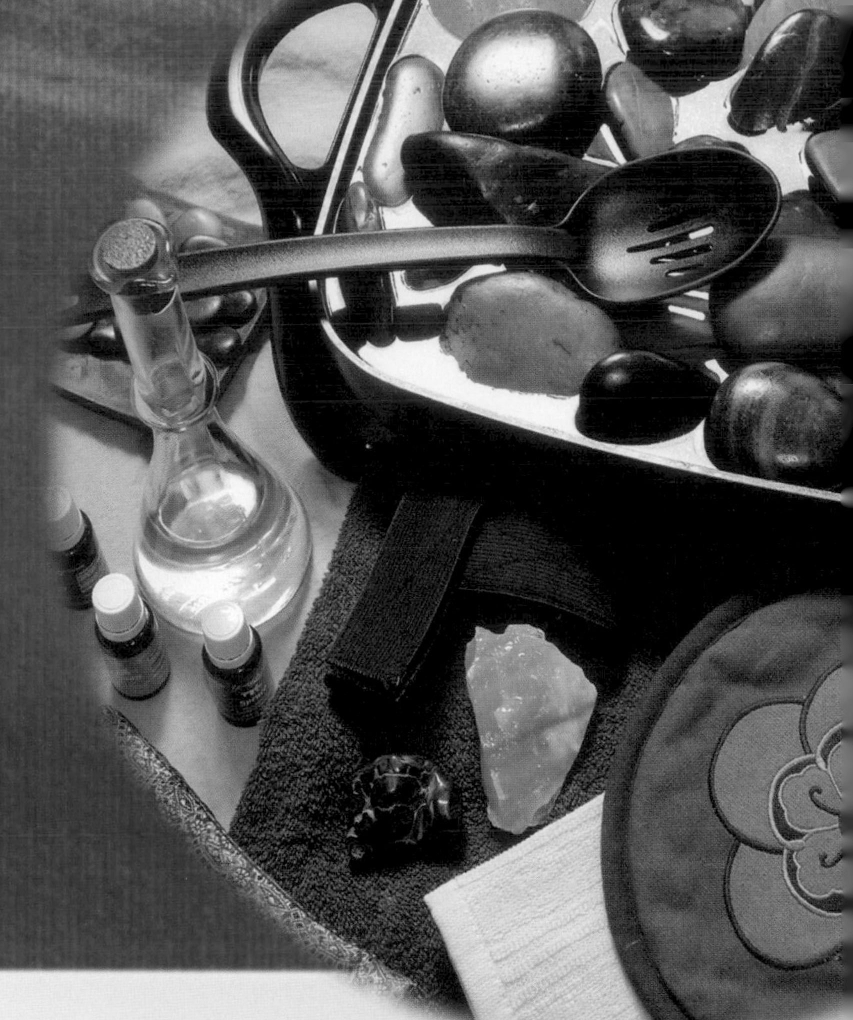

Outline

Equipment
- Massage Table
- Stone Table and Covers
- Electric Skillet

Accessories
- Slotted Spoon
- Bowls
  - *Bowl for Cold Stones*
  - *Bowl for Smallest Stones*
  - *Bowl for Spare Stones*
- Pitcher
- Pads and Wraps
  - *Pillowcase*
  - *Towels*
  - *Oven Pockets*
  - *Stone Wrappers*
  - *Eye Mask*
  - *Sand Bags*
- Oils
  - *Essential Oils*
  - *Massage Oil*

Unnecessary Items
- Wheeled Cart
- Skillet Lining
- Thermometer
- Fish Net
- Stone Bags
- Wooden Spoon
- Rubber Gloves

Setting Up the Stone Table
- Placement of the Stone Table
- Organization of Items on the Stone Table
- Using Shelves in Place of a Stone Table

Setting Up the Therapy Space for Hot Stone Massage
- Flooring
- Ventilation
- Access to Electricity
- Access to Running Water
- Providing Hot Stone Massage Outdoors

Objectives

After reading this chapter, you should be able to:

- Identify the necessary equipment and accessories for performing a hot stone massage.
- Set up the equipment and accessories for maximum efficiency and client comfort.
- Describe the alterations that may need to be made to the flooring, ventilation, and access to electricity or running water in the therapy space.

Key Terms

Stone wrapper: Elastic Velcro strap used to hold stones in place.

Stone table: The table on which the stones, skillet, and accessories are placed.

The proper equipment and accessories for administering a hot stone massage will make working with the stones much easier, especially when the environment in the massage room is suitable and supportive for giving a hot stone massage. With the proper paints and brushes, an artist can focus on the painting. In the same way, with the right equipment and accessories available and effectively arranged in a healing space, you will be able to focus without distractions on the massage.

This chapter provides instructions for establishing an efficient workplace for practicing hot stone massage and explains exactly what equipment is necessary, how this equipment is best organized, and what alterations you may need to make to your workspace. The chapter also identifies equipment that is not necessary and explains why. By following the guidelines in this chapter, you will be able to create a functional, safe, and healing environment for performing hot stone massage. By the way, the most essential pieces of equipment for performing hot stone massage, the stones themselves, are not discussed here! Instead, we reserve all of Chapter 4 for a detailed discussion of the composition, acquisition, and care of your stones.

Table 3-1 Equipment and Accessories Checklist

Use this checklist to make sure that all equipment and accessories are in place before beginning a hot stone massage.

Equipment and Accessories for Hot Stone Massage	Amount
Massage Table	1
Stone Table	1
Polyurethane Cover	1
Electric Skillet (large)	1
Slotted Plastic Spoon	1
Medium Plastic Bowl	1
Small Ornate Bowl or Plate	1
Large Plastic or Wood Bowl	1
Large Pitcher	1
Fabric Strip/Pillowcase	2
Large Towels	2
Hand Towels	2
Oven Pockets	2
Stone Wrappers	2 sets
Eye Mask	1
Sand or Grain Bags	1-2
Essential Oils	2-4
Massage Oils	3 bowls
Chopped Ice	Small bag
Stones	55

EQUIPMENT

The equipment and accessories needed to perform a hot stone massage are listed in Table 3-1. The section below describes each item in more detail and explains why each is helpful for a flowing, effective hot stone massage.

Massage Table

As with traditional massage, a sturdy, comfortable massage table is necessary for performing hot stone massage. If you are already offering massage professionally, then you already own this piece of equipment. If, however, you have only recently been certified as a massage therapist, you must acquire a massage table before offering hot stone massage. That is because it is impractical to perform an effective hot stone massage on a bed, on the floor, or in a chair. The only exception to this would be for clients who are confined to a bed or wheelchair, but such cases require further adaptations.

Any table that is designed for massage therapy is sufficient. There is no need for a special waterproof table.

Stone Table and Covers

For optimum access to the stones and other small accessories, they should be placed on a covered table near the massage table (Fig. 3-1). I refer to this as the **stone table** so that it is not confused with the massage table. This table should be large enough to fit all the equipment on it, with room for some of the stones to be laid out as well, yet not so large that it takes up the space you need for giving a massage. The size of the working space will determine how large the stone table can be, but it should be no smaller than 3 feet wide by 1.5 feet deep, and it does not need to be any larger than 5 feet wide by 4 feet deep. If room allows, the best dimensions for the stone table are 4 feet wide by 3 feet deep.

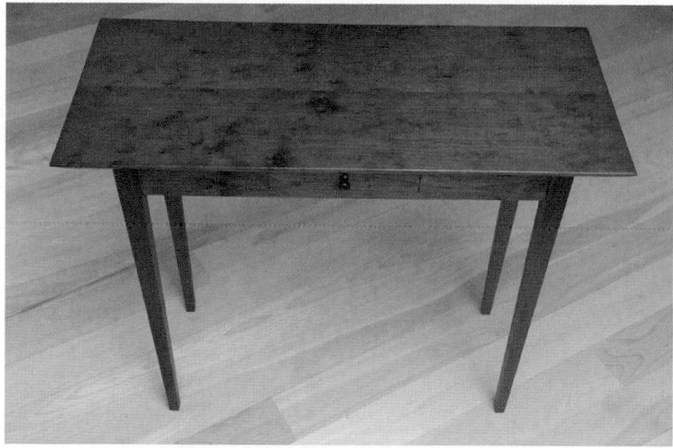

Figure 3-1 Table for Holding Stones. This small wooden table, shown without its polyurethane cover, is ideal for holding the stones. It was made by Master Woodworker Carlos Steybe, of Four Elements Design, Eldorado Springs, Colorado.

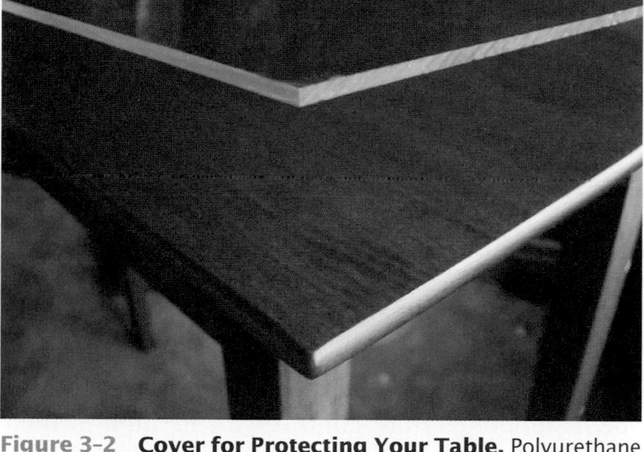

Figure 3-2 Cover for Protecting Your Table. Polyurethane cover on wooden table. Because it has been so well protected, this table still looks new after 7 years of use.

The height of the stone table is very important. If it is too high or too low, it will cause strain on your body and could lead to fumbling or dropping the hot stones. The ideal height for a stone table is approximately waist high when you are standing.

Stone tables need to be sturdy. The stones, along with the water in the skillet, are very heavy and a rickety table could collapse. Because the stone table is always covered, its appearance is not as important as its build.

If a stone table is made of wood, a polyurethane cover is needed to protect it. Otherwise, it will become wet from the stones, and the constant moisture will warp the wood over time. The polyurethane also provides some protection from heat.

A piece of polyurethane, about 0.25 inch thick, as shown in Figure 3-2, can be cut to fit the exact size of the stone table. Once cut, simply place the piece of polyurethane on top of the wooden stone table. Then, cover both the table and the polyurethane with a thick towel or piece of terrycloth to prevent moisture from seeping around the edges of the plastic cover. This soft-top cover will also serve to reduce the noise of the stones against the table. I have had my wooden table covered with this double layer for about 7 years now, and it is still in perfect condition. If the table is not wooden, then no polyurethane cover is needed. You will still need to cover it with a towel, however, to absorb moisture and reduce noise.

Electric Skillet

The accepted technique for heating stones is to submerge them in water in a "pot" with an electric heating device that can be regulated. There is some debate among practitioners of hot stone massage as to the best piece of equipment for doing this. Some stone companies insist on the necessity of using one of their specially made stone skillets. Some hot stone therapists choose to use a turkey roaster to heat their stones, whereas others use a crock pot. I recommend using an electric skillet, as shown in Figure 3-3.

Therapists who favor a turkey roaster point out that it is large and deep and can, therefore, hold a lot of stones. I don't find this to be an advantage. To the contrary, having too many stones in the skillet at once makes it harder to locate the desired stones, and when there is excessive depth, it's hard to reach in and get the stones. In addition, a turkey roaster is dark inside, exacerbating the lack of visibility. In

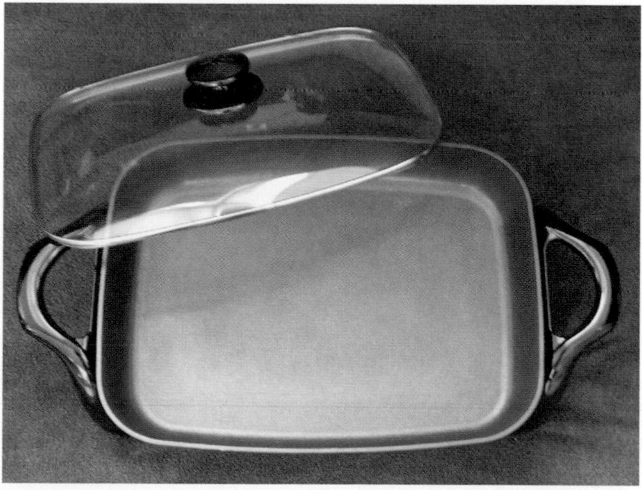

Figure 3-3 Skillet for Heating the Stones. An electric skillet is optimal for heating stones.

contrast, in a large but shallow skillet, an entire kit of 55 stones is visible and easily accessible.

I also strongly recommend against using a crock pot, because not only is its stone accessibility impaired, but it takes a considerable amount of time to heat the stones, and its limited range on the thermostat makes temperature control virtually impossible. Nor do I see a need for an exclusively designed, expensive stone skillet as promoted by several distributors. These skillets do not offer any advantages over a traditional electric skillet and are three times more expensive. They are also not available in stores.

A simple electric skillet works very well. It has adequate temperature control with its built-in thermostat, heats up rapidly, holds an adequate number of stones, offers easy access to the stones, and is comparatively inexpensive (Fig. 3-4). It is also durable—I have used mine for over 7 years.

Electric skillets usually come in two sizes. The small one is 12 inches square, and the large rectangular one is 16 inches by 12 inches. Both of the skillets are 4 inches deep. I highly recommend the large skillet for therapists who are planning to use stones comprehensively in their massage. For therapists who think they might just add a few stones here and there in a traditional massage or other healing modality, a small-sized skillet is sufficient.

CAUTION

As electric skillets age, the temperature regulator may malfunction, and even though it says it is on warm, it could actually be on high. If your water is boiling when the skillet is set to warm, check to see if your regulator has become faulty. For the few therapists I know that this has happened to, the skillet manufacturers were willing to replace the temperature regulator at no charge, even though the skillet was many years old. In addition, as a precaution against fire, always make sure you have turned off and unplugged your skillet at the end of each day.

TIP

Of several manufacturers, General Electric, Presto, Rival, and Black & Decker all make sturdy, attractive, cast-aluminum, and Teflon-coated electric skillets with built-in thermostats, at an affordable price.

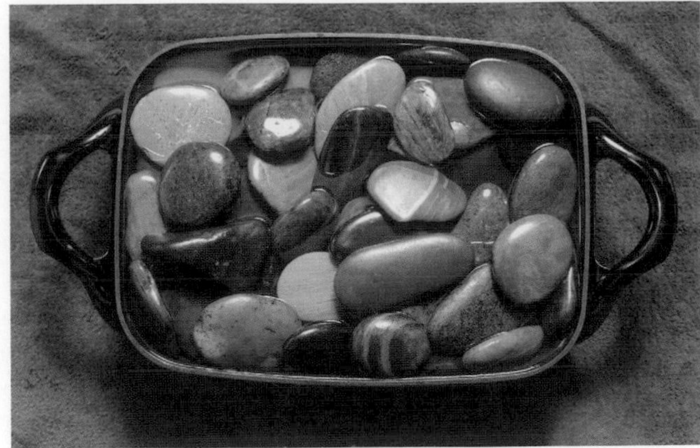

Figure 3-4 Stones in Skillet. Notice how many stones this large-sized skillet can hold and heat.

ACCESSORIES

Several smaller accessories will help make your hot stone massage go more smoothly. These include a slotted spoon, various bowls, a pitcher of water, different types of pads and wraps, and both essential oils and massage oil.

Slotted Spoon

A deep, slotted plastic spoon is necessary for safely removing stones from the skillet. The depth ensures that the stone will not fall out and back into the skillet, splashing you with hot water, and the slots allow the hot water to drain back into the skillet, preventing you from being burned (Fig. 3-5). The drainage also keeps the water that comes onto the stone table to a minimum. I prefer plastic to metal or wood because metal spoons make a scraping sound against the skillet, and wooden spoons wear out from the constant moisture.

TIP 

Look for a plastic spoon that is somewhat stiff and sturdy so that the weight of the stone doesn't bend it, but not so stiff that it won't offer slight flexibility. A spoon like this can be purchased at any store that sells kitchenware.

Bowls

Three types of bowls are needed for holding stones during the massage—one for holding chilled stones, one for holding tiny stones, and one for holding spare stones.

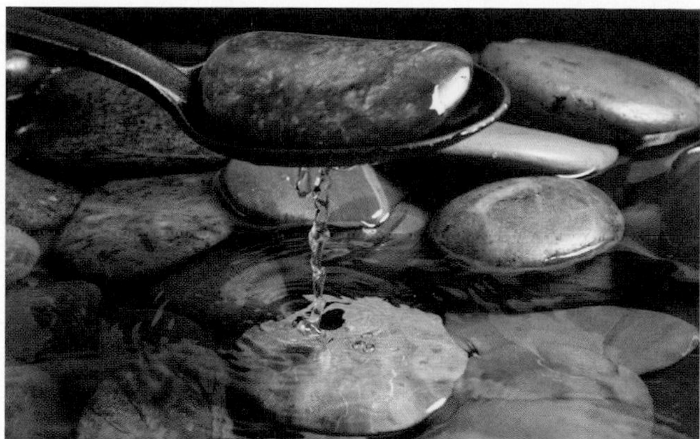

Figure 3-5 Slotted Spoon for Removing Stones from Skillet. A deep slotted plastic spoon with a sturdy but flexible handle is useful for handling hot stones. The slots allow the hot water to drain back into the skillet before the stones are removed.

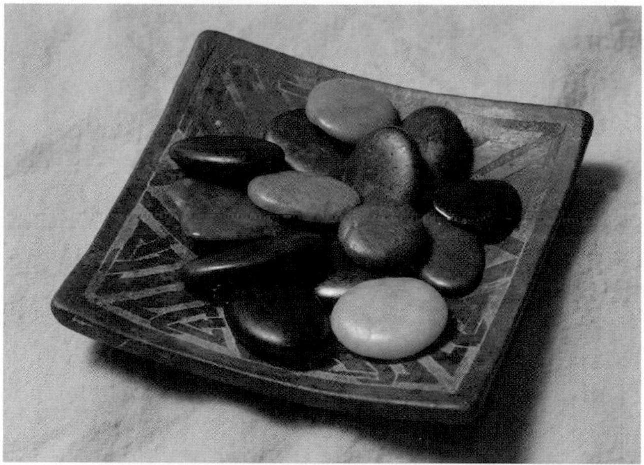

Figure 3-7 Small Bowl or Curved Plate. Tiny stones are more readily accessible during the massage if they are stored in a small bowl or curved plate.

Bowl for Cold Stones

You will need one medium-sized plastic bowl for storing both ice water and cold stones during the massage (Fig. 3-6). This ice water is also used for dipping hot stones into when you need to cool them quickly. This bowl needs to be plastic rather than metal, glass, or porcelain, as these can cause a clanking sound from the stones, and they might chip or break. A plastic bowl is light, quiet, and nonbreakable and can be purchased inexpensively at any store that sells kitchenware.

Bowl for Smallest Stones

A small bowl or curved plate, as shown in Figure 3-7, is useful for storing the smallest stones. If tiny stones are mixed in with larger stones in the skillet, it will be almost impossible to find and extract them at the moment you need them. Small stones heat quickly, so when you need them, you can pour them from their little bowl into the slotted spoon and dip it for a few moments in the hot water. A small bowl or plate can be purchased at any store that sells kitchenware. This bowl can be made of plastic, ceramic, or glass, as these tiny stones do not make much noise, and the small stones don't pose the problem of breaking when placed back into the bowl.

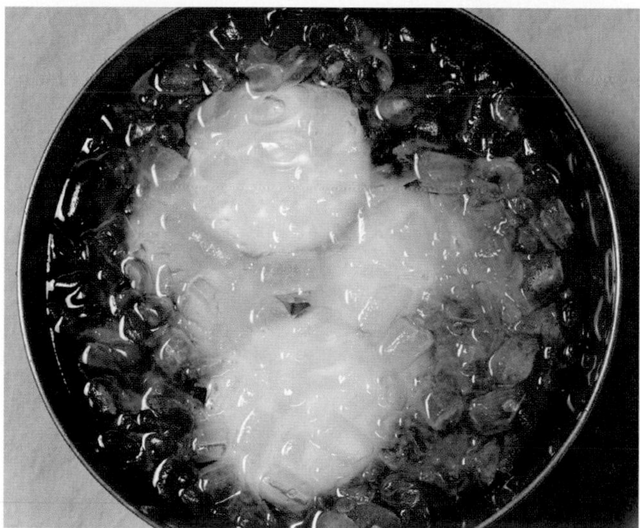

Figure 3-6 Bowl for Storing Stones. A medium-sized plastic bowl like this one is useful for storing cold stones and ice water.

Bowl for Spare Stones

A medium- to large-sized bowl made of plastic or wood is helpful for storing spare stones beneath or near the stone table. You'll need a place to store stones outside of the skillet for several reasons. If you find yourself collecting many stones to augment your original collection, you'll eventually have too many to fit easily in the skillet at the same time. Additionally, you need a place to store unusual stones that you don't use often, such as extra large stones and uniquely shaped stones, so that they don't take up room in the skillet when they are not being used. Stones require only a few minutes to heat up in hot water, so if you use a little foresight, the client need not experience any delay in the flow of the massage while you heat a spare stone.

Pitcher

A large pitcher of cold water is needed close by for refilling the water in the skillet as it evaporates throughout the session. I usually need to replenish the water in my skillet at least twice within one hot stone massage. Pitchers can be ceramic, clay, metal, or plastic, and they can be as inexpensive and simple or as expensive and decorative as you choose (Fig. 3-8).

The pitcher of extra cold water is also helpful for cooling water in a skillet that has become too hot. I also use it for cooling the bowl of cold water where I store my cold stones. Because I dip stones that are too hot to use in the bowl of cold water, it eventually becomes too warm to keep the chilled stones cold. Adding additional cold water to this bowl cools it back down. A large pitcher of cold water will last for a full day of hot stone massage.

Pads and Wraps

A variety of pads and wraps are used for protecting the client's skin from the heat of stones you place on the body. They also serve to secure the stones in place, especially on areas where the stones could not possibly remain without assistance.

Pillowcase

A pillowcase folded in half, or a narrow strip of soft fabric, is useful for placing over or under the stones when they are situated along either side of the spine beneath the supine client (Fig. 3-9). The reason for a narrow strip of fabric, rather than a wide towel the same size as the client's back, is that in the three-dimensional method that I teach, the client is never asked to sit up for me to remove the stones beneath the body. Instead, I roll the client onto his or her side, remove the stones and the fabric, and then lay the client back down again. If the fabric is too wide, the client's body will still be partially on top of it when I roll the client to the side, and I won't be able to remove it. In contrast, it's easy to remove a folded pillowcase or a narrow strip of fabric.

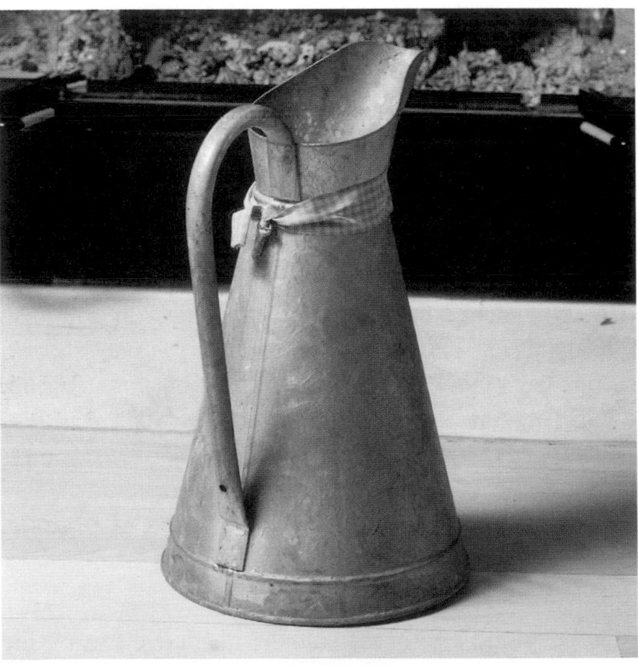

Figure 3-8 Pitcher for Storing Water. A pitcher is necessary for holding extra cold water.

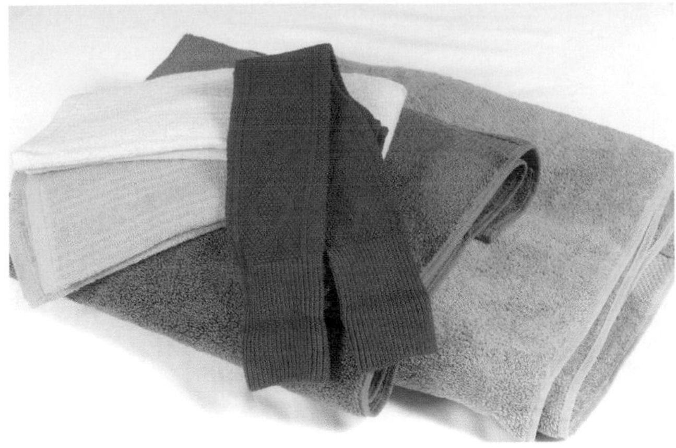

Figure 3-9 Towels and Socks for Covering Stones. Large towels are used for covering stones on the top of a client, small towels or strips of material are used for covering stones beneath the back, and socks are used to contain stones and use as a "hot pack."

TIP 

Pillowcases are also wonderful for wrapping up several stones and using them as a hot or cold pack that can be easily moved from place to place on the body. Line four stones in the center of a pillowcase and fold either side around the line of stones, as if you were folding a burrito. You can wrap this "stone pack" around areas that would normally pose difficulty for placing several stones at once, for instance, around the neck, thigh, arm, or buttocks, tucking the ends of the wrap under the body to keep the stones in place.

Towels

Towels are necessary items for a hot stone massage. Two large bath towels and two hand towels should suffice, although there is always room for variation based on personal preference. As mentioned earlier, you will need to place one large, thick towel on the stone table beneath the skillet, covering the entire table so that the water from the stones does not completely drench the table and so that the stones don't clank against the table. A large towel is also useful for covering the client's entire back and buttocks. You can lay the towel directly on the client's skin with very hot stones placed on top of it, and then fold the edges of the towel over the stone layout to help lengthen their heat retention.

Put hand towels under or over smaller stones to help regulate the heat as well as to keep the stones from slipping. You can double or triple the towel beneath very hot stones and remove one layer at a time as they begin to lose their heat. Small towels can also be used to cover and prolong the heat in the stones that are out of the skillet and on the stone table waiting to be used. Of course, towels can be purchased anywhere bathroom and linen supplies are sold.

Oven Pockets

One safety concern with hot stone massage is that stones placed and left on the body can transmit a significant amount of heat in just a few minutes. An oven pocket (also called an oven pad or hot pad), is a wonderful way to contain such placement stones when they are too hot to place directly on the skin or on the sheet. Most oven pockets have one side that is thin and one that is thick (Fig. 3-10). This feature will help you regulate the temperature of stones left in place on the body.

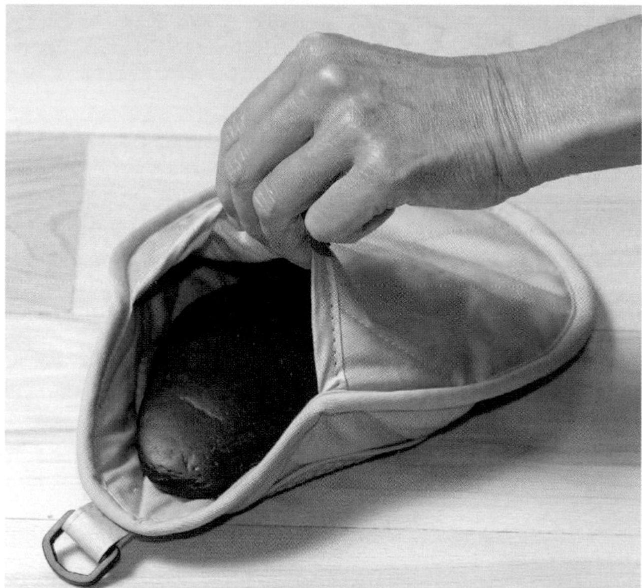

Figure 3-10 Oven Pockets for Reducing Heat and Securing Stones. Oven pockets serve to hold a stone securely in place. Ones with two different sides of thickness offer two options in temperature control for placement stones.

You can also use an oven pocket to keep a stone in place on the client's body. Turn its opening according to the curves in the body so that the stone will not roll out. Oven pockets can be purchased at any store that sells towels or kitchen items.

TIP 

When the stone is first placed on the body and is at its hottest temperature, turn the oven pocket face up with the thicker side against the body. As the stone begins to cool, turn the oven pocket over to its thin side. And then, as more time elapses and the stone cools even more, take it out of the oven pocket and place it on the sheet. Eventually, the stone will have lost enough of its heat that it can be placed directly on the client's skin.

Stone Wrappers

Stone wrappers are elastic Velcro straps useful for fastening one stone at a time to the bottom of the client's feet (Fig. 3-11). One stone on the foot makes it feel as if many stones surround it. I have often had a client ask me where I got the "stone booty." The elastic in the wrapper helps to hold the stone snugly but not too tightly. The straps can also be used to attach stones to the forearms, ankles, or knees.

Some practitioners advocate placing a sock over the foot with the stone; however, a sock does not hold the stone snugly in place and it takes longer to

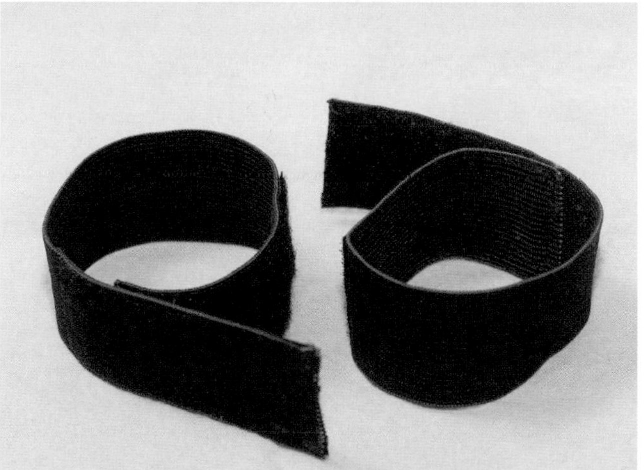

Figure 3-11 Stone Wrapper. Stone wrappers offer another method for holding stones snugly in place. One stone held securely against the foot can give clients the impression that they are wearing a stone booty.

remove and replace the sock for each stone change. Other practitioners use a stretchy, self-adhesive bandage, but you can reuse this only a few times before it loses its stickiness, and it can get tangled and stuck to itself. In contrast, Velcro straps never get tangled, they are long-lasting and sturdy, and will never open with the weight of a stone against them, no matter what position the client is in. In addition, you can switch stones that have cooled down for new warm ones without having to remove the straps to do so. You can make these stone wrappers yourself, or purchase them ready-made from a supplier (see Appendix B).

Eye Mask

Eye masks not only help to keep light out and relax the client's eyes, but they are also very helpful in keeping stones placed on the face from falling off during massage (Fig. 3-12).

CAUTION

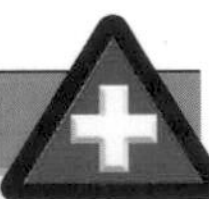

When using an eye mask to cover stones placed on the eyes, be careful not to tighten the mask too much or it could press the stones into the eyes or face. It is also easy to forget stones are beneath a mask, and they can get left on the client too long. A warm or cold stone feels wonderful, but a stone that is the exactly the same temperature of the body can eventually feel annoying. So, if you use an eye mask, remember to remove the stones when they have lost their preferred temperature.

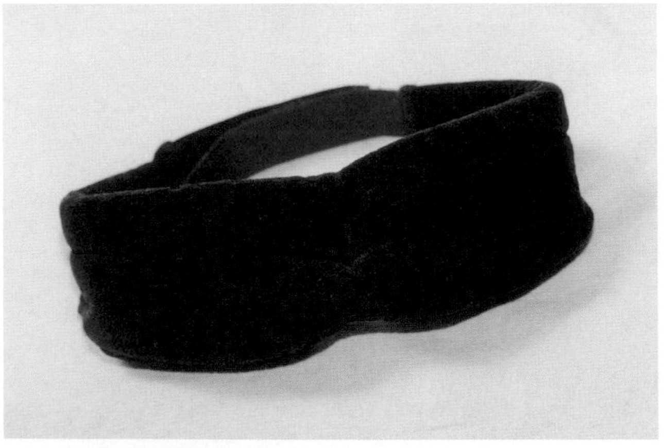

Figure 3-12 Eye Mask. An eye mask is useful for holding stones that are placed on the eyes, and third-eye, in position.

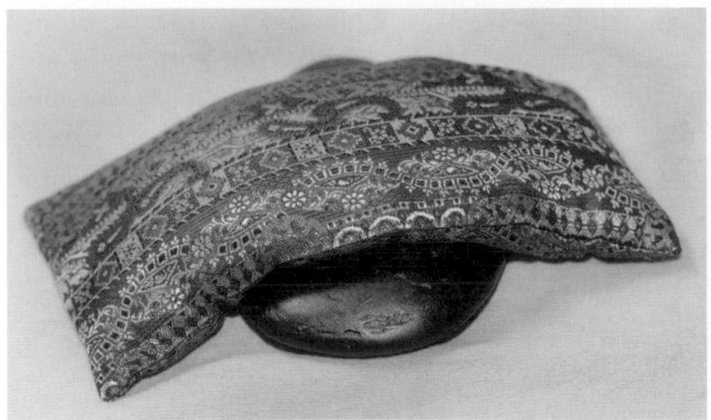

Figure 3-13 Sand or Grain Bags. Sand or grain bags help to create a comforting compression that deepens the penetration of the heated stone. They can also help to hold stones on precarious parts of the body.

Sand Bags

Sand bags are very helpful in creating compression and holding a stone in place on body joints and curves. Elbows, knees, and the curve of the upper back or chest benefit greatly from the weight of a small sand bag, which can keep a warm stone from sliding off the body while simultaneously exerting gentle pressure on the stone, deepening its heat and effect (Fig. 3-13). Clients report that having a stone pressed slightly against the body with the gentle weight of a small sand bag is comforting and soothing. Sand bags can be purchased at stores that sell massage, bath, or beauty supplies, and they are fairly easy to make.

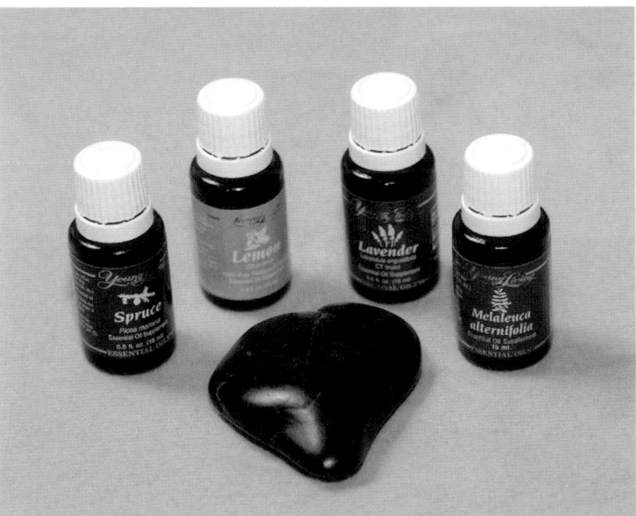

Figure 3-14 Essential Oils for Disinfecting and Soothing. A few drops of essential oil can be used to disinfect the water and add a soothing aroma to the air.

Oils

If you have been using essential oils and massage oils in traditional massage, you will find both old and new uses for them in hot stone massage.

Essential Oils

Adding 2 to 3 drops of essential oil to the water in the skillet as the stones are heating serves to disinfect the stones and create a pleasing aroma in the air. Different oils have different properties: Eucalyptus opens the sinuses; lavender relaxes the nervous system; peppermint calms the digestive system; lemon stimulates the brain; fir, spruce, and pine are grounding; and tea tree kills bacteria. All of these particular essential oils have disinfectant qualities for treating the stones as well (Fig. 3-14).

Although all essential oils may look alike, they vary greatly as far as their aroma and therapeutic value. A low-grade essential oil is often made with some synthetic ingredients and from very few flower petals or plant particles. These oils can have an acceptable smell but do not have healing properties. A therapeutic-grade essential oil is extracted from thousands of petals and plant particles taken from the purest of flowers and plants. Not only do they smell much closer to the essence of the flower or plant from which they are diffused, but they also have healing properties as well. It is important to use a therapeutic-grade essential oil when giving a hot stone massage. Not only can low-grade oils have an adverse effect on sensitive clients, but they also inhibit the therapeutic value of the session.

Essential oils are sold in many health food stores, pharmacies, and body shops, but these are generally low-grade oils. Therapeutic-grade essential oils are difficult to find in stores but can be ordered through distributors, such as the one listed in Appendix B. For more detailed information on the types, qualities, and effects of essential oils, see the books listed in the Suggested Readings in Appendix F.

> **TIP**
>
> Be sure to ask clients if they have a sensitivity to aromas before using an essential oil or a scented massage oil.

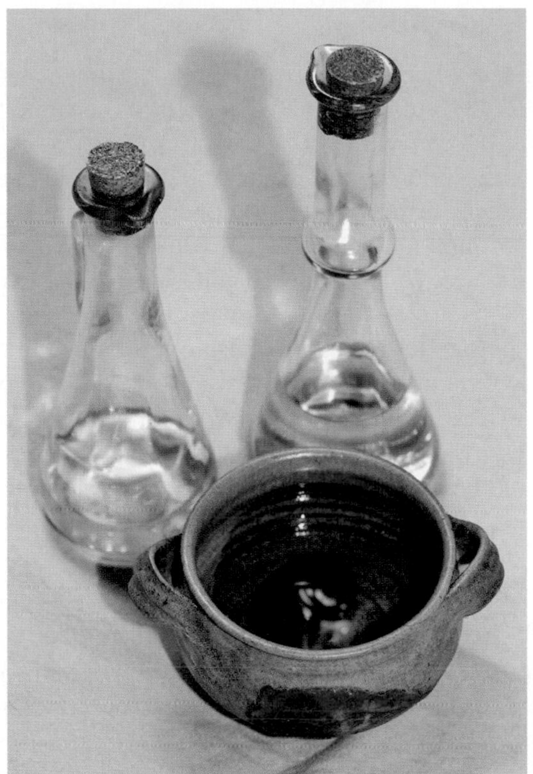

Figure 3-15 **Massage Oils in Bottles and in a Bowl.** You can pour oil into a small bowl for easy access. A small hot stone dropped in the bowl prewarms the oil.

Massage Oil

Massage oil, rather than cream or lotion, is the preferred lubricant when using hot stones, as it applies quickly and offers optimal glide. Scented massage oils, when applied to hot stones, create a nice aroma in the air. Almond oil or an almond oil mixture is a good oil to use because it has more viscosity than other massage oils and doesn't cause the stone to slip or slide too quickly. Using a small "soup" bowl for your oil allows you to dip your hand in quickly to access the oil. Dropping a small warm stone in the bowl of oil will pre-warm the oil for when you massage with your hands (Fig. 3-15). Massage oils can be purchased at a health food store, body shop, or online at one of the many massage supply Web sites.

UNNECESSARY ITEMS

Many distributors either include the following items with their stone kits, or promote them as necessary or very useful additions. In truth, these items are not necessary for performing an effective hot stone massage.

Wheeled Cart

At first, a wheeled cart seemed like a brilliant idea to me. Why go running back and forth to the stone table when you can wheel it with you around the room? But, unfortunately, the reasons that a wheeled cart is impractical become quickly apparent. For a cart to move around a massage table freely, there needs to be ample space, which is rare in a massage room. Even in a spacious room, maneuvering with an extension cord trailing from the skillet is a constant problem. Finally, it is very difficult to wheel a cart around on a carpeted floor or one with rugs. Because padding on the floor is a necessity for hot stone massage (see later discussion), it would be nearly impossible to move the cart.

Skillet Lining

Many therapists recommend lining the skillet with a white towel to make the stones easier to see and to lower the clanking sound when replacing stones in the skillet. I considered this, but after I tried it several times, I found that the towel simply would not remain on the bottom of the skillet unless there were always enough stones to weigh it down; otherwise, it just floated to the top and got caught in my spoon. I liked the idea so much, however, that I tried putting a white rubber nonslip mat inside the skillet. Unfortunately, that also floated to the top when enough stones were removed. I thought of spraying the skillet with a thick coat of white Teflon to increase the coating that was already in the skillet and thus minimize the clanking sound, but I couldn't find a spray that worked. So, finally I surrendered to the fact that stones do make a slight clank when returned to the skillet, and I began to think of that sound as music—and I enjoy it!

Thermometer

I see no need for a thermometer when electric skillets have a built-in thermostat. Although a thermostat is not as precise as a thermometer, it is sufficient for the purpose of hot stone massage. In fact, I recommend that you develop a sense of what temperature is too hot or too cold by relying on your sense of touch, rather than on an outside source. Stopping to take the water's temperature throughout the session is just another unnecessary interruption in the flow. If the stones or water feel too hot to touch, turn down the thermostat. Discussion on accurate temperatures can be found in chapter 5.

Fish Net

When I first heard of using a fish net to store the tiny stones in the hot water in the skillet, I thought it might be a good idea. But then I realized that tiny stones, which are used mostly between the toes or on the eyes, heat up in only 5 seconds. If they are heated for much longer than that, then you have to wait for them to cool before you can use them. So, there is no real benefit in storing the smallest stones in the skillet in a fish net. It just takes up room and gets in the way. If instead, the tiny stones are left in a small bowl near the skillet, as recommended earlier, they are just as accessible, and they are not getting overly hot. I also find it easier to take the stones out of the spoon after they have been dipped in the hot water, rather than removing the stones from a fish net.

Stone Bags

Some hot stone practitioners promote using several mesh bags to organize and place the stones in the skillet. The bags then have prearranged spots in the cooker. Their reasoning behind this is that it supposedly saves time away from the client and organizes their stones into layouts for above and below the body, for massage sequences, and for the tiny stones. In addition, they keep some specific stones loose.

The reasons I do not promote this method will become more clear to you as you read about my method of stone management in later chapters of this book. Briefly, most stones are multipurpose and having them in a particular bag would limit their accessibility to me for other purposes. When I have access to all my stones, I can easily choose the ones I want to use for each part of the body I am working on. And, again, tiny stones do not need to be heated for more than a few seconds to be used.

Wooden Spoon

Of course I generally prefer a wooden spoon to a plastic one, as I love to use materials from nature; however, the spoon used for a hot stone massage is dipped into hot water so often that, if it is made of porous material such as wood, it will break over time. I went through three wooden spoons in a year, and since then, I have had the same plastic spoon for 5 years. Also, wooden spoons rarely come with a deep ladle; instead, most are nearly flat. With a flat design, it is much more difficult to secure the stone in the spoon. This is a case where synthetic materials simply work better.

Rubber Gloves

As long you're using a slotted spoon to remove the stones from the skillet, there is no need for you to wear rubber gloves. Having to put on rubber gloves each time you take a stone out of the skillet and remove them each time your hand makes contact with the client's body is extremely time consuming. It also creates unnecessary interruption in the flow of a hot stone massage.

TESTIMONIAL

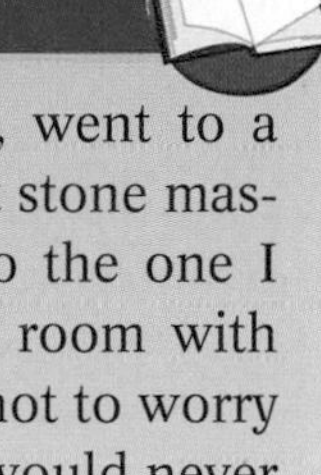

I had a client who, while traveling, went to a high-end spa and signed up for a hot stone massage, expecting to get one similar to the one I give her. The therapist came in the room with rubber gloves on and told my client not to worry about the gloves because her hands would never be making contact with the client's body. Only the stones would be touching her, she said. My client was shocked, being accustomed to the combination of hand with stone, so she endured a very disappointing, sterile session.

SETTING UP THE STONE TABLE

The way in which the equipment is organized will either enhance or hinder the efficiency of administering a hot stone massage. When all the pieces of the puzzle are in place, the working environment enhances the massage rather than interfering with it. I have found that the following set-up works quite well in my therapy room, which is rather small. With some planning, lack of space does not necessarily lead to disorganization.

Placement of the Stone Table

Place the stone table to the side of your massage table, and towards the middle, approximately 3 feet away. This location offers optimal access to the stones when you are on the side of the massage table closest to the stone table, and it also offers equal access from the head and foot ends. The only side that is at a disadvantage with this location is, of course, the opposite side of the massage table, but there is no escaping having at least one portion of the table less accessible than the others.

When the stone table is placed at the head or foot of the massage table, it is only easily accessible to that end of the table. From all other sides, you will need extra time to reach the stones. As you have not yet worked with stones, the few seconds of extra time may sound trivial, but once you have learned my system for stone management, you'll recognize that locating the stone table on the side increases the efficiency and flow with which you handle the stones, allowing the task to become more of dance than a chore.

Organization of Items on the Stone Table

All of the equipment and accessories discussed in this chapter are shown as they are laid out in my workplace in Figure 3-16. To arrange your items as I do, place your skillet of stones in the back center of the table, with the cold stone bowl sitting to its left, filled almost to the brim with ice water. Keep the slotted spoon either in the skillet or in the front of the skillet. Remove some stones from the skillet and place them on the stone table directly in front of the skillet. The smallest stones sit to the right in a small bowl or curved plate for easy access. Place the stone wrappers and essential oils on the left side in front of the cold stone bowl where there is space.

The pitcher with cold water and your spare bowl of extra stones can be stored beneath the stone table for easy access. Hang the oven pockets from hooks or Velcro loops off the side of the stone table. This is just one possible arragement of items. Feel free to improvise. As long as these items are easily accessible and don't interfere with or impede the flow of your

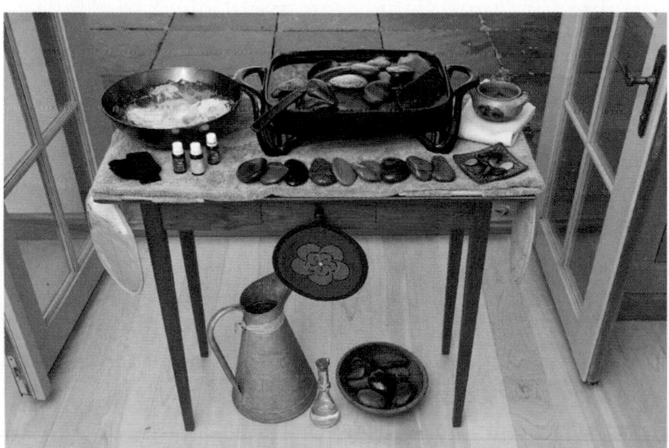

Figure 3-16 Ready to Begin. This photo shows a complete set-up of all equipment and accessories just prior to beginning the massage.

stone management, it doesn't matter exactly where each sits.

Except for the first 15 minutes when I am heating the stones, I keep the lid of the electric skillet tucked in the back, between the table and the wall, as I do not use it again during the session. After the client leaves, I put it back on the skillet while I boil and clean the stones. Of course, the lid is always left on the unplugged skillet overnight and on days when I am away from my practice. I also keep a lid over the bowl of cold stones to keep out dust and insects when I am not using it.

Using Shelves in Place of a Stone Table

If you cannot fit an appropriately sized stone table to either side of your massage table, then you might want to consider installing two heavy-duty wall shelves. These should be at least 1.5 feet deep so that the skillet will fit on them, and at least 3 feet long to hold your stones and other supplies. The shelves should, ideally, be installed waist-high to preserve your back and the proper management of the stones. Some accessories can hang from hooks on the wall or the edge of the shelf. You will also need to be sure that there is an electric outlet nearby and that the cord for the skillet is fixed to the wall so that it does not get in your way. Certainly, it is not ideal to need to install shelves in a therapy room, but it is a workable option for very small spaces.

SETTING UP THE THERAPY SPACE FOR HOT STONE MASSAGE

To ensure that your therapy space is safe and comfortable for your clients, you might need to alter the flooring, ventilation, and access to electricity and running water before offering hot stone massage.

Flooring

If the therapy space has hardwood flooring, a tile floor, or smooth linoleum, you will need to place a large rug, soft mats, or carpeting around the massage table. This is to reduce noise, as stones tend to roll off the client and the massage table during a hot stone massage and will cause a loud crashing sound if they hit a bare floor. This jarring sound could easily destroy all of the relaxation induced by the stones. When you are choosing floor coverings, look for rugs or mats that are soft and plush, rather than a grass or fiber mat. When stones fall, they are usually no longer wet or very hot, so you do not have to worry about moisture or burning; however, they will most likely have oil on them, so using a rug that can be washed would be ideal.

Ventilation

Ventilation is an essential consideration when giving a hot stone massage. Steam from the stones in the skillet warms the room, and heat from the stones applied to the body warms the client. To promote your clients' and your own comfort, your space should have either a window or a door that opens to the outside. If there is no access to either of these, a quiet fan with a low setting can be used to create some ventilation without too much breeze. An air conditioner generally makes the space too cold and uncomfortable for a client to receive a massage, even with hot stones; thus, I would not recommend using one for purposes of ventilation.

Access to Electricity

When setting up your space for performing hot stone massage, the location, availability, and capacity of electrical outlets are important considerations. It is best to have an outlet close enough to the skillet so you can avoid the use of an extension cord. Extension cords are potential hazards: You or your client could easily trip over a long, unsecured cord, and an extension cord may lower the resistance of circuit breakers, increasing the risk of fire. However, if one is required, use a heavy-duty cord and be sure it is compatible with a three-prong plug. It may be advisable to hire an electrician to create a separate outlet for the skillet. This is an important detail to attend to before beginning to use hot stones professionally.

TIP 

If your therapy room is in a shared workplace where there are a number of electric appliances in use, check to be sure that when the skillet is plugged in and turned on, it will not overload the circuit in use. The total must not exceed the rating of the circuit that is shown on the circuit breaker that feeds the workplace. If this is the case, you might need to have an electrician install a separate circuit for your skillet.

Access to Running Water

It is also necessary for the therapy room to have convenient access to running water. It is ideal, albeit unusual, to have a sink in the room itself, but if that is not possible, a shared restroom or other source of running water must be accessible. Running water is needed because the stones need to be cleaned and the skillet water needs to be replaced each day. In addition, the water in the skillet as well as the ice water in the cold stone storage bowl needs to be replenished throughout each session. Incidentally, if your workplace does not have a refrigerator, you will need to bring with you enough ice to fill the cold stone storage bowl each day.

Providing Hot Stone Massage Outdoors

Although performing a hot stone massage outdoors is challenging logistically, it does add the dimension of nature's beauty to the massage (Fig. 3-17). When the weather is nice and you have a client who would like to be outdoors, consider bringing your set-up outside. You will need to allow extra time to carry your table, skillet, stones, bowls, water, and all accessories outdoors. In addition, you'll need an extra heavy-duty extension cord if it must travel a long distance from the outlet.

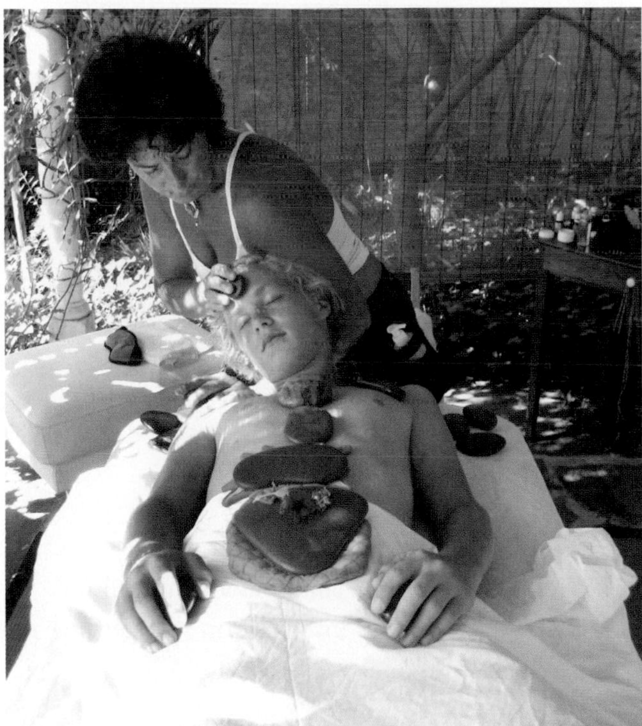

Figure 3-17 Doing Hot Stone Massage Outdoors. Even though giving a hot stone massage outdoors can be logistically difficult, when it is possible, it offers a whole other dimension to the session.

Should you choose to do hot stone massage outside, be sure that the weather looks like it will hold, as it takes several minutes to return all of your equipment inside. You also need to be sure the ground is level so that the skillet is stable and the water inside of it is level. Also, be sure that both you and your client will be able to endure the weather conditions. If it is hot outside, clients may sunburn, sweat too much to keep the placement stones in place, or overheat. If it is cloudy, you run the risk of rain. Thus, doing hot stone massage indoors is the easiest and most practical approach. That said, when you are able to provide a hot stone massage outside, it can be a truly spectacular experience for you and your client.

SUMMARY

Effective hot stone massage requires some equipment and accessories not needed for traditional massage. These include a set of stones; a small, sturdy table for holding stones; an electric skillet for heating the stones; and other smaller supplies such as a slotted plastic spoon, pitcher, several bowls, towels, pads, and wraps.

Essential oils are used to disinfect the stones, add a pleasing aroma to the therapy space, and enhance the therapeutic quality of the session. Massage oil is required rather than cream or lotion.

Some items recommended by manufacturers, including a wheeled cart, skillet lining, thermometer, fish net, stone bags, wooden spoon, and rubber gloves, are not needed.

Place your stone table to the side, rather than at the end, of the massage table. The skillet, slotted spoon, essential oils, bowl with ice water and chilled stones, and small bowl with tiny stones should all be able to fit on the stone table, leaving enough room for the stones. The pitcher of spare water, towels, oven pockets, bowl of spare stones, and stone straps can be stored either under or near the stone table.

If you do not have room for a stone table in your therapy space, then you can install wall shelves. Two waist high shelves at least 1.5 × 3 feet are necessary, and they need to be near access to an electric outlet.

It is important to have plush padding, such as carpet or rugs, on the floor beneath and around the massage table to soften the sound of the stones that inevitably fall during the massage.

Ventilation is important in order to not overheat your clients during a hot stone massage. If there are no windows are doors that access the outside, then a small quiet fan is recommended.

Electricity is also a concern for giving a hot stone massage. Outlets need to be near the electric skillet to avoid use of extension cords, if possible. The circuits need to be strong enough to handle the current of the skillet.

Your space requires access to running water so that you can replenish the water throughout the massage. You'll also need to replace the water between massages.

Once all of this equipment has been acquired and set-up and the room has been altered appropriately, you are closer to being ready to begin practicing hot stone massage. However, the main piece of equipment needed to do this is still missing—the stones! Chapter 4 will help you to take the next step into coming to know and acquire your stones.

REVIEW QUESTIONS

TRUE/FALSE

1. A special type of massage table is required for doing hot stone massage.

   Circle: True False

2. A stone table refers to a table that only the stones sit on.

   Circle: True False

3. A deep plastic slotted spoon has more advantages than a flat wooden one.

   Circle: True False

4. Essential oils and scented massage oils should always be used in a hot stone massage.

   Circle: True False

5. Rubber gloves are essential accessories for handling the hot stones.

   Circle: True False

MULTIPLE CHOICE

6. An essential safety accessory is:
   a. A specialized lining to absorb some of the heat in the electric skillet
   b. Rubber gloves to protect your hands
   c. A thermometer to monitor the temperature of the water in the skillet
   d. Sand bags to ensure that your wheeled cart doesn't move during treatment
   e. None of the above are essential safety accessories
7. The stone table is ideally placed:
   a. At the center side of the massage table, about 3 feet away
   b. At the head of the massage table, about 3 feet away
   c. At the head of the massage table, against the wall at least 4 feet away
   d. At the foot of the massage table, about 3 feet away
   e. At the foot of the massage table, against the wall at least 4 feet away
8. A therapy room used for hot stone massage must have:
   a. A window that opens to the outside
   b. A sink in the room itself
   c. Hardwood floors
   d. Access to electricity
   e. All of the above
9. Essential oils are particularly useful not only for creating a pleasing aroma, but also for:
   a. Helping the stones glide smoothly
   b. Disinfecting the stones
   c. Increasing the therapeutic effect of the massage
   d. Both a and b
   e. Both b and c
10. Placing your oil in a small bowl is useful for:
    a. Eliminating the interruption of getting oil from a bottle
    b. Creating aromatherapy
    c. Accessing the oil by dipping your hands
    d. All of the above
    e. Both a and c

SHORT ANSWER

11. Before using the electric skillet, it is important to make sure it will not ______________________ ______________________.

12. To prevent fires, always ______________________ the skillet at the end of each day.

13. It is important to have some ________________ in the therapy room so that the client will not become overheated.

14. It's best to add ______ to the cold water in the cold stone bowl to prevent it from getting too warm.

15. Four accessories that can help to hold the stones in place on various parts of the body are: ________________, ________________, ________________, and ________________.

Answers to Review Questions can be found in Appendix D.

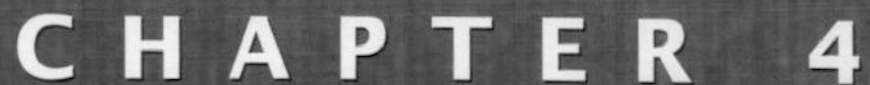

CHAPTER 4

The Stones

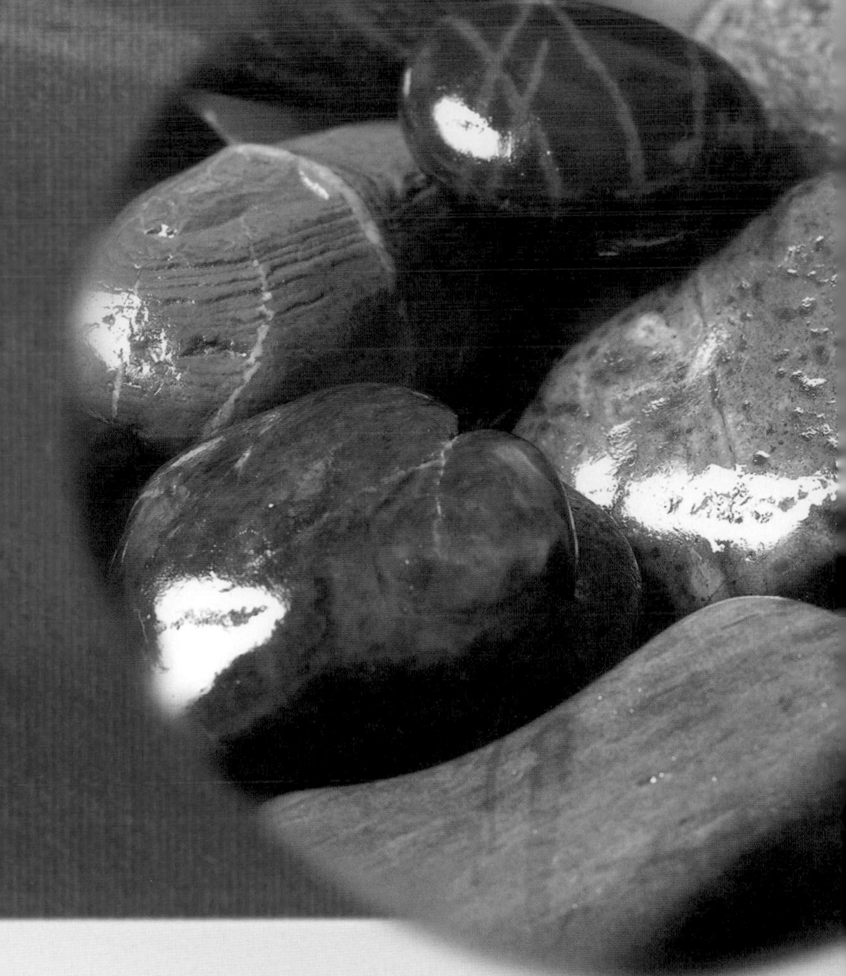

Outline

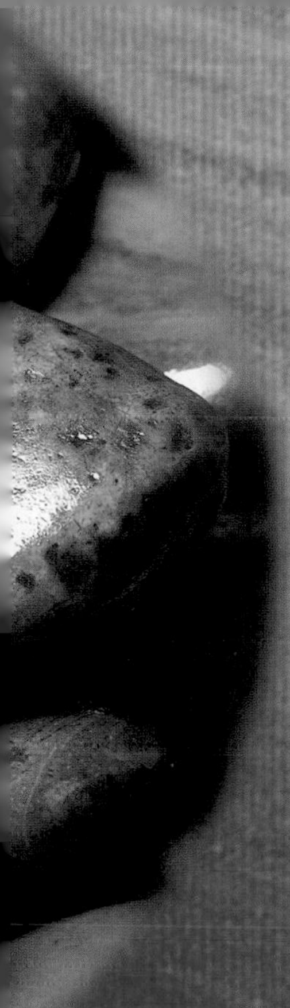

"The love of stones is deeply implanted in the human heart, and the cause of this must be sought not only in their coloring and beauty, but also in their durability. All the fair colors of flowers and foliage, and even the blue of the sky and the glory of the sunset clouds, only last for a short time, and are subject to continual change, but the sheen and coloration of stones are the same today as they were thousands of years ago and will be for thousands of years to come. In a world of change, this permanence has a charm of its own that is eagerly appreciated" (1).

George Frederick Kunz, author,
The Curious Lore of Precious Stones

Objectives

After reading this chapter, you should be able to:

- Classify stones as igneous, sedimentary, or metamorphic.
- Describe the unique properties of different types of stones.
- Identify stones as appropriate for either working massage or static placement.
- Group stones by size.
- Identify the number of stones of each type appropriate for a complete set.
- Explain how to acquire a set of stones appropriate for use in hot stone massage.
- Explain how to cure, store, strip, clean, clear, and recharge stones.

Key Terms

Basalt: A dark-colored extrusive igneous rock with small fine-grained crystals that forms as a result of rapid cooling on the earth's surface.

Crystal: A regular polyhedral form bounded by plane surfaces that are formed by a repeating internal arrangement of atoms. Crystals are found within mineral stones.

Extrusive: A type of igneous rock that is formed as magma erupts from a volcano and pours, as lava, onto the earth's surface, where it cools rapidly.

Granite: An intrusive igneous rock generally light in color, high in silica, and composed of large, coarsely grained crystals that result from slow cooling in the earth's interior.

Igneous rock: Type of rock that arises from the cooling and solidification of molten matter from the earth's interior.

Intrusive: A type of igneous rock that is formed within the earth's interior from magma trapped in pockets within a magma reservoir and cooled slowly.

Jadestone (or jade): An extremely tough, fine-grained metamorphic stone consisting of jadeite or nephrite.

(Continued)

Key Terms *(Continued)*

Lava: Molten rock that has erupted from an active volcano.

Limestone: A sedimentary rock composed chiefly of the mineral calcium carbonate derived from the remains of marine animals.

Magma: Naturally occurring molten rock material generated within the earth and capable of intrusion and extrusion, from which igneous rocks are derived.

Marble: A rock formed by the metamorphic recrystallization of limestone or dolomite.

Metamorphic rock: Type of rock that is formed through the transformation and change of pre-existing rocks due to heat, pressure, or changes in chemical environment.

Mineral: A naturally formed element or compound having a specific and definite range in chemical composition and a characteristic crystal form.

Molten: Melted state of rock.

New England seastone: A conglomerate metamorphic granitic stone consisting mostly of mineral composites such as granite, feldspar, magnetite, dark- or light-colored quartz, and ore.

Placement stones: Stones that are used for static placement on the body.

Quartzite: A metamorphic rock formed from the sedimentary rock sandstone that has been heated and recrystallized during metamorphic processes.

Rock: Any naturally formed aggregate or mass of mineral matter making up an appreciable part of the earth's crust.

Sandstone: A classic sedimentary rock that is formed from the cementing together of sand-sized grains. Quartz is the most abundant mineral in sandstone.

Sedimentary rock: A stratified soft rock that is formed by the consolidation of transported sediments derived from the physical and chemical breakdown of pre-existing rocks or from chemical precipitation from solution.

Semiprecious gemstones: An arbitrary designation of a gemstone of lesser value than a diamond, ruby, or emerald. Some examples are jasper, jade, and turquoise.

Slate: A metamorphic rock that is formed from the consolidation of shale, a sedimentary rock composed of fine silts, clays, volcanic dusts, or other very fine-sized grains of rock.

Tool stones: Concave, arched, or pointed stones used to massage the body in a specific manner.

Working stones: Stones that are actively used to massage the client.

Rocks and stones (small pieces of rock) are formed by a variety of geological processes, which in turn produce varying properties. When you understand and appreciate these properties and the relative advantages and disadvantages of different types of rock, you'll be able to choose the stones that are appropriate for you to use in hot stone massage. This chapter begins with a description of rock origins, composition, and qualities. This geological information will also give you a better idea of where, geographically, you can find the stones you are seeking.

As part of your preparation for hot stone massage, you'll also need to know the different categories into which to group the stones as you are creating your stone kit, or learning how to organize a kit you've purchased. This chapter will, therefore, help you understand the different uses for the various types, sizes, shapes, and textures of the stones.

You'll also need to know how to care for the stones you purchase or find. Thus, this chapter ends with a detailed discussion on how to cure, store, clean, clear, and recharge your stones. This not only assures their proper upkeep, but also shows appreciation for the sacredness of the stones and gratitude for their many benefits.

"Stones are the vessels through which the love and compassion of the therapist can freely flow."

Michelle Helms, hot stones therapist

TYPES OF STONES

Geologists classify rock in one of three categories based on the way it has been formed: igneous, sedimentary, and metamorphic. The geological information in this section describes each category of rock and the particular types of stones within each category. It is based on my own research as well as numerous oral and written communications with geologists Ric Breese and Omer Raup of Boulder, Colorado. I am indebted to them for providing me with an accurate lay description of the geological processes that have created the stones we are so blessed to be able to use in hot stone massage.

Igneous Rock

Igneous rock, sometimes referred to as *fire rock* (from the Latin *ignis* meaning fire), is formed by the cooling and solidification of **molten** rock (**magma**), either within or on the surface of the earth. When this process occurs beneath the earth's surface, the resulting rocks are known as **intrusive** igneous rocks. When the process occurs on the earth's surface, the rocks produced are called **extrusive** igneous rocks. When magma cools slowly within a magma reservoir, its crystals are often large and prominent. This feature reflects the growth potential associated with slow cooling, and the surface of the natural, unpolished rock is consequently coarsely grained. On the other hand, when magma rises from a magma chamber and, by means of volcanic eruption, pours as **lava** onto the earth's surface where it cools rapidly, it exhibits smaller, more finely grained crystals. Thus, its natural, unpolished surface is relatively smooth to the touch.

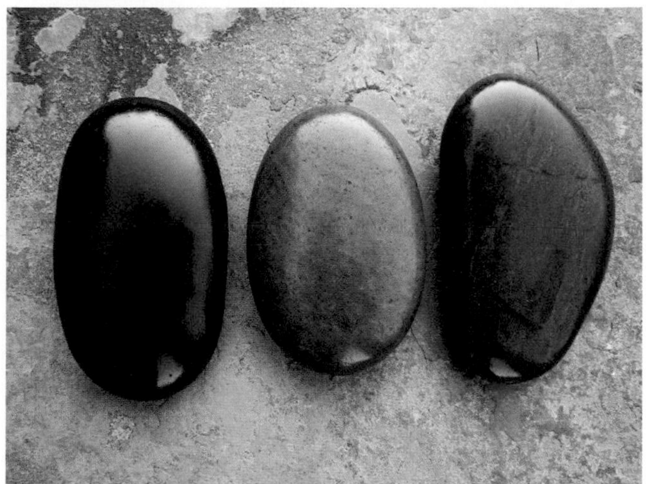

Figure 4-2 **Basalt.** Notice how finely grained and smooth the surface of basalt appears. This comes from the quick cooling following ejection from a volcano and from years of tumbling in rivers and oceans. These extrusive igneous stones were all found on beaches in Baha, Mexico.

Granite

One of the better-known and common intrusive igneous rocks is **granite,** a light-colored rock composed chiefly of silica-rich minerals such as quartz, feldspar, and mica (Fig. 4-1). Because of its coarse-grained texture, granite is not widely used for hot stone massage, although some therapists do use weathered ones for exfoliation and cooling.

Basalt

One of the better-known and common extrusive igneous rocks is **basalt,** a dark-colored, fine-grained lava composed primarily of minerals such as feldspar and pyroxene with or without olivine. The basalt we most commonly see is black; its dark color derived from the abundant presence of such elements as iron and magnesium (2). Basalt can also be found in gray and greenish blue colors, depending upon the ratio of its mineral content. A variety of colors is shown in Figure 4-2. Because of its appealing colors, high retention for heat, and smooth texture, which can offer an optimal glide, as well as its abundant availability and relatively low cost, basalt is one of the most popular and widely used stones for hot stone massage.

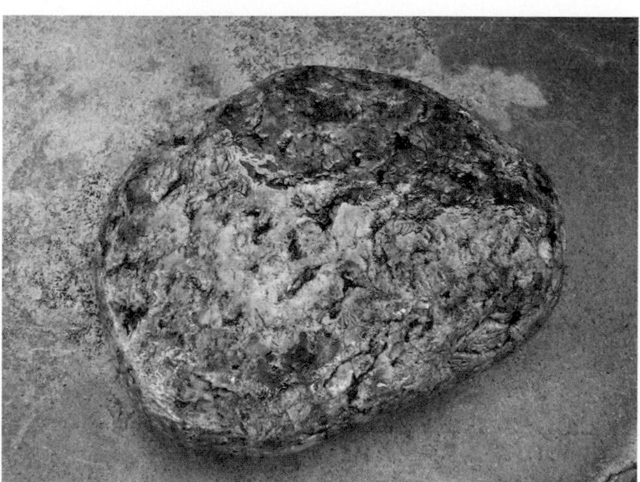

Figure 4-1 **Granite.** Notice the coarse texture of these light-colored intrusive igneous stones. They can be useful for both exfoliation and cooling during a stone massage.

Transported blocks and cobbles (small, rounded stones) of basalt rock can be found in oceans, rivers, and lakes near locations of past volcanic activity, such as in Mexico, Arizona, and Hawaii. A beach where basalt stones are found in Mexico is shown in Figure 4-3. A typical river in Colorado where basalt stones are found is shown in Figure 4-4. The tumbling of these stones in the ocean's waves or a river's current further enhances the natural smoothness of basalt stones. Some therapists have found basalt to be too slippery for them to get a good grip on the stone. I have not found this to be the case, unless they have been mechanically tumbled.

Sedimentary Rock

Sedimentary rock is formed by the cementing of transported mineral and rock grains. These grains may be derived from the physical and chemical

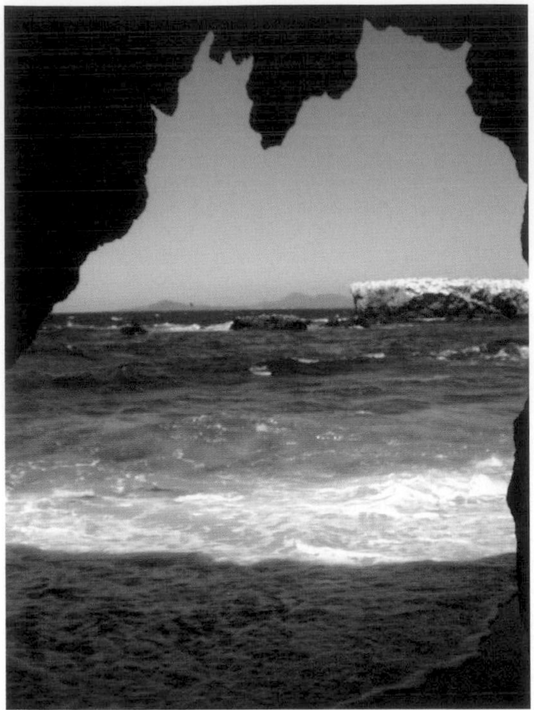

Figure 4-3 Ocean Location Where Basalt Is Found. A beach in Mexico where basalt stones can be found after being nicely tumbled by the waves' constant movement.

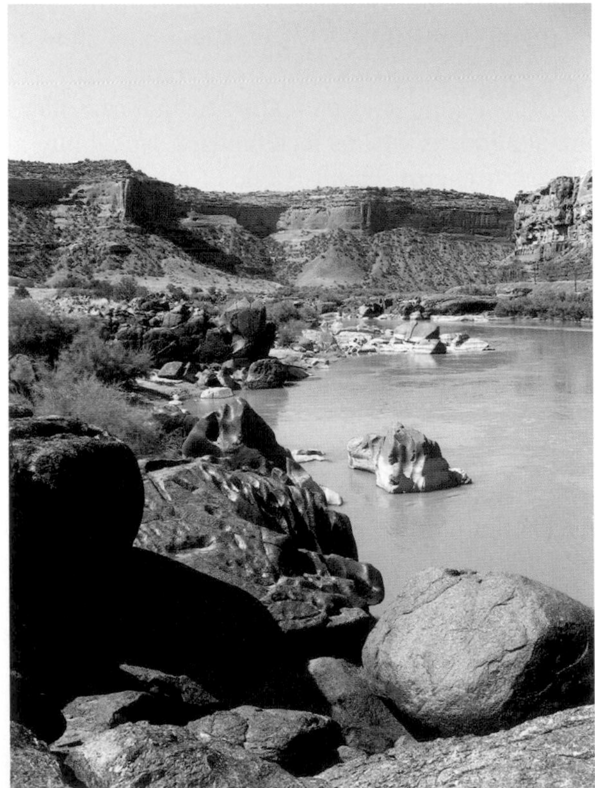

Figure 4-4 River Location Where Basalt Is Found. Basalt can also be found in rivers. The force of the current pounding over the rocks naturally smoothes them.

breakdown of pre-existing rocks, or from chemical precipitation and accumulation of mineral grains from a solution such as seawater or lake water. Thus, characteristic features of sedimentary rocks are their grainy composition and/or stratified bedding layers. **Sandstone,** formed by the cementing of sand-sized grains, and **limestone,** comprised chiefly of calcium carbonate derived from chemical precipitation and/or by the remains of marine animals, are two of the more common types of sedimentary rock (3).

Because it is relatively soft and easily broken, sedimentary rock cannot, in general, withstand the tumbling forces of a river or an ocean and tends to break down and/or to dissolve over time. Likewise, sedimentary rock tends to crack, break, and flake apart in the hot water and pressure used to give a hot stone massage. For this reason, it is not very reliable and is rarely used for giving a hot stone massage.

Metamorphic Rock

Metamorphic rock is formed through the transformation of pre-existing sedimentary or igneous rocks, or older metamorphic rocks by heat, pressure, or changes in chemical environment. These forces can greatly change the rock's original appearance, texture, and mineral content. Such conditions of extreme heat and pressure that result in metamorphism can be found where mountains are being, or have been, uplifted and where the earth's great tectonic plates have collided (4).

Geographically, metamorphic rocks are widely distributed. They exhibit a beautiful range of color and foliation banding that reflects their history (Fig. 4-5). Transported and water-worn blocks and

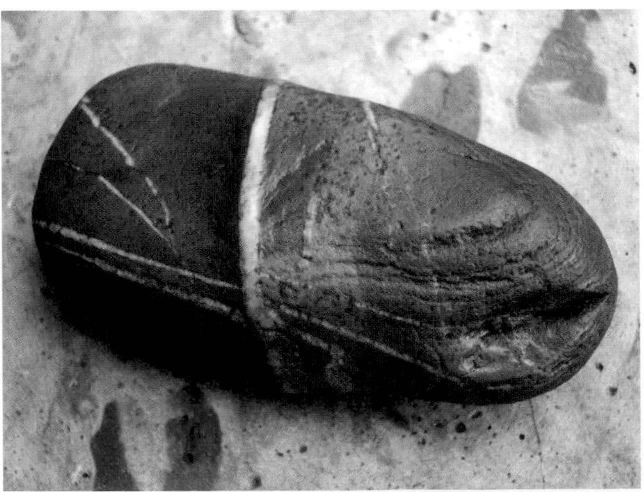

Figure 4-5 Foliation Banding on a Metamorphic Rock. Foliation banding reveals the stone's history.

cobbles of metamorphic rocks can be found along many rivers and ocean beaches worldwide. Among the common metamorphic rocks are quartzite, marble, slate, and jadestone. New England seastone is a lesser-known type. All of these are wonderful for use in hot stone massage, as they have a smooth texture, are dense, have a high retention for heat and/or cold, and are abundantly common in useful sizes. Each of these metamorphic rocks is discussed in more detail next so that you will be more knowledgeable in using them for hot stone massage.

Quartzite

The metamorphic rock **quartzite** is formed from the sedimentary rock sandstone that has been heated and recrystallized during metamorphic processes (5). Quartzite commonly exhibits a smooth and some what satiny sheen, and it often retains some of the straight and curved lines left over from the stratification of the original sandstone. These stones can be quite striking with their inherent sedimentary designs and variations in color. The wide color range of quartzite stones includes, but is not limited to, brown, orange, buff, red, green, and black, as shown in Figures 4-6 through 4-10. The minerals limonite, hematite, or ferric iron are responsible for the buff, brown, and red colors. Glauconite grains or ferrous iron, in sufficient quantities, can create the color green (6). Quartzite can be found as transported and water-worn blocks and cobbles in many Western rivers, such as the Colorado River, as well as on many ocean beaches.

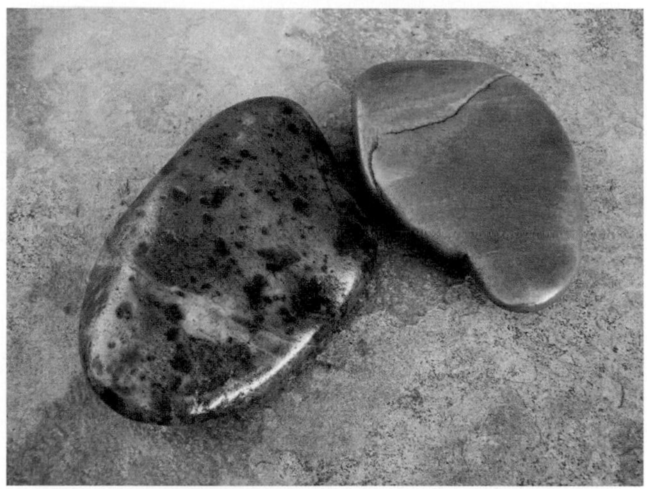

Figure 4-7 Orange and Buff Colored Quartzite Stones. Notice the mixture of speckles and lines from past sedimentary deposits in this orange quartzite. The stratification lines are very faint in this buff quartzite stone.

Marble

Marble is formed by the metamorphic recrystallization of limestone or dolomite. Whereas limestone is a marine or lake sedimentary rock composed chiefly of calcium carbonate, dolomite is a magnesium-rich carbonate rock formed as magnesium alters preexisting limestone. Either of these two rock types can form marble when subjected to heat, pressure, or chemical processes. If the limestone subjected to metamorphic processes was nearly pure calcium carbonate, the resulting marble is white, as shown in Figure 4-11. If other layers, such as sand or clay, exist

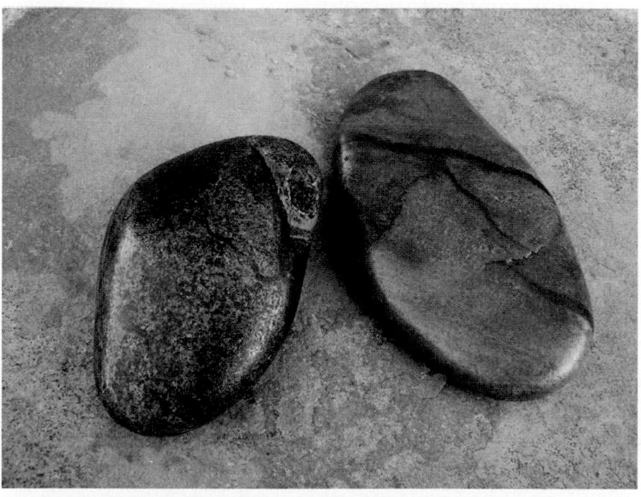

Figure 4-6 Brown Quartzite Stones. Beautiful and prominent stratification designs shown in two metamorphic quartzite stones.

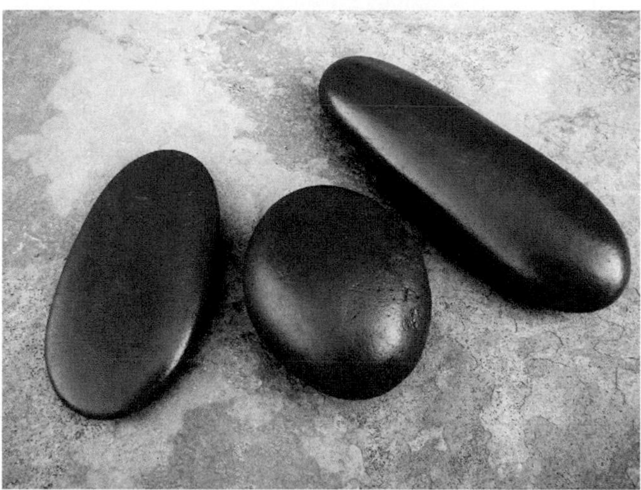

Figure 4-8 Red Quartzite Stones. There are no visible stratification lines in these metamorphic red quartzite stones.

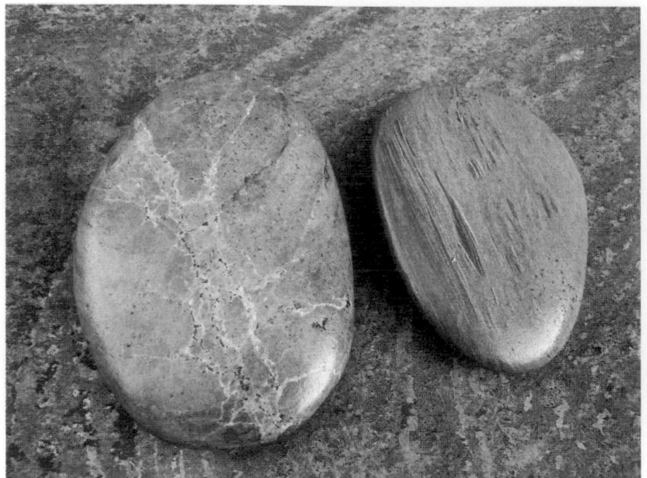

Figure 4-9 Green Quartzite Stones. Notice the different stratification lines in each of these green metamorphic quartzite stones.

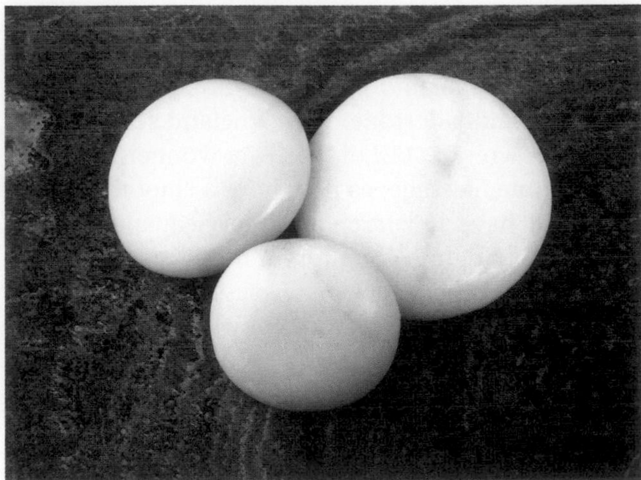

Figure 4-11 Polished White Marble. Once limestone, this metamorphic rock is now dense, smooth, and solid. It must be polished, as its natural state is too rough to use. This marble was mined in Marble, Colorado.

in the limestone, the marble takes on other colors and it can also exhibit a flow banding that adds to its attractiveness.

A brief description of the origin of marble given by geologist Ric Breese may be of some interest.

"Marble is derived from the heat and pressure generated by the intrusion of hot bodies of magma into limestone-bearing rock bodies or alternatively from the heat and pressure associated with the uplift of limestone-bearing mountains due to continental drift and the shifting, collision, and subduction of the earth's great tectonic plates. Theoretically, when limestone is pure and contains only calcium carbonate, the formation of marble simply involves recrystallization of calcite. The chemistry of metamorphism is more complex and can produce a broader suite of minerals when the limestones are impure or when the carbonates contain abundant dolomite."

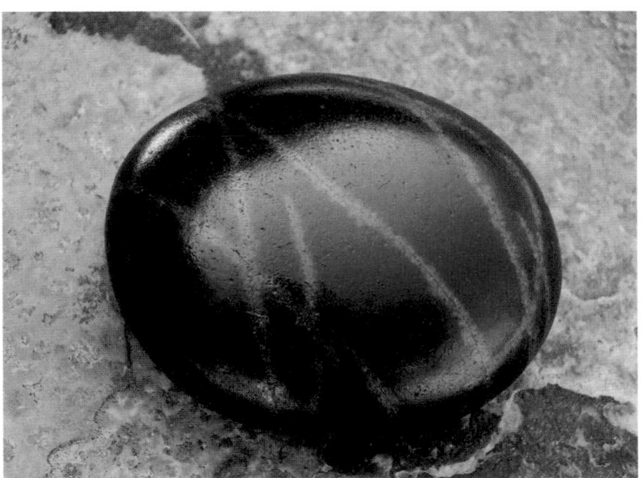

Figure 4-10 Black Quartzite Stones. The white stratification lines in this black metamorphic quartzite rock were etched by an artist called nature.

Marble is rarely found naturally as small rounded pieces ready for use in massage. It must be mined, mechanically cut, shaped, and tumbled, all of which contribute to its cost. Once tumbled, marble's smoothness and density make it a wonderful stone to use for both hot and cold stone massage, but you must be willing to use an artificially tumble-polished stone and pay the higher price for shaping. In the United States, marble is quarried in Colorado, Vermont, Tennessee, Missouri, Georgia, and Alabama.

Jadestone (Jade)

Jadestone is a term that is used broadly to describe a stone that encompasses a wide variety of hard, green minerals, including California jade, Mexican jade, and other rock types. True jade is an extremely tough, fine-grained metamorphic gemstone consisting of jadeite or nephrite. Jadeite is rarer than nephrite and considered more precious. Jadestone is a lower grade of jade containing more nephrite than jadeite. Both jadestone and jade have an unevenly distributed color ranging from deep green to a dull or greenish white, but can occur in many other striking colors, such as lavender.

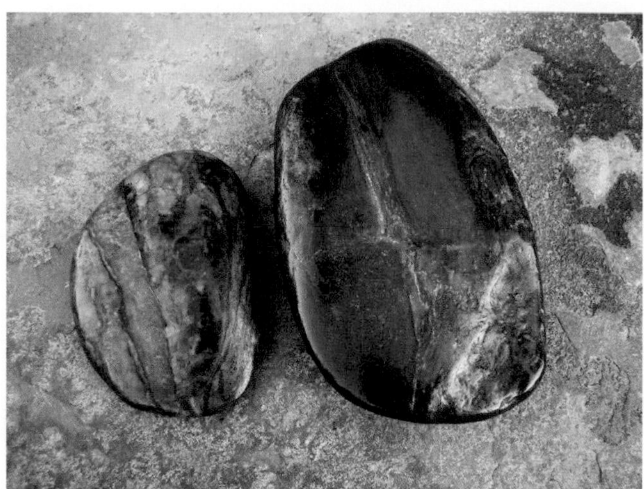

Figure 4-12 Unpolished Jadestone. Even though this natural metamorphic jadestone has not been mechanically polished, it still has a nice smooth feel to the skin and is quite beautiful.

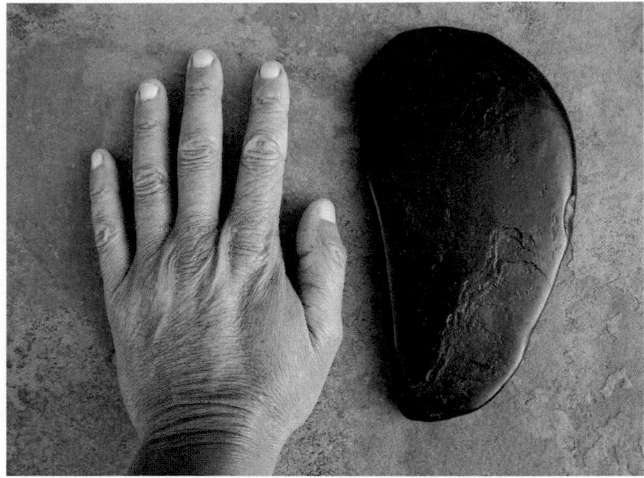

Figure 4-14 Slate. The lightness of slate allows it to be placed on a tender belly or back without creating too much pressure.

Nephrite deposits have been found in China, New Zealand, Russia, Guatemala, the Swiss Alps, and Big Sur, California. Jadeite is found in China, Russia and Guatemala, but the best stones come from Burma, now known as Myanmar (7). Jade has a mystical symbolism around it and is said to help one relax, love, and become more balanced.

The jadestones that I use are from Jade Cove, in Big Sur, California, where the cliffs of these ancient mountains now meet the ocean shores. Most of the jadestone found there is rough and requires polishing to be used in hot stone massage, but some of the pieces that are naturally weathered are smooth enough to use without being polished (Fig. 4-12). Although I much prefer naturally tumbled stones, the beauty and healing powers of the jadestone more than make up for any slipperiness that I must contend with when I use polished jadestone (Fig. 4-13). Because jadestones are hard to find and fairly expensive to buy, they are not practical for an entire stone set, but it is wonderful to add a few to your collection as a special treat.

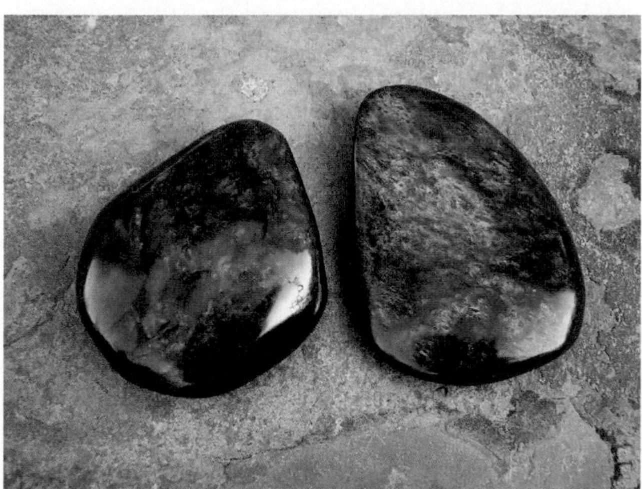

Figure 4-13 Polished Jadestone. Notice the smooth and compact nature of these magnificently veined polished metamorphic jadestones. Their beauty and power make the slippery polish worth it.

Slate

The metamorphic rock **slate** is formed from the consolidation of shale, a sedimentary rock composed of fine silts, clays, volcanic dusts, or other very fine-sized grains of rock. Slate is a hard, dense, and fine-grained, low-grade metamorphic rock that easily splits into thin, flat-surfaced slabs, as shown in Figures 4-14 and 4-15. Slate is commonly found in areas where shale has been subjected to heat and pressure during the process of mountain building (8).

Because it can flake, slate is not an ideal massage stone; however, its large, flat, and smooth surfaces and the thinness of its slabs make it useful as a

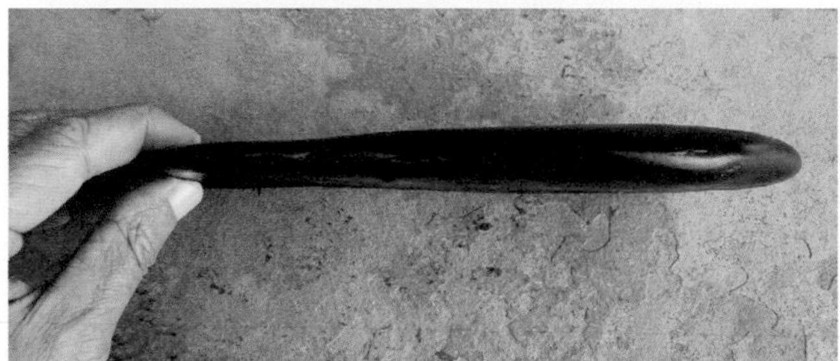

Figure 4-15 Side View of Slate. Notice the thinness of this large piece of slate.

placement stone during a hot stone massage. It can be challenging to find a placement stone for the belly or low back that is large enough to cover a significant area of the body without being too thick and heavy. Although some clients really enjoy the pressure of a heavy stone, not all do. Slate provides width without too much weight. Slate is more commonly found in the mid-Atlantic and northeastern states transversed by or bordering on the Appalachian Mountain chain.

New England Seastone

New England seastone is a designation of a particular stone used by two stone healers living in New England, Karyn Chabot of Sacred Stone Healing and Carollanne Crichton of Healing Stone Massage (9). They reportedly find these stones along New England shorelines with high surf. They describe them as metamorphic stones consisting mostly of mineral composites such as granite and feldspar, often mixed with magnetite or quartz (Fig. 4-16). They often come in various shades of gray, but they tend to get much darker after they are submerged in water and oil. New England seastones are smooth, but offer a bit more texture than basalt stones; thus, they provide greater grip in massage. However, they are neither as flat nor as accessible as basalt and thus are a less popular stone for hot stone massage.

Minerals, Crystals, and Semiprecious Gemstones

A **mineral** is an inorganic, solid substance with a specific and definite chemical composition, and a characteristic **crystal** form. The rocks we've been discussing are aggregates of one or more minerals. The crystals that minerals form have a regular polyhedral structure bounded by plane surfaces that are created by a repeating internal arrangement of atoms (10). The names of crystals reveal the mineral in which they are formed; for example, a smoky quartz crystal, a rose quartz crystal, or an amethyst crystal.

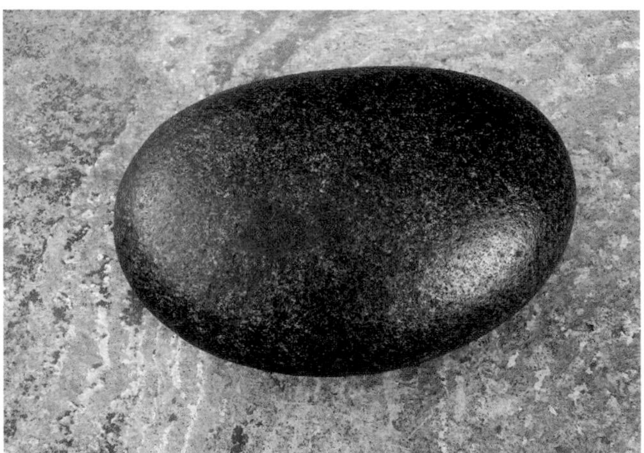

Figure 4-16 New England Seastone. While the New England seastone is almost as dark as black basalt, it is neither as smooth nor as flat.

Gemstones refer to minerals that have high value and can be cut and polished for use as an ornament or jewelry. The value of gemstones is indicated by the terms precious and semiprecious. The term **semiprecious gemstone** is an arbitrary designation of a gemstone of lesser value than a diamond, ruby, or emerald. Some examples of semiprecious gemstones are jasper, garnet, jade, and turquoise.

While not useful for gliding along the body in a hot stone massage, crystals and semiprecious gemstones can be placed on the body over energy vortices such as chakras. Table 4-1 identifies some of the stones that correspond to each chakra, along with the energetic qualities they are purported to elicit or enhance. Figures 4-17 through 4-19 provide an example of a mineral stone for each chakra.

CATEGORY, SIZE, SHAPE, AND QUANTITY OF STONES

Before you set out to collect or purchase your stones, it is helpful to know the different categories of stones and the size, shape, and texture that are desirable for each of the various groups. The proper size and shape of the stone has a great deal to do with both the size of your hand and the part of the body on which the stone will be used. The ideal texture of the stones depends on the category it is in and also varies with personal preference. The amount of stones required to perform a hot stone massage also varies with each therapist, but generally a set of 50 to 55 stones is a good starting point. When first learning to use the stones, you may want to employ only about 30 and add more as your comfort level grows. Eventually, you may supplement your stone kit so that you have 50 in the skillet and 25 (or so) in your spare stone bowl. The amounts I recommend for each category are based on a total of 55 stones. I categorize the stones into three main groups: working stones, tool stones, and placement stones.

Working Stones

Working stones are the stones I use to do most of the general massage strokes on the client. They make up

Table 4-1 Chakras and Their Corresponding Stones

Chakra Center*	Color*	Energy Focus*	Stones
1st Chakra Base, Root Located at the base of the spine	Red, black	Stability, grounding, physical energy, will, security.	Hematite Black Obsidian Black Tourmaline Red Zincite Garnet Smoky Quartz
2nd Chakra Sacral Located below the navel	Orange, blue-green	Creativity, healing, sexuality and reproduction, desire, emotion, intuition.	Orange Calcite Vanadinite Carnelian Blue-green Turquoise Blue-green Fluorite
3rd Chakra Solar Plexus Located at solar plexus, below breastbone	Yellow	Intellect, ambition, personal power, protective.	Citrine Yellow Jasper Golden Calcite
4th Chakra Heart Located in the center of the chest	Pink, green	Love, compassion, universal consciousness, emotional balance.	Rose Quartz Tourmaline Watermelon Tourmaline Green Aventurine Malachite Jade
5th Chakra Throat Located at the neck above collar bone	Blue	Communication center, expression, divine guidance.	Sodalite Blue Calcite Blue Kyanite Angelite Blue Turquoise
6th Chakra Third eye Location centered above eyebrows, at medulla	Indigo	Spiritual awareness, psychic power, intuition, light.	Lapis Lazuli Azurite Sugilite
7th Chakra Crown Located at the top of the head	Violet, golden-white	Enlightenment, cosmic consciousness, energy, perfection.	Amethyst White Calcite White Topaz

Source: *Used with permission from www.bestcrystals.com.

the majority of the stones in my collection. Most of them are more or less palm-sized, as shown in Figure 4-20. I group them by size, ranging from small stones to medium stones, with a few large stones (one of which can be seen in Figure 4-21).

Working stones can be flat or somewhat thick, round or oblong, or any variation thereof. A perfectly round or symmetrical shape is not as desirable as many therapists are led to believe. What is more important is that the size and shape of the stones match your hand and the shape of the body part you're working on. When a working stone is in your palm, your fingers should be able to reach around the edges of the stone enough to make contact with the client's skin along with the stone as you massage. Thus, a stone that is as large as or larger than your hand is generally too large to comfortably and effectively use as a working stone, although exceptions are made for the occasional long broad strokes on larger areas of the body.

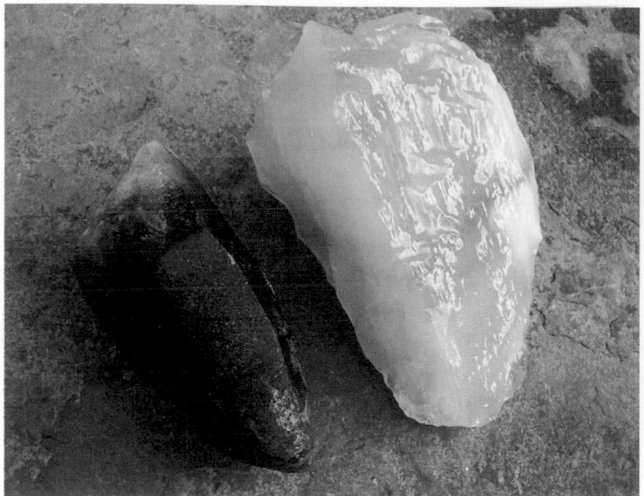

Figure 4-17 Smoky Quartz and Orange Calcite. These mineral stones are typically placed on the first and second chakras, respectively.

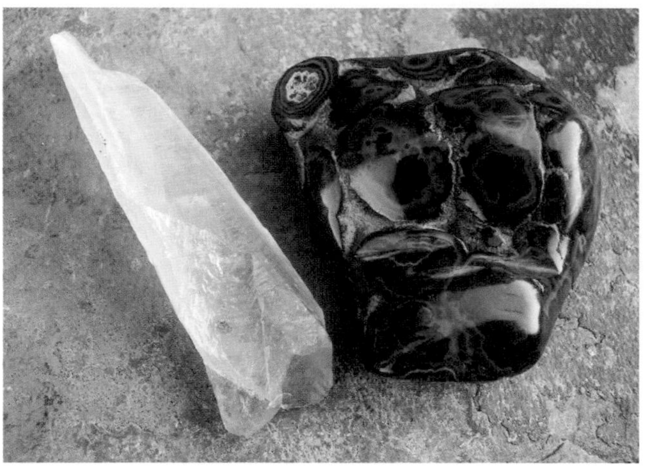

Figure 4-18 Golden Calcite and Malachite. These mineral stones are typically placed on the third and fourth chakras, respectively.

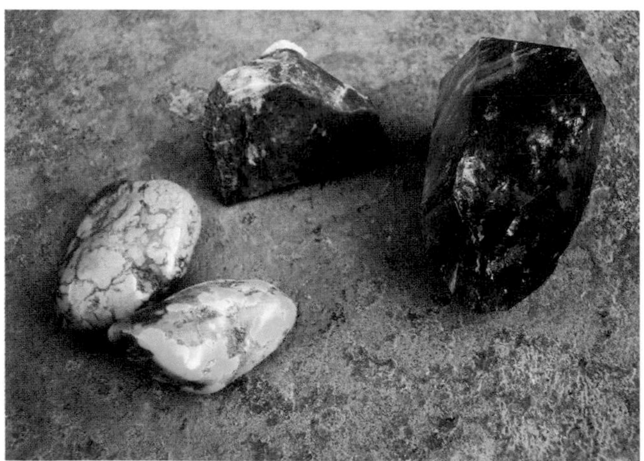

Figure 4-19 Turquoise, Lapis Lazuli and Amethyst. These mineral stones are typically placed on the fifth, sixth, and seventh chakras, respectively.

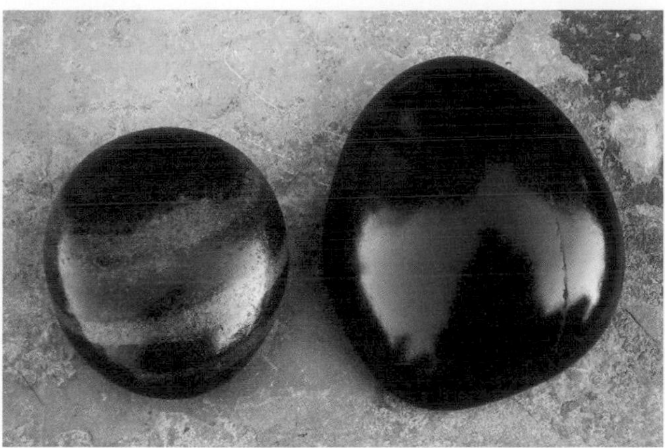

Figure 4-20 Small and Medium Round Working Stones. Small working stone are great for massaging the face and neck. Medium round working stone are great for massaging the arms and calves, chest, and abdomen and, placing along either side of the spine.

Here are some guidelines for assembling your working stones:

- Small working stones range from 1.5 to 2.5 inches wide and long. Use them to massage your client's face and neck. I recommend having eight small working stones in your kit.
- Medium round working stones are approximately 2.5 to 3 inches round, and not too thick. Use them to massage your client's arms, shoulders, calves, and feet. I recommend having 14 medium round working stones in your kit.
- Medium oblong working stones are approximately 3 to 4 inches long by 2 to 3 inches wide and are of both thin and medium thickness. Use them to

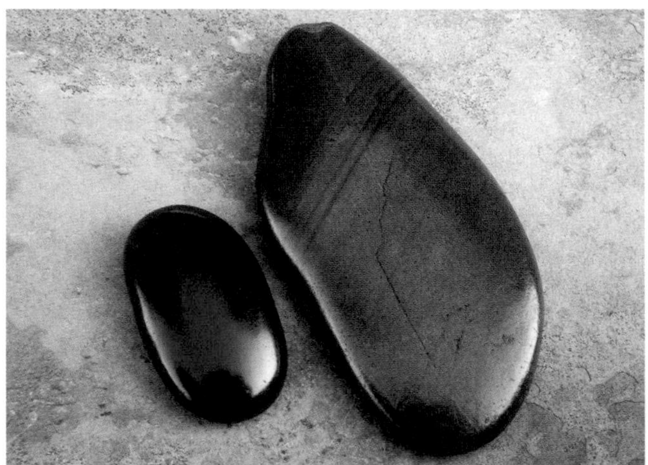

Figure 4-21 Medium Oblong and Large Working Stones. Medium oblong working stone are great for massaging the thighs and placing on the feet. Large working stones are great for massaging the back and placing on the sacrum or abdomen.

massage your client's chest, legs, back, and buttocks. I recommend having 12 medium oblong working stones in your kit.

- Large working stones range from 4 to 5 inches long and are either flat or thick. Use them to massage your client's abdomen and back. I recommend having only two large working stones in your kit.

Thus, quantities recommended for working stones are: 8 small, 14 medium round, 12 medium oblong, and 2 large, totaling 36 stones for your working stones.

Tool Stones

Tool stones are stones with special shapes that are used as devices to accomplish a particular technique. Although tool stones are also used to massage the body, they are used in such a specific manner that they merit their own category. The techniques performed with tool stones will be discussed in great detail in Chapter 9; however, I will identify their purpose, size, and shape briefly here.

Tool stones can either be pointed, concaved, curved, or thin-edged:

- The pointed tool stone should fit comfortably in your hand and have a point that is not too sharp or too blunt, as shown on the left side of Figure 4-22. Use pointed stones to work on trigger points or areas of immense tension that require deep specific penetration.
- The concave tool stone should be rounded on one side and smoothly indented on the other as shown on the right side of Figure 4-22. The indentation does not have to be drastic to work well on angular bones. It, too, should fit nicely in the curve of your hand. Use concave stones to accommodate angular bones such as elbows or ankles.

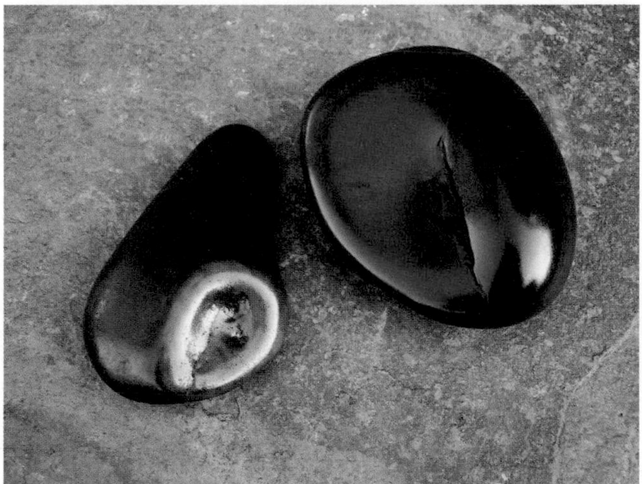

Figure 4-22 Pointed and Concave Tool Stones. A pointed stone allows deep specific penetration on trigger points. A concave stone helps to manipulate over and around angular bones.

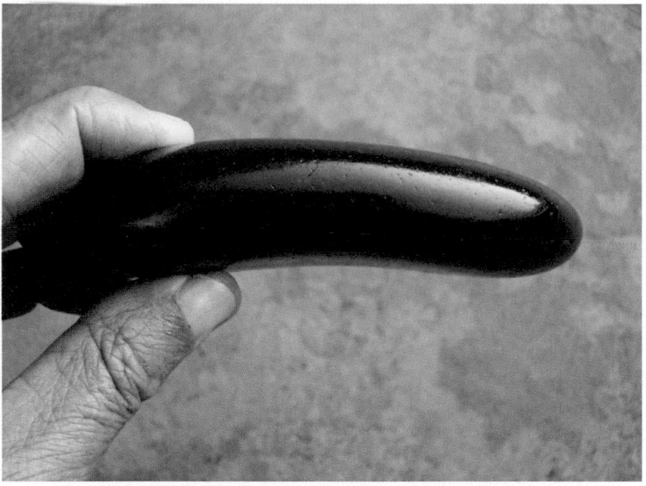

Figure 4-23 Curved Tool Stones. A curved stone can slide down either side of the spine without touching the vertebra. It also matches the shape of curved parts of the body.

- The curved tool stone should be medium sized with a slight arch either on the side or bottom (Fig. 4-23). Like the concave stone, it should fit nicely in your palm. Use curved stones to slide over the spinal column without touching the vertebrae and getting both sides of the erector muscles at once.
- The thin-edged tool stone should be large enough so that your two hands can grab the edge at the same time, but not so large that it can't be used on small areas of the body. Use stones with a narrow edge as shown in Figure 4-24, to do cross fiber friction in the lateral groove along the spine.
- The versatile tool stone (Fig. 4-25) should include several facets of the various different tool stones.

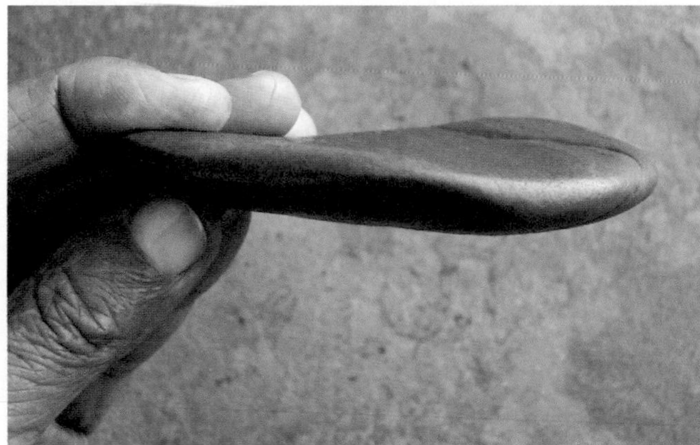

Figure 4-24 Fine-Edged Tool Stone. A finely edged stone makes it possible to use cross fiber friction in the lateral grove of the spine.

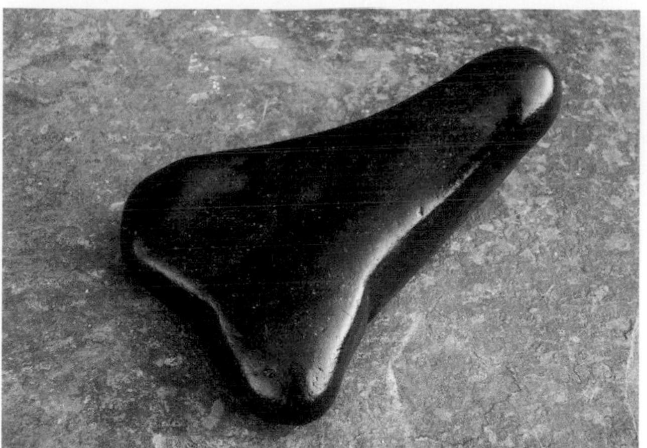

Figure 4-25 Versatile Tool Stone. This stone is versatile in that it has a point, a curve, and a concave end, so it can be used for several purposes.

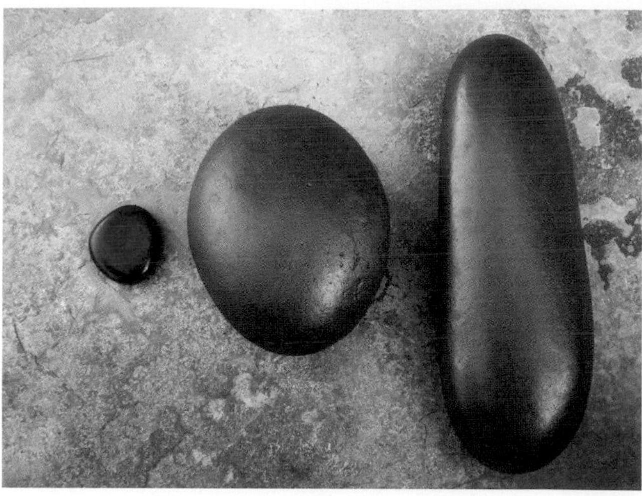

Figure 4-26 A Variety of Placement Stones. Tiny stones fit perfectly between the toes. Medium round thick stones fill in the gap beneath a face down hand. Large cylindrical stones fit nicely beneath the arch of the neck.

Although more difficult to find, the versatile tool stone is ideal, as it uses less space in your stone skillet and accomplishes many of the tasks of quite a few different stones.

I recommend having a total of four specific tool stones, one of each shape; however, if you are lucky enough to find a versatile tool stone, you can minimize the amount of tool stones required. A few of your working stones may be versatile enough to double as tool stones. Thus, don't limit yourself to just using your designated tool stones as your only tools.

Placement Stones

Placement stones are stones that I place on the body. They are static and remain in place until I remove them (or they fall off!). I rarely use them to massage. All working stones can become placement stones in that they can be left under or on top of any part of the body during the massage as the heat in the stone diminishes. But these stones are, nonetheless, sized and categorized as working stones, as that is their main purpose.

The stones that are used just for placement alone are either much larger or smaller in size than working stones. Placement stones can be as large as 1 foot by 1 foot for the abdomen and back, and as small as 1 inch long by 0.25 inches thick for the toes. A range of sizes exists between these two extremes to accommodate other areas of placement. I separate the placement stones into four groups:

- Tiny placement stones are approximately 1 to 1.25 inches long, by 0.5 to 0.75 inches wide and 0.25 inches thick (Fig. 4-26). You can use them for placing between the toes and fingers as well as on the third-eye and cheeks. I recommend having 10 tiny placement stones in your kit. Note that small working stones can also be used for throat chakra placement; however, they will not add into your numbers for placement stones as they are already counted in the working stones.
- Medium thick placement stones are approximately 3 inches round and thick like a potato (Fig. 4-26). You can use these for placing under the hands and knees of your client when they are supine. I recommend having two medium thick placement stones in your kit. Medium oblong working stones can also double as placement stones for the scapula, along the spine, the solar plexus, and feet.
- Large cylindrical placement stones should be approximately 5 to 7 inches long and 2.5 to 3.5 inches wide with a depth ranging from 2 to 3 inches (Fig. 4-26). They can be used to place under your client's neck, occipital ridge, or upper shoulders. I recommend having only one cylindrical shaped placement stone. Large working stones can also double as placement stones for the heart chakra and sacrum. It's nice when you can find ones triangularly shaped to match the shape of the sacrum or heart.
- Extra-large placement stones range from 6 to 12 inches long or wide and no more than 1 or 2 inches thick (Fig. 4-27). These stones can be shaped round, oblong, or any variety in between the two. You can place these stones on your client's abdomen or back, as long as they are not too heavy. I recommend having two extra-large placement stones in your kit.

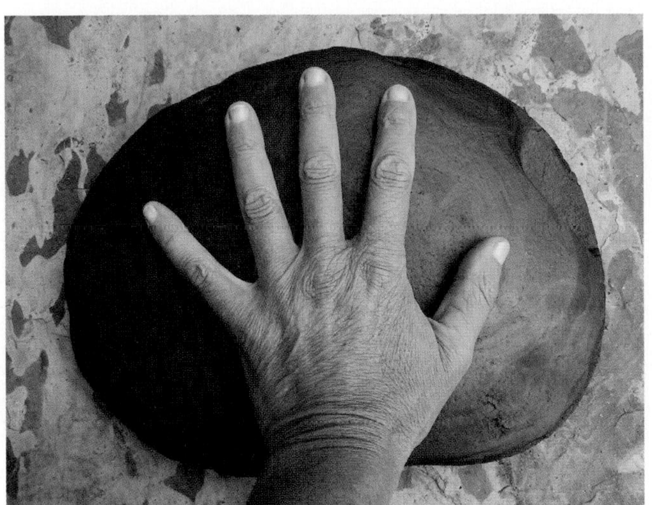

Figure 4-27 Extra-Large Placement Stone. Extra-large stones that are thin and thus, not too heavy feel wonderful when placed on the belly or beneath the lower back.

Thus, the quantities recommended for placement stones are: 10 tiny stones, 2 medium round thick, 1 large cylindrical, and 2 extra-large, totaling 15 placement stones.

When placing stones, take special care to try and match the shape of the stone as well as the size to the area where it is being placed. For instance, the tiny stones that go over the eyes feel better when they have a slight curve to them. Small stones that are placed on the throat chakra should have a slight roundness to them to drop into the cavity below the Adam's apple. The medium oblong stones that strap to the feet fit better when there is a slight curve to the stone. Stones that line either side of the spine feel nicer when they are matched in height from their opposing side. If you are lucky enough to find a large flat stone that is heart-shaped, it is a sweet touch. Paying attention to these subtle aesthetics can have an effect on your client as well as the relationship you have to the art of placement.

Table 4-2 is an easy reference guide to the size, shape, and number of stones in each category, along

Table 4-2 Stone Chart

Category Name	Size and Shape	Location or Purpose	Amount 55 total
Tiny stones (placement)	1-1.25 inches long, 0.5-0.75 wide, and 0.25 inches thick	Place between the toes and fingers, on the eyes, third-eye and cheeks	10
Small stones (working/placement)	1.5 2.5 inches wide and long	Use to massage face and neck Place on throat chakra	8
Medium round (flat) stones (working)	2.5-3 inches round, not too thick	Use to massage the arms, feet, calves, shoulders and to do flowing placement	14
Medium round thick stones (placement)	3 inches round and thick like a potato	Place under hands and/or behind knees of supine client, groin-prone	2
Medium oblong stones (working/placement)	3-4 inches long by 2-3 inches wide and are of thin and medium thickness	Use to massage the chest, both sides of legs, back and buttocks. Place on feet, solar plexus, scapula	12
Large cylindrical stone (placement)	5-7 inches long and 2.5-3.5 inches wide and 2-3 inches deep	Place under the neck, occipital ridge, or upper shoulders	1
Large stones (working/placement)	4-5 inches long, are either flat or thick	Use to massage abdomen and back Place on heart and sacrum	2
Extra-large stones (placement)	6-12 inches long or wide, and no more than a few inches thick	Place stones on the abdomen or back	2
Tool stones (working)	Pointed, concaved, arched, or thin edged stones	Use to massage trigger points, around boney protuberances, in grooves	4

with the location or purpose of the stone. Remember, however, not to get too caught up in certain stones only being "allowed" to be used for certain areas. These are merely recommendations and guidelines. Ultimately, you will find what works best for you.

TEXTURE OF STONES

A smooth texture is important for both working and placement stones. They feel good against the client's skin, and they allow the stone to glide easily along the body. I prefer stones that are naturally shaped and tumbled by oceans and rivers, rather than ones that are cut, shaped, and artificially tumbled. The rapid mechanical tumbling or polishing of a stone can be likened to the sun burning one's skin. The process interferes with the matrix of the stone, weakening its electromagnetic field and lowering its healing potential (11). The geological processes that cause stones to become smooth occur over thousands of years; to me, it seems disrespectful to subject a stone to a mechanical tumbling process that smoothes it in minutes. In addition, stones that have been tumbled by rivers and oceans over centuries feel better in your hands. Stones that have been mechanically tumbled are extremely slippery when they are oiled. This makes it difficult to move slowly with the stones and get the resistance needed against the skin to go deep. A stone that has a natural coat offers a better grip and allows you to work as slowly and deeply as you and your client desire.

Sometimes, as in the case of jade and marble, I do make an exception and use a stone that has been mechanically tumbled, either because it would be unusable otherwise or because it is simply beautiful and seems to call out to me. It is important to be open to all possibilities when working with the stones. As another example, a stone with a slightly coarse texture can be useful as a gentle exfoliating agent for the face, back, or feet and can help bring additional blood to a stagnant area. Some clients actually enjoy the alive, refreshing feeling that comes from a slightly rough stone that is carefully scrubbed against their skin. With experience, you will discover the texture of stone that works best for you and your clients.

ACQUIRING STONES

Before you can perform hot stone massage, you'll need to acquire an appropriate set of stones (Fig. 4-28). You can collect your stones yourself or purchase a commercial stone kit through one of the numerous massage stone representatives. There are advantages and disadvantages to either approach.

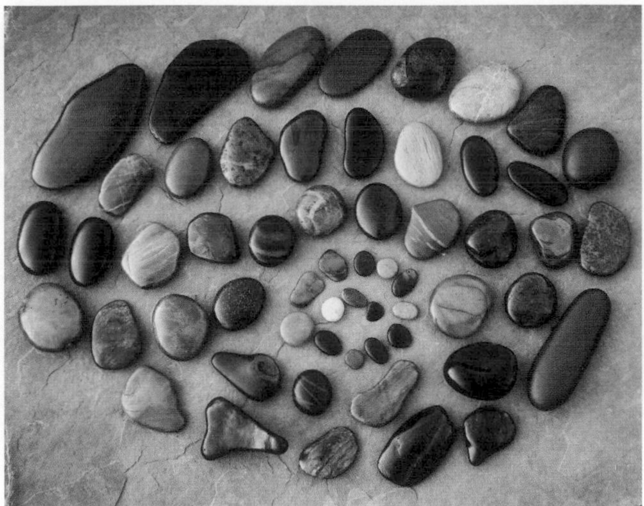

Figure 4-28 Stone Set. This photo shows one example of an appropriate set of stones to use in a hot stone massage. Notice the variety of colors, shapes, types, textures, and sizes. These stones were hand-selected by the author from the banks of the Colorado River and the beaches in Baha, Mexico.

Collecting Stones

By collecting your own set of stones, you will end up with a much more personalized collection, tailored to your particular hand size, intended uses, and sense of aesthetics. Many therapists have expressed feelings of deeper kinship to their stones when they have found them on their own (Fig. 4-29).

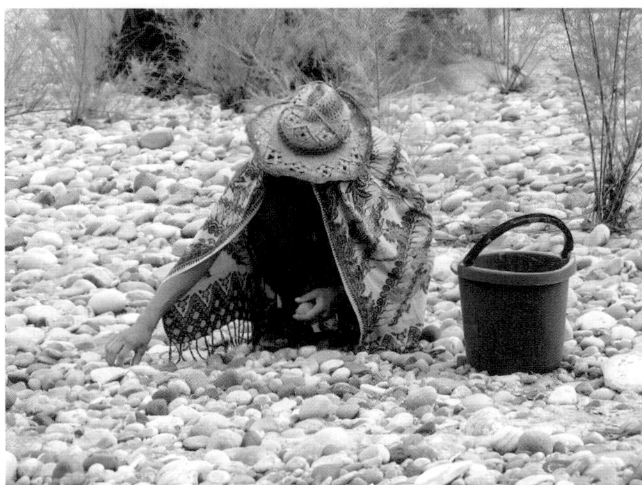

Figure 4-29 Collecting Stones. Selecting the proper stones for you is a personal, sometimes arduous and yet very satisfying experience.

If you decide to collect your own stones, schedule ample time to collect them. Do not expect to walk on a beach and find 50 stones of appropriate size, shape, and composition just lying there. In order to acquire an appropriate set of 50 or so stones, you'll have to sort through hundreds, if not thousands. It can take days to collect just a starter set, and the process can be ongoing for years. Watch out! Once your search for stones begins, it can be all consuming, and you might find yourself bent over looking at the ground everywhere you walk.

TIP 

It is important to bring along a sturdy container with strong handles for carrying the stones. Stones get heavy very quickly, and what might begin as a stroll for a few can swiftly turn into an expedition leading to dozens. You certainly want to avoid having stones spilling out of the little bag that you thought would be sufficient!

When collecting stones, look for particular sizes and shapes that will match joints and regions of the human body, as well as particular types, textures, and colors. In addition, seek stones that are aesthetically appealing to you. Stones have their own personality and beauty, and it is fine to choose a stone for no other reason than that you like it! Before removing a stone from its environment, silently ask its permission to take it, and wait mindfully for an answer. If any internal conflict, discomfort, or anxiety arises within you, consider the possibility that the stone should remain in its majestic environment and that a different stone might be a better choice.

TIP 

I acquired my favorite stone by listening rather than looking. One day, I was at a river and seemed to feel pulled toward a certain spot. I began digging there and found a stone that took my breath away. It was kidney-shaped, very flat, and golden brown, with a streak down the middle. Velvety smooth, it had a feel to it like no other stone I had ever found. Because it was buried under sand, I would have missed it had I relied solely on my eyes. Instead, I listened with my heart.

There have also been times when returning to a riverbed I have been visiting for years that I notice a familiar stone that seems to acknowledge my return and communicate to me, "Now I am ready to go!" I also make a point of removing only a few stones from each small area so that it does not seem decimated.

If you can collect your stones close to your home, this will create a comradeship with the land where you are living. It is also easier and more affordable. My stone kits are made up primarily of stones I find on the banks of the Colorado River, the pebble shores of Mexico, and the Big Sur coastline, as I either live in or frequently visit these areas. However, there is nothing wrong with traveling to seek out the stones desired. It is more time-consuming and costly, but makes for an interesting and fun vacation. There are ample areas to choose stones from, each offering a unique quality of stone.

When looking for stones in a riverbed, it is best to go to an old river that is wide and flat and has offered the stones time for weathering. The lower sections of the Colorado River in Colorado, Utah, Arizona, and even into California have a good selection of basalt and metamorphic stones. Areas around the volcanoes in Hawaii, large lakes such as Lake Superior, and ocean shores in Baha, Mexico, New England, Canada, Alaska, and Big Sur, California, also supply a wonderful selection of basalt and metamorphic stones.

TIP 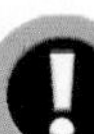

Ask people who have collected stones where they found them. You will be surprised at just how many stone havens exist.

Some people choose to try and collect all their stones at one time, while others take their time and collect them little by little over a period of time. You can begin learning to do hot stone massage with a small number of stones at first, say 15 or 20, and then build up to a full set as you gain experience. Whatever the collection process, it is critical to have stones to practice with while you are learning the techniques of hot stone massage. It is not uncommon for students to forget most of what they have learned in a hot stone class, because they were not able to practice at home. Thus, acquiring a set of stones, be it small or large, is the first step that must be taken before beginning a hot stone massage class.

Purchasing a Stone Kit

As discussed previously, finding stones is not a speedy process. It often requires travel, time, and lots of back bending to sort through thousands of stones to find the right sizes and shapes. Many therapists choose to purchase their stones so that they can begin practicing hot stone massage immediately. The most obvious advantage of purchasing stones is that the work of collecting is done for you.

When purchasing a stone kit, be sure that it includes the various types, shapes, and sizes needed to perform a hot stone massage. Many stone kits on the market have generic stones that are not hand-selected. They also tend to be all one type and color of stone, which not only limits their utility, but is also unappealing to the eye. When researching the stones available on the market, I purchased several kits. Unfortunately, the vast majority of the stones they contained were of the wrong size, shape, or texture for massage. Hundreds of them now grace my garden.

There are a few stone companies, listed in Appendix B, that do hand-select their stones and pay careful attention to the types, shapes, sizes, and colors best suited for giving an optimal hot stone massage. If you do not have the time or live in a location convenient for collecting your own stones, then I recommend ordering a kit through one of these companies and then supplementing over time with stones you find on your own. If you decide to order a stone kit from a distributor, if possible, first speak to someone who has already ordered from that company. You should also call the distributor and discuss the stones they offer. Don't rely on photos in a magazine or a Web site to determine if the stones are appropriate for you. Many photos of stone sets are enhanced and often do not reflect what will actually be delivered.

TIP

When calling distributors to ask about their stones, make sure you determine the sources, exact shapes and sizes, and how many stones are included in their kit. Ask about the availability of tool stones, if their stones are naturally tumbled, if they have any variation in color, and if they are pre-oiled.

CARING FOR STONES

Once the stones have been acquired, it is then time to learn how to care for them. When you care for your stones properly, you will be able to use the same stones for as long as you desire. You will never have to replace them.

TESTIMONIAL 

I once taught a hot stone massage class at a high-end spa on a remote island in the West Indies. I had dragged hundreds of pounds of stones with me to this island, as the spa personnel had not been able to find the appropriate stones on the island. The spa manager was pleased and excited when she saw all the stones I had brought, and looking up at me with a wide-eyed expression, she innocently asked, "How long will the stones last?"

I paused before answering, not sure what she meant. I asked for clarification: "You mean, how long does the heat last in the stones?"
She shook her head and said, "No, I mean how long will the stones last?"

I was stupefied. I had never been asked this before. Realizing the absurdity of the question but not wanting to offend the manager, I jokingly said, with an air of mock concern, "Well, these particular stones have been around for a millennium, so they just might be on their last legs. Who knows, by the end of the class we may discover that they've all vaporized!"

By now, she had caught on to the absurdity of her question and laughingly said, "Okay, so we won't have to order more stones anytime soon, huh!" The truth is that stones, unlike almost everything else on earth, will last.

Curing Stones

Whether stones have been collected or purchased, the first step in caring for them is to cure them by steeping them in oil and applying heat. When stones have been cured, they retain the oil within them and require only a light touch-up of oil each time they are used. Stones that are not cured remain dry to the touch; thus, a therapist using uncured stones has to wrap the stones with oil each time before using them. This slows down the flow of the massage considerably.

You need to cure your stones only once, just before the first time you use them. The only time the process needs to be repeated, is if the stones become dried out and/or sticky. This will happen if they are stored out of water for too long.

The process of curing stones is as follows:

1. Wash stones with warm water.
2. Dry both sides overnight.
3. Oil stones generously with a rich almond oil (with a nice scent).
4. Bake stones in an oven (not in a skillet) at 350°F for 15 minutes. Stones should not be placed in water when baking, but rather laid on a cookie sheet or in a cake pan dry with only oil on them.
5. Remove from the oven and cool on towels overnight.
6. Oil both sides of the stones again the next day and cover with plastic.
7. Wait a few days and oil stones for the third time.
8. Place stones in water to store or use.

Storing Stones

Once stones have been cured, they must be stored either in water or an airtight plastic bag; otherwise, the oil will congeal and they will become "gunky" or sticky. It is best to store the "hot" stones in water in the covered skillet they will be occupying when giving a hot stone massage, and the "cold" stones in a covered plastic bowl with water. All stones can rest in the water endlessly with no harm to them just as they would in a river. In fact, storing the stones in water not only keeps the oil on them nice and smooth and prevents them from drying out, but it also simplifies the beginning of the massage, as the stones are already in the skillet ready to be heated and go to work.

If the stones must be transported and be out of water for longer than 3 or 4 days, they must be sealed in an airtight plastic bag. This will keep them moist and prevent them from getting sticky. If, by chance, the stones were cured and mistakenly left out for an extended period of time or were burned in a waterless skillet, they will need to be stripped of their oil, and the curing process will have to be repeated. Stripping is discussed in the next section. It is best, however, not to leave stones in plastic bags for prolonged periods of time, as doing so can affect their vibrational frequencies and can cause them to mold. If stones are not going to be used at all for a very long period of time, it is best to strip them of their oil and let them rest outside in a natural environment.

Stripping Stones

To strip stones, simply put them in a large old pot on the stove, cover them in water, and boil them with a gentle detergent for approximately half an hour, or until there is no discernible presence of oil. Once this state has been reached, simply begin the curing process over. The stripping process should not be done in the massage skillet because it coats the device used with residual oil and soap.

Cleaning Stones

Clean the stones after every use and at the end of each day. In between massages, all that is necessary to clean the stones is to boil them in the skillet for approximately 3 to 5 minutes. Cold stones need to be boiled as well. Include them in your final boiling and then return them to their cold stone bowl.

I do not recommend using antibacterial soap or spa disinfectants for cleaning, as it is unnecessary and breaks down the oil coating on the stones. There are no skin-passing bacteria that can survive in boiling water; however, if you still feel additional sanitation is required, add a few drops of disinfecting essential oils, such as lavender, lemon, fir, tea tree, or eucalyptus, to the water in the skillet and let it boil with the stones (Fig. 4-30). Do this between every hot stone massage given in one day. The water does not need to be changed until the end of each day, unless of course hair or oil is accumulating in it, in which case you should change the water before the next use.

At the end of each day, unless only one hot stone massage was given, the water in the skillet needs to be emptied and replaced. One way to speed this process along is to remove each stone from the skillet

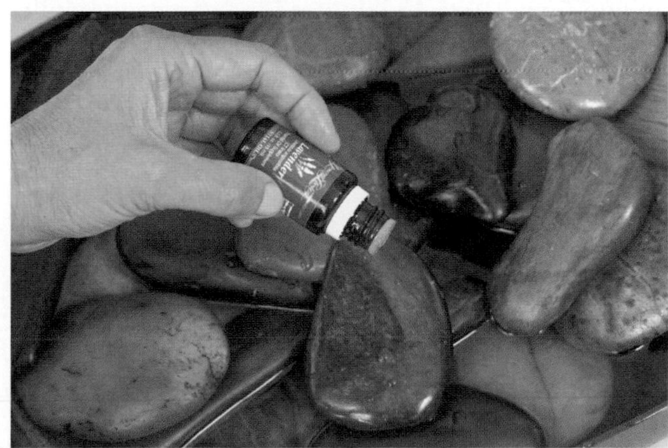

Figure 4-30 Disinfecting the Stones. Adding a few drops of essential oil to the boiling water will further disinfect the stones at the end of a session.

during the last 5 minutes of the last client's massage. As you remove each stone from the skillet, place it on top of or along-side the client's body.

TIP 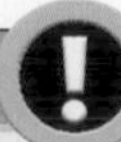

Always ask the client's permission before doing this, as having an entire skillet full of stones on the body at once could be slightly intimidating and claustrophobic. However, with the client's approval, this technique can bring great joy and save you time at the end of a long day. My clients who have received this treatment have reported that they found it soothing. They could handle the weight and heat because they knew the stones would only be there for a few minutes.

Once you have placed all of the stones on or near your last client, unplug the skillet and take it away to empty the water. While the client is relaxing with the stones, wash the skillet and then return to your office with the clean skillet. Refill the skillet halfway with fresh clean water. Turn the skillet back up to high and remove the stones from the client one by one, cleaning each one with a small towel before placing it in the water. If the stones are heavy with grime, you can clean them individually with rubbing alcohol. After all the stones have been returned to the skillet, add a few drops of a disinfectant essential oil and allow the water to boil the stones for 3 to 5 minutes, releasing the fragrance of the essential oil in the treatment room while your client is getting dressed. After you return to the treatment room to say goodbye to your client, all you have to do is turn off and unplug the skillet and leave. If you don't include the cocoon treatment as part of your massage, then you must plan an additional 10 to 15 minutes for cleaning the skillet and stones after the last client leaves.

TIP 

Be sure the skillet is turned all the way off and unplugged at the end of each day in order to avoid burning the stones or causing a fire.

Clearing Stones

Because stones have been embedded in the earth for so long, and some contain iron-bearing minerals such as magnetite, they can take on some of the magnetic attributes of the earth's magnetic field. The stones not only offer energy to us, but they receive energy from us as well. Acting like magnets on a subtle level, stones can absorb negative energy from the client's physical and energetic fields. The use of stones can be helpful in drawing out repressed emotions, deep sorrow and pain, and in polarizing imbalances allowing for transformation if the client is ready for it (11). After a period of heavy use, however, the stones can begin to feel "full" and need to be cleared out of all the human energy they have absorbed.

After the stones have been cleaned, a simple way to clear the stones is to place them in a large bowl of fresh cold water with a cup of sea salt and leave them outside overnight under a full moon. This can be done year round, as the seasons will not alter the effect the moon has on the stones. The difference of how the stones feel the next morning is astounding. This ritual is best done monthly if the stones are being used frequently. Otherwise, base the clearing schedule on the amount of use the stones are getting.

For additional clearing in between the monthly moon ritual, a quartz crystal can be placed in the cold skillet with the stones as they rest over night. Be sure to remove the crystal before turning the skillet on the next day.

Even though mineral stones are not used to massage clients, they still absorb energy from the client's chakras where they are placed. Place them in their own bowl of fresh water, with or without salt, to avoid the oil from the massage stones. I have a small waterfall mist-maker bowl that I place my crystals and gemstones in, as shown in Figure 4-31, and allow the water to circulate over them for an entire evening.

Smudging your stones with white sage is another way to clear them of the energy they have absorbed. Simply light the sage and direct its smoke over the stones using a feather fan or your hand. This is best accomplished when the stones are out of water.

Recharging Stones

In nature, stones may tumble down a river, crash under waves, or sit on a sunny shore. In contrast, stones that you choose to assist you in massage have become, in a sense, "doers," and they need to have their energy recharged as humans do. After the stones have been used for a while, they might have a "tired" feeling to them when you use them. The precise quality is hard to describe, but you will be able to feel it as you become more and more attuned to the

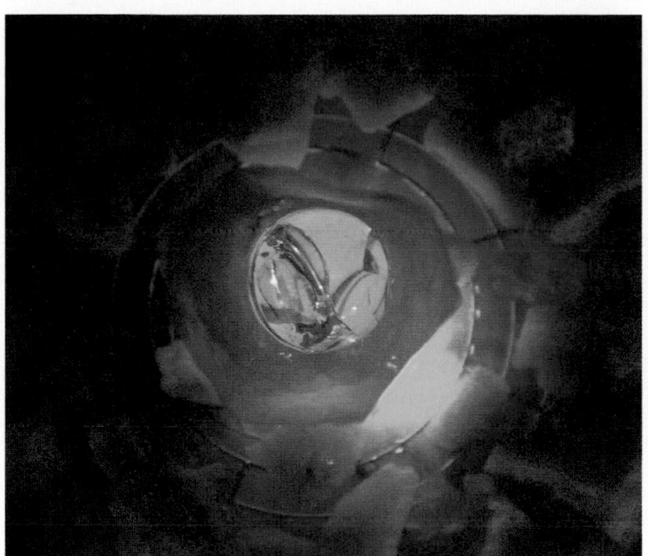

Figure 4-31 Clearing Crystals. Mini waterfall and mist maker used to clear the energies from tired crystals and gemstones.

energy of your stones. Thus, in addition to clearing your stones, you should recharge them. This will revitalize their energy.

The simplest and most effective way to recharge stones is to lay them out on a blanket in the sun and leave them there all day. As long as weather permits, this can be done year round. Bring them inside in the evening and store them once again in water. See if you notice a difference the next time you use the recharged stones.

Another method for recharging stones that has been suggested is to place the stones out in a thunder and lightning storm to recharge their energy. Although this sounds good, I have yet to have the courage to run outside in the middle of an electric storm with my stones! I prefer the sun, but feel free to experiment with the elements and let me know your results.

SUMMARY

The three main classes of stone are igneous, sedimentary, and metamorphic. Igneous rock is formed as a result of magma solidifying either within or on the surface of the earth, forming rocks such as granite, which is coarsely grained, and basalt, which is finely grained. Sedimentary rock is formed by the cementing of transported mineral and rock grains and has characteristic features such as grainy composition and/or stratified bedding layers. Two common forms of sedimentary rock are sandstone and limestone. Metamorphic rock is formed through the transformation of pre-existing rocks due to heat, pressure, or to changes in chemical environment. Some examples of metamorphic rock are quartzite, marble, jadestone, slate, and New England seastone.

Basalt, quartzite, marble, jadestone, and New England seastone are all useful stones for performing hot stone massage because of their smooth textures, heat retention, accessibility, and beauty.

A stone kit should contain approximately 36 working stones, 4 tool stones, and 15 placement stones, totaling 55 stones. Working stones are used to massage your client. Tool stones are used for specific techniques within the massage. Placement stones are simply placed on the body for warmth.

Stones are best when they have a naturally smooth texture and have not been interfered with by artificial tumbling. However, stones like marble, that must be artificially tumbled, outweigh the disadvantages of the tumbling by their beauty and usefulness in massage.

To acquire a set of stones for hot stone massage, you must either collect them or purchase them. When collecting your stones, be sensitive to which stones are asking to stay and which are willing to go. Choose only a few stones from each area. If you purchase your stones from a distributor, make sure to ask the questions listed in this book to assure getting the stones that you want.

Once you have acquired your stone set, take some time to be with and get to know your stones. If they have not been cured, then follow the procedures in this chapter. Once you begin using your stones, be sure to store, clean, clear, and recharge them properly so that they will remain radiant and full of good energy for as long as you use them. Treat your stones with the same respect you do your clients or a loved one and they will serve you well in return.

REVIEW QUESTIONS

TRUE/FALSE

1. Jadestone is the same thing as the semiprecious gemstone jade.

   Circle: True False

2. The constituents of marble were once on the ocean floor, even though the rock is found in mountains.

   Circle: True False

3. Stones have a limited life span and will work for massage for only so long, even if they are well taken care of.

   Circle: True False

4. It is a good idea to collect lots of stones from one area.

   Circle: True False

5. The size of the stones you use should reflect the size of your hands as well as the size of the area of the body they are working.

   Circle: True False

MULTIPLE CHOICE

6. Stones that form deep within the earth and are cooled slowly have which properties:
   a. Smoothly textured fine grain
   b. Very sharp edges
   c. Roughly textured large grain
   d. A dark color
   e. Both b and c
7. Some common metamorphic rocks are:
   a. Jadestone
   b. Marble
   c. Quartzite
   d. Both b and c
   e. All of the above
8. Marble is formed by:
   a. Volcanic activity
   b. The recrystallization of sandstone
   c. The uplift of limestone-bearing mountains
   d. Man-made factories
   e. b, c, and d
9. The fourth chakra corresponds with the heart and the following mineral stones:
   a. Rose quartz
   b. Watermelon tourmaline
   c. Garnet
   d. Both a and b
   e. All of the above
10. When collecting your own set of stones, which of the following is true:
    a. Look for them in young, narrow, rough rivers
    b. Look for them in areas of past volcanic activity
    c. Look for them in old, wide, calm rivers
    d. Both a and b
    e. Both b and c

SHORT ANSWER

11. The 4 main categories of rock are: ____________ ________________, ______________________, and ______________________.
12. Rocks that are formed by magma cooling deep within the earth's interior are called __________ __________ rocks. A common rock of this type is ______________.
13. Rocks that are formed by magma cooling on the earth's surface due to volcanic eruption are called __________ __________ rocks. A common one is___________.
14. Rocks formed by the cementing of transported mineral and rock grains of pre-existing rocks are called ___________. Two common ones are __________ and __________.
15. Stones should be stored in ____________ when using them regularly and in a ____________________ when traveling or not in use for a period of time.

MATCHING

a. Stripping c. Clearing e. Recharging
b. Curing d. Cleaning

16. Cooking the oil into the stone to seal it in. ______________
17. Leaving stones in cold water with salt under the full moon. ______________
18. Leaving the stones on a blanket in the sun. ______________
19. Boiling stones with soap to remove the gunky oil. ______________
20. Boiling stones in between sessions with a disinfecting essential oil. ______________

Answers to Review Questions can be found in Appendix D.

CHAPTER 5

Heating and Cooling the Stones

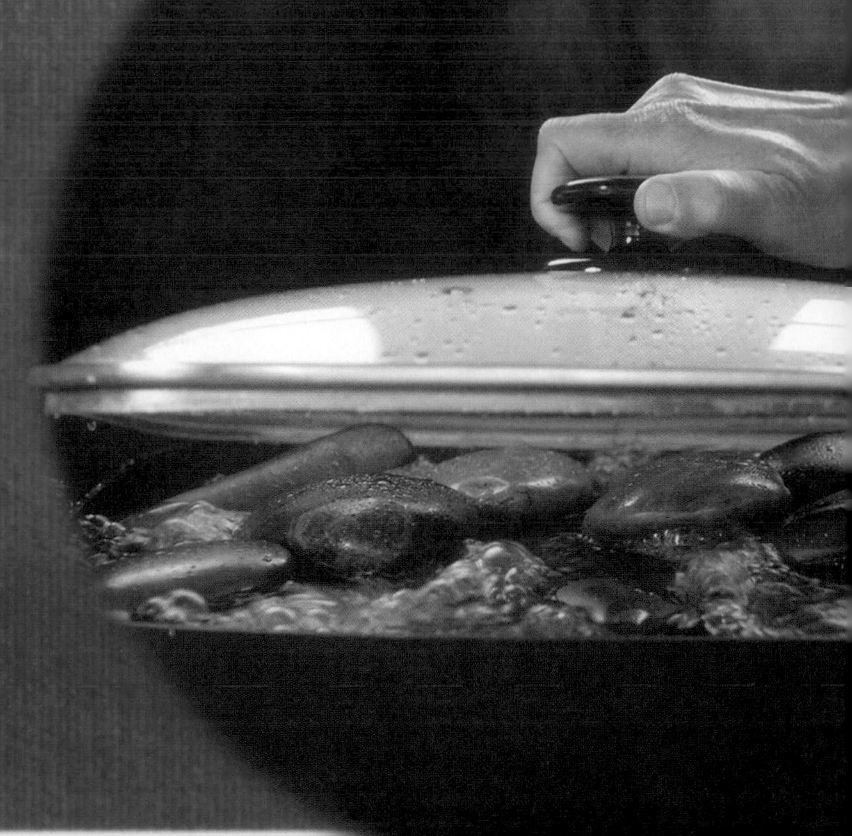

Outline

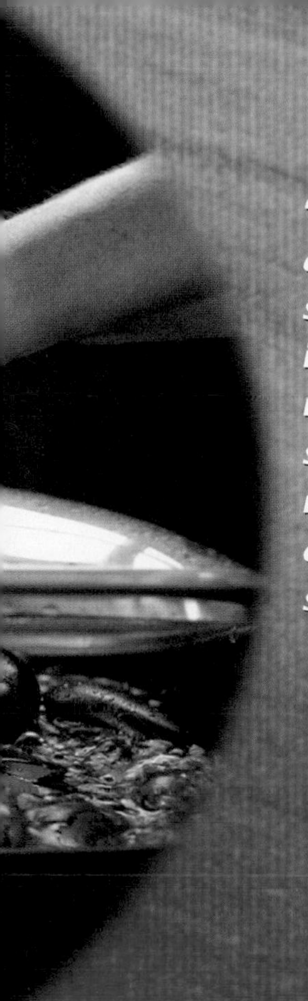

"Managing the temperature of stones is a subtle art. When a therapist is overly conservative and uses only warm stones in an effort to avoid burning the client, the massage is boring. But if the stones that are used are too hot, the massage is torturous. Finding the temperature at which the stones are fractionally below being too hot gives clients a most satisfying experience with waves of deep warmth percolating down their bodies. These are the hot stone massages worthy of mmm's and ahhh's!"

April Moon,
Three-Dimensional Hot Stone Massage
Practitioner and Instructor

Objectives

After reading this chapter, you should be able to:

- Demonstrate the safe use of a skillet for heating stones.
- Identify the amount of time and the temperatures necessary for heating stones.
- Demonstrate the safe and efficient removal of stones from the skillet.
- Describe the proper temperatures for working stones.
- Describe the temperatures necessary for placement stones.
- Explain how to regulate stone temperature.
- Identify which stones are best used for hot and cold.
- Explain how to chill stones and keep them cool.
- Identify the ideal ratio of cold stones to hot stones.
- Discuss when to use cold stones in the massage and when to avoid their use.
- Identify how to introduce cold stones into the massage.

Key Terms

Infrared temperature gun (also called an *optical pyrometer*)**:** A tool that measures temperature by aiming its infrared laser beam at an object.

Thermal emanation factor: The measured length and rate of time in which a stone gives off heat.

No matter how skillfully you work with your stones, if they are not the proper temperature for each client, the massage will be a disappointing, boring, or jolting experience. That's why you need to develop a sense for the right temperature of stones. Although it is challenging, this is one of the most important aspects of a hot stone massage. With practice and experience using the stones, you'll develop a "sixth sense" for the exact temperature that is just right for each region of the client's body. However, until that sixth sense is strong, you can rely on the specific guidelines in this chapter to help you administer the proper temperature.

This chapter will discuss the many considerations in heating the stones, including working with the skillet, the appropriate temperature for working and placement stones, the relative sensitivity of different body parts to heat, and the length of time stones can be expected to retain their heat. This chapter will also discuss the use of cool stones, including how to cool them, when to use cold stones during the massage, and when to avoid using them. Over time, this information will become internalized, and you'll develop a feel for what is required for each client in the course of a hot stone massage.

HEATING THE STONES

There are a variety of methods for heating stones, some dry, most wet, but for reasons explained in Chapter 3, I recommend using a large electric skillet, as shown in Figures 3-3 and 3-4. The following information will enable you to work effectively with your skillet as you develop that sixth sense in managing the temperature of your stones.

Using the Skillet to Heat Your Stones

An electric skillet is a fairly simple heating device; however, you'll find the following guidelines helpful for its safe use and care.

Safe Use of Your Skillet

The lid of the skillet has a plastic shield that juts out to one side; be sure that it is facing the side of the skillet where the thermostat device plugs in.

CAUTION

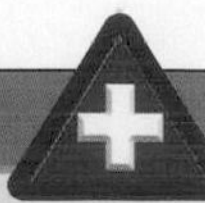

It is important to have that plastic shield over the thermostat device to prevent water spilling on the electric circuitry of the skillet, as this could cause an electrical short or other fire hazard.

It is also vital to have the thermostat device pushed all the way into the skillet. If it is pushed only part of the way in, the light will come on, but the skillet will not heat up. This could make for an unexpected delay in the start of a hot stone massage. As skillets age, the thermostat device can become defective. If the water is boiling when the thermostat is set on warm, the thermostat device needs to be replaced.

TIP

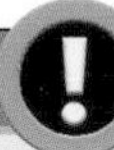

New skillets may come with defective thermostats, and they need to be checked before use.

The Teflon lining the skillet's interior serves to quiet the stones when they are returned to an empty skillet. Avoid using implements like sharp metal spoons or scouring brushes that could scrape it off. Be sure, however, that you do thoroughly scrub off the residue that builds up on the sides of the skillet at the end of each day, before replacing the water. A gentle sponge and detergent will do the job.

Keep the lid on the skillet only while you are heating the stones from cold to hot. After they are heated, remove the lid and keep it off throughout the massage.

CAUTION

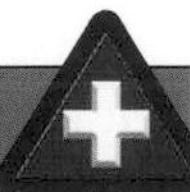

Be careful when removing the lid! The water that precipitates and collects on the inside of the lid is extremely hot and can stream off and burn you.

Replace the lid between sessions for boiling and cleaning stones as well as at the end of the day.

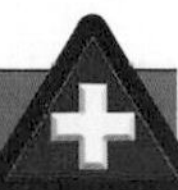

CAUTION

It is critical to remember to turn the skillet off and unplug it at the end of the day, as the stones can burn, and even worse, a fire could result. I recommend leaving a note near the skillet or on the door saying, "Turn skillet off!" It has alerted me many times when I was in a rush to leave.

Time and Temperature for Heating

When the stones are cold and the water in the skillet has not yet been heated, the fastest way to heat the stones is to cover the skillet and turn the thermostat all the way up to high. Be sure the water fills the skillet so it will immerse as much of the stones as possible. This speeds up the heating process. It takes approximately 15 to 20 minutes to go from completely unheated water and cold stones to stones that are hot enough to use for massage. After the stones have reached boiling and are hot, turn the skillet down to warm. On most skillets, warm is approximately 160°F. This is a good temperature to maintain the stones in the skillet throughout the massage. Even though this temperature is hotter than the temperature that will be used for massage, the extra heat allows the stones to sit outside the skillet for an extended period of time before becoming too cold to use. This is essential for the stone management system that will be discussed in Chapter 7.

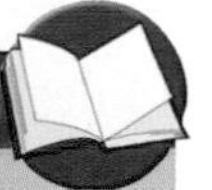

TESTIMONIAL

Many hot stone practitioners assert that if a stone is too hot to comfortably take out of the skillet with your hand, then it is too hot to use on your client. They recommend keeping all stones in the skillet at a temperature of approximately 130°F. This approach works only if you will always be going directly from the skillet to the client's skin. As explained in detail in Chapter 7, there are important reasons for having the stones hotter than you can immediately use one at a time. For now, be assured that it is beneficial to both you and your clients to have the stones hotter than most practitioners recommend.

As time elapses, you may need to turn the thermostat down slightly to adjust for water that has evaporated, or up slightly after adding a large amount of cold water to maintain the proper volume of water. The only time the skillet needs to be turned to high again is for the 3-minute boiling that you will do to clean the stones in between sessions. Immediately after the cleaning is complete, the skillet should be turned back down to warm for the next massage, or off if there will be an extended period of time before the next session.

Removing Your Stones from the Skillet

It may seem trite to focus on the exact way a stone should be removed from the skillet, but your technique for stone removal makes a big difference.

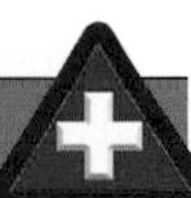

CAUTION

Never grab stones from the skillet with your hands. As just noted, they are too hot to comfortably touch at this temperature.

If the water is at a temperature that allows you to reach in with your hands and remove stones without pain, then it is too cool to keep the stones warm for an extended period of time after removal.

TIP

Water that is at the proper temperature for effective stone management is too hot to comfortably reach into.

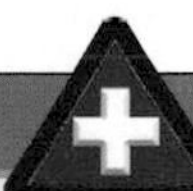

CAUTION

Never make immediate contact to the client's skin with a hot stone that has come directly from the skillet. Special care must be taken when a hot stone is making initial contact to the skin. This will be discussed in greater detail in Chapter 7 in the Stone Entrance section.

A slightly deep and wide slotted plastic spoon is the best tool for removing stones because it is easy to use, offers quick removal, and protects your hands. The slots in the spoon allow the water to drain back into the skillet, as shown in Figure 3-5. Let all of the water from the spoon drain back into the skillet before moving the spoon from the skillet to the stone table. Holding the spoon over the skillet for approximately 1 to 2 seconds will allow the water to fall through the slots. If you take the spoon away from the skillet immediately, you risk burning your hand or arm, and too much water will accumulate on the stone table and soak the towel. After a few massages, the towel will be so drenched that the stones on it will cool too quickly. In addition, the water will drip from the soaked towel onto the floor.

Managing the Temperature of Your Hot Stones

A different temperature is needed for working stones that glide along the body versus placement stones that sit stationary directly on the skin, and placement stones that will be inserted into an oven pocket or placed on top of a towel. In addition, each part of the client's body, as well as each individual client, has a different level of sensitivity to heat. These considerations are discussed in the following sections.

Temperature Ranges for Placement and Working Stones

Table 5-1 gives the temperature range for placement stones (on the skin) and working stones on various parts of the body from most sensitive to least sensitive. The table does not include the temperatures for placement stones that go inside or on top of a cover, as these can be as hot as the layers of cover will permit. The temperatures in this table were based on research that I conducted on a group of 20 clients. The range for each area of the body represents the variation in different people's tolerance for heat. I measured the temperature of the stones with an **infrared temperature gun** (or *optical pyrometer*), a device that uses a laser beam to measure temperature. Even if you don't have such a device to measure your own stones' temperatures, it is still useful to have the numbers in Table 5-1, as they'll give a sense of which areas of the body can handle more or less heat.

Even more useful than my statistics on the ideal temperatures of stones is the sense in your own hands of what temperature is good for a placement versus a working stone. This takes time and experimentation to develop. Generally speaking, the temperature of a working stone should be approximately 15 degrees higher than that of a placement stone that is placed directly on the skin.

Table 5-1 Temperatures Appropriate for Placement and Working Stones

Part of Body	Placement Stone	Working Stone
Eyes	100-105	NA
Third eye chakra	100-110	NA
Feet	103-105	115-120
Face	107-110	120-125
Throat chakra	107-112	NA
Heart chakra	107-112	120-125
Solar plexus chakra	107-112	120-125
Belly chakra	107-112	125-130
Groin chakra (thru sheet)	110-115	NA
Neck (inner)	110-115	125-130
Arm (inner)	110-115	125-130
Thigh (inner)	110-115	125-130
Buttocks	112-120	128-130
Back of legs	112-120	128-130
Neck (outer)	115-120	128-130
Hands	115-120	128-130
Thigh (outer)	115-120	128-130
Arm (outer)	115-120	128-130
Back	115-120	128-130

Use the following guidelines for temperature evaluation:

- If you can comfortably hold a stone in your hand for no more than approximately 5 seconds before having to switch hands, it is a good temperature for a working stone.
- If you can hold a stone in your hand for more than 5 seconds and it still has heat in it, it is useful as a placement stone against the skin.
- If a stone is tepid, it should be put back in the skillet.
- If a stone is too hot to hold for even 5 seconds, you should either wait longer before using it, cool it off manually, or place it in a protective shield such as an oven pocket before placing it on the body.

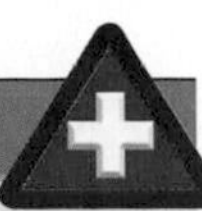

CAUTION

Be sure that placement stones are dry if you are putting them on the sheet or towel that is over the client's body. Otherwise, the stone will cause the sheet or towel to become wet. The heat from the stone will slowly permeate a dry towel or sheet, but the heat will penetrate a wet sheet or towel much too quickly and result in the stone feeling too hot for the client.

TIP

If you are not sure if the temperature of a stone will work as a working stone or a placement stone, try it out on yourself before you use it on your client.

Be aware, though, that your tolerance for heat might differ from that of your client. For example, if you have a high tolerance for heat and the stone feels perfect for you, it might be a bit too hot for your client—or just right. The only way to find out is to ask. Once you learn both your own and your client's tolerance for heat, you will be able to better judge what temperatures to use with your client by trying the stone out on yourself.

Maintaining Your Client's Comfort

Stay aware of your clients' comfort level with the temperatures of the stones. Compliant or stoic clients may say that the stones being used for massage are not too hot, when in actuality they are too hot for them.

TIP

Watch the client's body language. If they startle, flinch, inhale quickly, pull away, or grip their hands into a fist when touched with a working stone, the stone is too hot for them, regardless of what they say. If this is the case, lower the temperature of the working stones slightly by dipping them in cold water for a few seconds until they can be used without such a reaction.

The same holds true for static placement stones. It is common for clients to report that the temperature of a placement stone is fine initially, and then to discover that, when left in place for a few minutes, it becomes uncomfortably hot. Often, clients will not say anything about it because they are too relaxed and don't want to speak or because they are trying to be stoic—there are telltale signs that should suggest to you that a placement stone is too hot. For instance, clients might begin to wriggle around slightly, push the stone a bit higher or lower, move their hand off the stone, or try and lift the stone slightly off their body with the sheet. It is important to watch your client's reactions and not just rely on their words. As soon as I see a client doing any of these behaviors, I lift the stone and place another fabric layer beneath it.

Often, clients do not want to be seen as demanding and will wait until the last second before they complain that a stone is too hot. They might assume that they will adjust to the temperature and so they wait it out.

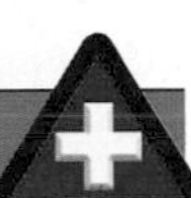

CAUTION

When a client does finally exclaim that a placement stone has become too hot, it is generally too late to wait even a few seconds before removing it. Instead, stop whatever you are doing at that moment and instantly remove the stone. If you are not sure which stone the client is referring to, then quickly remove all the stones in that area to play it safe.

When you take off all the stones because the client was too hot, the stone that was too hot will be obvious to you. Put the other stones back where they were, then put a second fabric layer under the stone that is too hot before replacing it. Alternatively, you can cool it by dipping it in cold water for a few seconds before drying and replacing it.

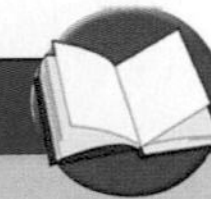

TESTIMONIAL

One of my students, Edye Rose, shared an experience of receiving a hot stone massage that almost turned her away from it for good. Her therapist had covered her back with hot stones, which readily became too hot. Even after Edye exclaimed that they were too hot, the therapist took her time, saying she would be there in a minute, just as soon as she finished getting new stones from the skillet. Meanwhile, Edye had to jump up off the table to knock the stones off her back, and she ended up with a slight burn from one of the stones. It took a great deal of convincing to get her to try another hot stone massage, but she did, and she loved it so much that she became a three-dimensional hot stone practitioner herself; one who is devoted to listening and responding readily to her clients' needs.

Regulating Stone Temperatures

Stone temperatures can be easily regulated. If a working stone is too cool to use for massage, put it back in the skillet for as little as 1 to 2 minutes (Fig. 5-1) and then use it to massage. If a working stone is too hot to use for massage, dip it briefly in cold water and then massage with it immediately, using long quick strokes until it has cooled down enough to be used in a slower fashion (Fig. 5-2).

If a placement stone is too hot to leave on the skin, you have several options. If it is very hot, you can put it in an oven pocket or over a towel and then place it. If it is just slightly too hot to place, you can massage with it momentarily to diminish its heat and then place it directly on the skin. You can also dip it for approximately 3 seconds in your bowl of cold water and then place it directly on the skin.

There should never be an extended period of time when a therapist has no stones to use. Once the water in the skillet is hot, a stone can heat up in a couple of minutes. And if a stone is too hot, it takes only a few seconds to cool it down.

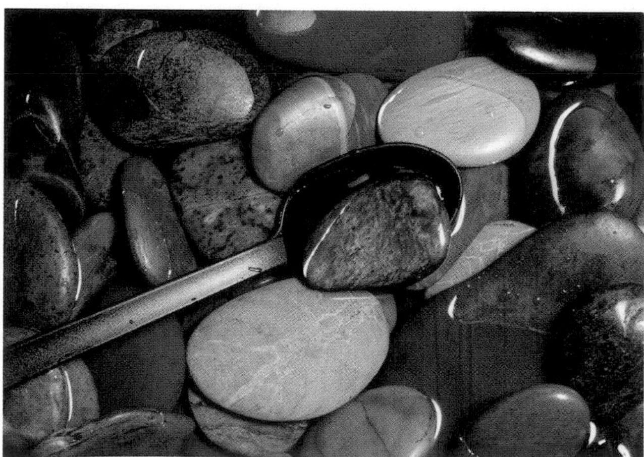

Figure 5-1 Reheating Your Stones. Return a stone that has lost too much heat back to the skillet for approximately 1 to 2 minutes for reheating and immediate use.

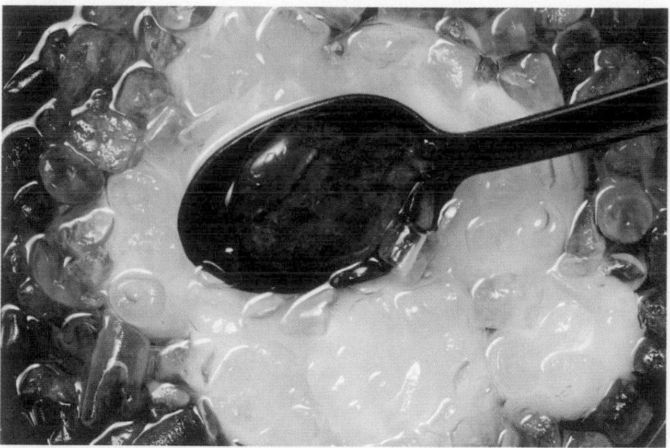

Figure 5-2 Cooling Your Stones. Dip a hot stone in cold water for 1 to 2 seconds to make it useable as a placement or working stone.

Understanding the Thermal Emanation Factor of Your Stones

A stone's **thermal emanation factor** can be scientifically defined as the measured length and rate of time in which a stone gives off heat. Knowing the thermal emanation factor of your stones will enable you to predict how long your stones will hold their heat.

Many claims have been made in books and videos as to which type and color of stone will hold its heat or cold the longest. However, my own experience, research, and experimentation have led me to believe that most of these claims are based on personal conjecture rather than hard data. For instance, the belief that black basalt holds heat the longest because it was formed from lava and is black proves not to be true. And the common claim that white marble holds heat the least because it is white is also false. I am not aware of any published empirical data, to date, on the thermal emanation factor of particular stones. And although the research I have done is cursory at best, it does provide exact figures on the thermal emanation factors of stones used specifically for hot stone massage.

Using my infrared temperature gun, I experimented with a wide selection of stones commonly used for hot stone massage to determine which stones actually did hold heat the longest and whether or not that duration was based on type, composition, color, or size of stone, as well as how long and at what temperature the stones were heated and the temperature and ventilation of the room. The experimentation took place over a 2-week period of time, with retesting each day, and an average was taken of all readings for each stone. Although the experiment was not extensive, its data are useful in helping to get some sense of how long particular stones do hold their heat under these specific conditions.

The stones included in the experiment were: black basalt, gray basalt, blue-green basalt, red quartzite, green quartzite, brown quartzite, slate, jadestone, and white marble. Examples of each stone are provided in Chapter 4. I used four categories for sizes of stones: large, medium-thick, medium, and small. Not all stones types were available in each size category, and when that was the case, I logged "nda" for "no data available."

I did four different experiments:

1. Waiting stones. This experiment tested the length of time a stone held its heat when simply sitting on a table, waiting in the wings, with no human contact whatsoever.
2. Placement stones. This experiment tested the length of time a stone held its heat when covered with a towel and placed on or beneath the body.
3. Working stones. This experiment tested the length of time a stone held its heat while being used to massage the body.
4. Cold stones. This experiment tested the length of time a stone held its cold while being used to massage the body. For this cold retention experiment, I only used two stones for comparison—black basalt and white marble.

The results from each experiment are discussed fully, with accompanying tables of my data, in Appendix E; however, a brief summary of my findings is as follows:

The three stones that held their heat the longest, as working, placement, and waiting stones, were (in order of first to last): brown quartzite (large), white marble (medium and small), and red quartzite (medium-thick). As working stones, these stones held their heat for approximately 30 seconds longer than the stones that came in last. As placement stones, these stones held their heat approximately four minutes longer than the stones that came in last. As waiting stones, these stones held their heat for approximately nine minutes longer than the stones that came in last (see tables in Appendix E). All of these cases represent a significant amount of time added to the duration the stones can be used or placed in a massage. Of the three, white marble takes first prize overall because, in addition to retaining heat well as a waiting and working stone, white marble also held its heat the longest as a placement stone.

And yet, even though these top three stones hold their heat for more time, there are still valid reasons for using other stones. For instance, large black basalt came in fourth place as both a waiting stone and a working stone and is much more accessible and inexpensive than marble; jadestone was close to basalt, is magnificent to behold, and is believed to have special healing powers; and even though white marble seems to hold heat the longest, its smooth, round shape is not found in nature. Because it is tumbled artificially, it is more expensive, less available, and has lost some of the energetic qualities found in a stone that has been naturally tumbled. In addition, there is some evidence that the larger and thicker the stone in general, the longer it will hold its heat. Thus, if some of the medium-sized stones that did not hold their heat as long were found in larger sizes, they would most likely hold their heat longer as well.

Thus, there is merit for using all kinds of stones. Knowing their thermal emanation factor will simply help you to make an informed decision about which stones to choose for your hot stone massage and why.

Determining How Long to Use Stones

The data collected in these experiments suggest that a static placement stone that is in a cover can hold its heat for 15 to 30 minutes, depending on the type and size of stone. A static placement stone that is placed directly on the skin, without being used as a working stone first, tends to hold its heat for approximately 10 to 20 minutes. A flowing placement stone (a working stone that is converted into a placement stone after losing its heat from use) will generally be on the lower end of the temperature range and will hold its heat usually no more than 5 to 10 minutes. Keep these times in mind to avoid leaving stones in place for too long.

CAUTION

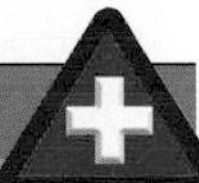

A cool stone is a hard stone.

When stones are the right temperature, the client does not perceive them as hard when lying on them; however, as soon as the stones lose too much heat, the client will feel their hardness as uncomfortable. Remember where and when you place stones and keep rotating them with new ones or simply remove them before their heat is gone.

TIP

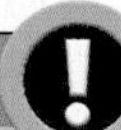

When first learning to do hot stone massage, it is a good idea to not place too many stones at once because you could end up having too many cold placement stones to deal with simultaneously.

Working stones can generally be used for only 30 to 50 seconds, depending on the type of stone, thickness, and size. You will rarely get a full minute out of a working stone. If you are massaging with the same stone for more than 1 minute, you are definitely using it for too long. A stone that is appropriately hot feels soft or invisible when used to massage the body, but a stone that has lost too much heat feels hard and boring to the client and will not be useful or therapeutic. When learning to do hot stone massage, students sometimes get attached to their stones and don't want to stop using them when their heat is no longer sufficient. I see this in every class I teach. Be careful not to use the stones for too long. It is better to have a slight interruption to get new hot stones than to keep working with lukewarm ones for the sake of not wanting to disrupt the flow. Flow is very important, but proper temperature is even more imperative. With experience, you'll find the right balance between temperature and flow.

TIP

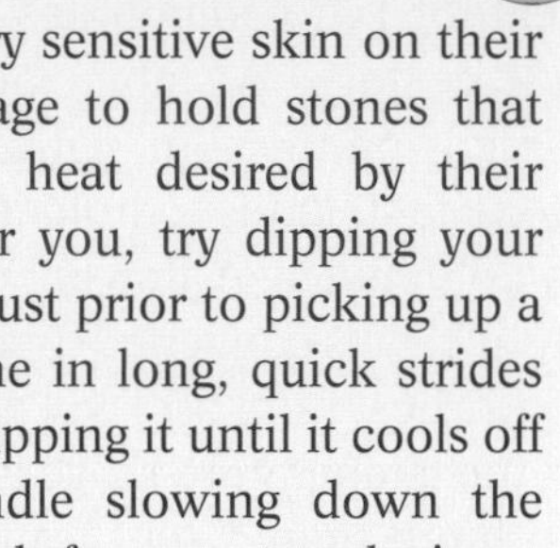

Some therapists have very sensitive skin on their hands and cannot manage to hold stones that contain the amount of heat desired by their clients. If this is true for you, try dipping your hands in the cold water just prior to picking up a stone. Then use the stone in long, quick strides along the client's body, flipping it until it cools off enough for you to handle slowing down the speed. If this doesn't work for you, try placing a small piece of cloth in the center of your palm between you and the stone to protect your skin. Over time, your hands will acclimatize and develop a capacity to withstand higher temperatures.

COOLING THE STONES

Using cold stones is an art in itself. Although cold stones have many therapeutic properties (see Chapter 2), if you do not use them carefully, their healing properties could be lost in the client's negative reaction to them. This section discusses how to cool your stones, the ratio of cold stones to use in a hot stone massage, and when and how to use cold stones.

Deciding Which Stones to Use for Cold

When determining which of your stones to use for cold stone massage, you should consider how long each type retains its cold temperature as well as the sensitivity level your client has to cold. In my own experiments, white marble, once again, took the prize, this time for its ability to retain cold. White marble retained cold temperatures five times longer than did black basalt, releasing its cold much more gradually (see Appendix E).

Marble's unusual ability to retain cold for so long is advantageous for prolonged use; however, it may feel too cold for clients who have a strong sensitivity to cold temperatures. For these clients, basalt may be less shocking and thus more useful. Also, because basalt can be found naturally tumbled and marble cannot, basalt may be the better choice for using as a cold stone. In the end, I think it is wise to be versatile and have both marble and basalt stones. You can then decide which stone is more appropriate to use for each particular client.

How to Cool the Stones

Some therapists like to store their cold stones in the freezer so that they are ready to use at any time. If you do this, have two sets of cold stones so that one is always in the freezer getting cold while the other set is in use. Frozen stones are extremely useful for acute injuries or inflammation, and they tend to hold their cold longer than stones that are not frozen; however, be careful with clients who have sensitivity to cold, as these stones may be too cold for them to endure.

Obviously, frozen stones are not an option if you do not have a freezer in your workspace. If this is the case, or if you choose not to use frozen stones because of their extreme temperature, another more common method for keeping stones cold is to place them in a plastic bowl with ice water on the stone table near the skillet as shown in Figure 3-6. The water can be kept cold by adding ice (or snow when it is winter!), or by refilling with cold water from a nearby sink, if there is one. Because this water doubles as the dunking water to cool off stones that are too hot, it will become warm toward the end of a massage, so you'll need to replenish it with fresh cold water and/or ice between sessions.

Ratio of Cold to Hot Stones

There are diverse approaches to determining the ratio of cold to hot stones, as well as varying situations that call for different amounts of cold stones to be used in a hot stone massage. Some therapists use cold stones as much as half the time during a hot stone massage, whereas others only use them infrequently for special situations. I like to weave them into a hot stone massage approximately 10% of the total massage time. Usually, I place cold stones on and around the eyes and on any areas of inflammation, and I work with cold stones in cases of stagnant energy and at the end of a massage if a client needs help "waking up." I increase my use of cold stones for clients who have acute injuries, who are experiencing a "hot flash," or who generally "run hot" and enjoy the sensation of cold stones.

I find that clients enjoy hot stones a great deal more than cold stones. But because of the therapeutic value of cold, especially with injuries, certain health conditions, and stagnant energy, I encourage clients to be open to cold stones. Many clients discover that they enjoy the feeling of the cold stones once they experience them. The thought of them is worse than the actuality! And I have some clients who naturally like cold stones as much as hot ones, especially when it is hot out or if we are massaging outside in the sun. Experiment with your clients to find out what the best ratio is for them.

When to Use Cold Stones in the Massage

Knowing when to introduce cold stones into the massage can make a big difference as far as the clients' enjoyment of them. Avoid beginning a hot stone massage with cold stones, unless a client is feeling extremely hot. Otherwise, cold stones are received best after the client has had some time to relax, approximately 15 to 30 minutes into the session.

CAUTION

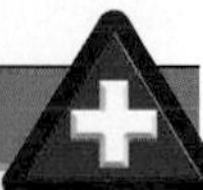

When clients are asleep or in a very deep state of relaxation, either avoid the use of cold stones until they are a bit more awake or use less extreme temperatures of cold.

How to Use Cold Stones in the Massage

As is true with heat, cold stones require special care when integrating them into a stone massage.

Initial Contact

Never make contact with a cold stone without previously warning the client and priming that area of the body with a warm stone. Take both a warm and a cold stone to the table so that the cold stone is nearby and there will be no break between the use of the warm one and the entrance of the cold one. Work the specified area with a warm stone and then, just before it loses its heat, warn your client gently that a cold stone is coming and then glide in with the cold stone. Begin gradually, using your fingertips, then the edge of the cold stone, and then the full surface of the cold stone. This method allows clients to receive the cold in a much more pleasant fashion.

Using Cold Stones Alone

After you have made contact properly with your cold stone, use it until it no longer feels cold. Bear in mind, however, that a stone that no longer feels cold to you may still feel cold to your client. I have occasionally taken a stone away that no longer felt cold to me and then made contact with it on another part of the client's body, only to have the client flinch and say, "Oh wow, that's still cold!" So, keep this in mind when using cold stones: They will almost always feel colder to the client than to you.

After a stone has lost its cold, you can replace it immediately with another cold stone without having to reintroduce a warm stone. Work with the cold stones like this, using one until it has lost its cold, and then immediately coming in with a fresh cold one until the area feels complete. It is also fine to use two cold stones at the same time once an area has been well primed (Fig. 5-3). It's a good idea to end the cold stone use with a quick run of a warm stone, just to leave the area feeling a bit more supple and relaxed.

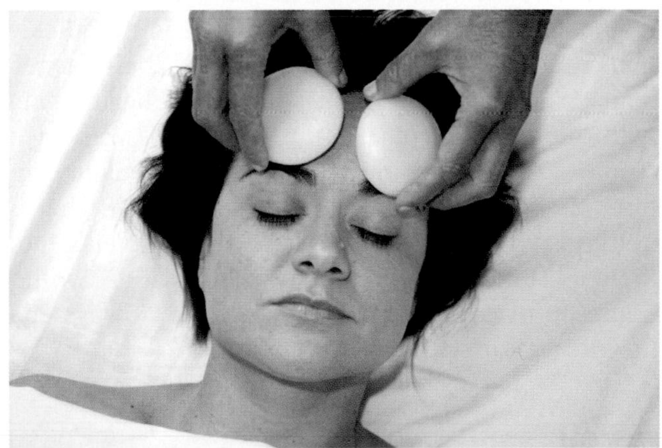

Figure 5-3 Using Two Cold Stones. Using two cold stones at the same time feels great after an area has been well primed.

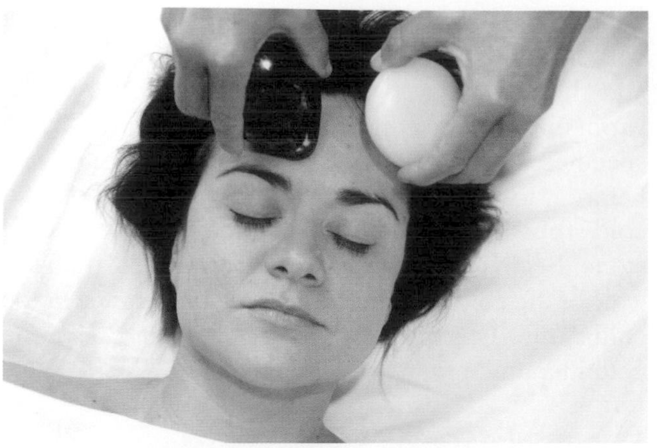

Figure 5-4 Alternating Hot and Cold Stones. Alternating a hot stone with a cold one is therapeutic for a variety of conditions and gives clients a pleasing sensation of vitality.

Alternating Cold with Hot Stones

An alternative to using cold stones by themselves is to repeatedly alternate cold and hot stones in the same area, as shown in Figure 5-4. As explained in Chapter 2, this thermo-cryotherapy is therapeutic for many conditions, unless heat is contraindicated. When heat is allowed, alternating cold and hot stones is a powerful tool for flushing an area of toxins by bringing lots of fresh blood and oxygen to the muscles and skin. Cold is also much easier for the client to handle when it is alternated with heat. The alternation creates a tingly, alive sensation that is very refreshing and rejuvenating. My clients seem to appreciate cold stones most when I use this alternating approach.

To alternate cold and hot stones, begin with a hot stone in one hand and a cold stone in the other. Do one stroke with the hot stone, then one with the cold stone, then hot, then cold, until both stones have lost their desired temperatures. Because of the contrast of temperatures, this will happen much more quickly than usual. When the stones have lost their desired temperatures, replace both stones and begin again with the hot stone, alternating the stones with each stroke. The contrast of temperatures eventually confuses the body and the clients lose track of what is hot and what is cold. This helps them to relax into the cold stones more than they would with a continuous run of cold stones by themselves. Always end the alternation with a warm stone.

SUMMARY

Developing a sense for the right temperature of stones is challenging, but it is essential for providing a safe and therapeutic hot stone massage.

To safely heat your stones, be sure the thermostat regulator on your skillet is covered by the lid and is pushed in all the way. When you remove stones from the skillet, be careful to let the hot water drain back into the skillet before placing them on the stone table. Be sure you turn off and unplug your skillet at the end of each day.

Heating your stones, starting with water and stones at room temperature, takes approximately 15 to 20 minutes, but once the water is heated, it only takes 1 to 2 minutes to reheat a stone that has become too cool to use.

Place the stones you want to use for your cold stones in a bowl with ice water. A stone that is too hot to use can be cooled quickly by dipping it momentarily in the bowl of iced water.

Different clients, as well as different parts of the body, will require different levels of heat. Placement stones that go directly on the skin must be less hot than working stones, which will be gliding along the client's skin. It is critical to maintain your client's comfort level by paying careful attention to signs that a stone is either too hot or too cold. Make any necessary adjustments immediately.

The stone's thermal emanation factor is the measured length and rate of time in which a stone gives off heat. The three stones that hold their heat the longest as working stones, placement stones, and as waiting stones are brown quartzite (large), white marble (medium and small), and red quartzite (medium-thick). White marble also holds cold the longest. Black basalt (large) is next in retaining heat and cold.

Learning which stones tend to hold heat and cold the longest will help you decide which stones to use and for how long. However, you should also base your stone choices on cost, availability, texture, beauty, and energetic state.

Stones should only be used in the massage as long as they maintain the desired temperature. Stones that are hot feel soft and invisible to the client, whereas stones that have cooled off too much feel hard and uncomfortable. Stones that are very cold also feel invisible to the client, after the initial entrance, as they are numbing. However as their coldness diminishes, they also feel hard and noticeable to the client. Don't sacrifice proper stone temperature because you are afraid to interrupt the flow of a massage. Although flow is important, proper temperature is more important.

Cold stones are very useful for areas of acute injury and inflammation as well as for cooling clients who are hot. However, most clients enjoy hot stones more than cold, and they enjoy cold for only a small portion of the total time. Cold stones can be used by themselves or alternating with a hot stone, and they should always be introduced into the massage gently and immediately following a warm stone.

Finding and maintaining the proper temperatures for your hot and cold stones throughout a hot stone massage takes time and practice, but it will eventually become second nature as your hands develop a "sixth sense" for what is the right temperature for each particular client.

REVIEW QUESTIONS

TRUE/FALSE

1. To learn the proper temperature for stones, therapists should use an infrared temperature gun throughout the massage.

   Circle: True False

2. As long as the thermostat device on the skillet lights up, the skillet is working properly and will heat the stones adequately.

   Circle: True False

3. Starting with warm water and cold stones, it will take approximately 45 minutes for a skillet that is set on high to heat up the stones.

   Circle: True False

4. As long as a stone can be held in the hand for more than 5 seconds, and it still has some heat left in it, it can be used as a placement stone.

   Circle: True False

5. A hot stone can be used as a working stone, as long as it has any heat left in it at all, even if it is tepid.

   Circle: True False

MULTIPLE CHOICE

6. Which of the following stones holds cold the longest?
   a. Black basalt
   b. White marble
   c. Jadestone
   d. Slate
   e. New England seastone

7. In general, which of the following types of stones hold heat the longest?
   a. Large, thick stones
   b. Large, thin stones
   c. Medium-sized stones
   d. Small, round stones
   e. Small, thin stones

8. Once the water in your skillet has reached boiling and the stones are hot and ready to use, you should:
   a. Turn the skillet off and unplug it for the duration of the massage
   b. Turn the skillet off and add about a cupful of ice water to cool the stones quickly so you can begin to use them immediately
   c. Turn the skillet down to warm/low for the duration of the massage
   d. Turn the skillet down to medium for the duration of the massage
   e. Keep the skillet on high and keep replenishing the water that boils off during the massage

9. A static placement stone that is covered can hold its heat for up to:
   a. 1 minute
   b. 5 minutes
   c. 10 minutes
   d. 15 minutes
   e. 30 minutes

10. Which of the following statements about cold stones is true?
    a. Cold stones should never be used alone, but always alternated with hot stones.
    b. Cold stones should be used to awaken a client who has fallen asleep during the massage.
    c. Cold stones are particularly useful for beginning the massage.
    d. Cold stones can be stored in a freezer or a bowl of ice water.
    e. Cold stones always feel colder to the therapist than they do to the client.

SHORT ANSWER

11. Because of the shocking nature of cold, it is important to pay attention to ________________ when first introducing a cold stone to the skin.

12. When using cold stones, it is best to ____________ clients before contact is made.

13. If heat is permitted, it is most advantageous to ____________________ cold with heat when working an injured or congested area of the body.

14. Stones are easiest to keep cool by placing in a bowl with ____________________.

15. A working stone should be approximately ______________ degrees hotter than a placement stone that goes on the skin.

MATCHING

a. Basalt
b. Thermal emanation factor
c. 10 to 20 minutes
d. Marble
e. 30 to 50 seconds

16. The length and rate of time in which a stone gives off heat. _____
17. This stone retained its heat longer than the other stone listed. _____
18. This stone did not retain its heat quite as long as three other stones that were tested. _____
19. Length of time a stone that is placed directly against the skin (without being used as a working stone first) holds its heat. _____
20. Length of time a working stone generally holds its heat. _____

Answers to Review Questions can be found in Appendix D.

CHAPTER 6

Placing the Stones

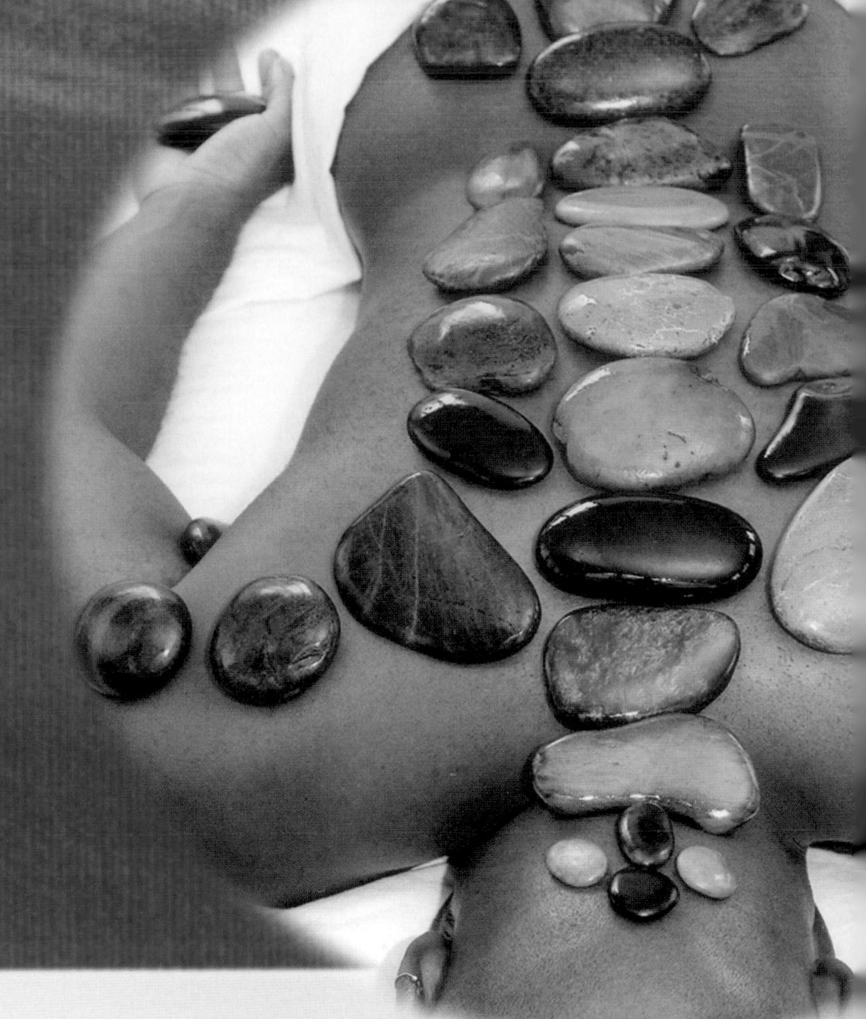

Outline

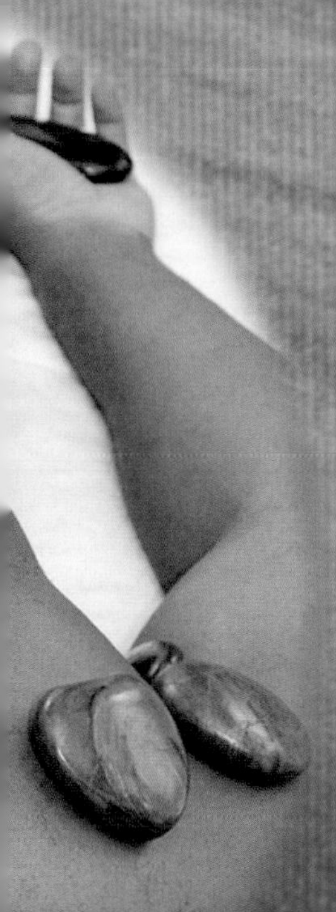

"Simply lying face up on a bed of warm stones with a few large ones placed on my heart and belly was all I needed to drop into an incredibly powerful deep rest. The stones on my body felt like many extra hands were holding me. Being massaged with the hot stones was the icing on the cake, but honestly, if all that happened was stone placement, I still would have been delighted. The stones, their radiant heat and earth energy, are healing all unto themselves."

Cedar Johnson, client

Objectives

After reading this chapter, you should be able to:

- Compare and contrast a static and a flowing placement of hot stones.
- Correlate specific placements with particular regions of the body.
- Explain the use of different devices for making placements.
- Describe static layouts of stones for both sides of the body in supine and prone positions.
- Explain how to remove placement stones without involving the client.
- Describe the relationship between working and placement stones.

Key Terms

Flowing placement: Use of warm working stones for placement on the body during the flow of a massage.

Static placement: Use of individual stones or layouts of several stones underneath or on the client's body before or during the massage. These stones are used solely for placement and not for massage.

This chapter discusses different methods of stone placement. It also provides directions for placing both individual stones and complex layouts of stones for the front and back of the body in supine and prone positions. Some of these placements are fairly encompassing; however, you need not feel that you must use these placements exactly as described. They are simply suggestions. Feel free to experiment and create new ways of placing stones. As long as you follow the guidelines for proper temperature discussed in Chapter 5 and avoid bony protuberances, you'll find that there is hardly a place on your client's body that would not enjoy the placement of a warm stone!

METHODS OF STONE PLACEMENT

There are two methods of stone placement, static and flowing. **Static placements** are stones or stone arrangements that are used solely for the purpose of placement, not for massage. These placements take some time and care to create and are usually done at the beginning or end of a massage. **Flowing placements** are dynamic, as they occur during the flow of the massage and incorporate working stones that have become too cool to use for massage.

Although you can create a static placement from time to time during the course of a hot stone massage, such placements usually involve fewer stones and a more simple configuration than the complex layouts done at the beginning or end. This is partly because it is difficult to massage extensively with a complex stone layout on the client's body and partly because layouts take some time to create and doing so interrupts the flow of the massage. Thus, complex static placements are best reserved as "bookends" for the massage.

If you place a protective layer, such as a sheet, towel, or oven pocket, over the stones you use for static placements, you'll protect the client's skin and you'll be able to use the stones at hotter temperatures. These stones will then hold their heat longer. As the heat dissipates, you can remove the fabric covering. For instance, in the case of an oven pocket that has different thicknesses of material on each side, you can start with the thick side down, then flip to the thin side, and then remove the stone from the oven pocket and place it on the sheet and eventually directly against the client's skin. This process prolongs the amount of time a stone can be left in place and still have heat. Thus, static placements are best placed initially with protective layers.

In contrast, flowing placements are always applied directly to the skin, as the stones you use for them are working stones that have cooled. Because flowing placement stones are not as hot as static placement stones, you cannot leave them in one place as long; however, they are more useful throughout the flow of a massage. Thus, there is a time and a purpose for both types of placements.

Static placement stones sometimes require accessories to hold the stones in place. Stones that are placed at a tilt on the chest can be put into an oven pocket and turned the right direction so that the stone will not fall out. The top fold of the sheet or a folded towel will also serve the same purpose. Stones that are placed on the feet need a device to hold them in place. Some practitioners use socks for this, but I prefer my stone wrappers made of wide elastic and Velcro (see Fig. 3-11), which keep the stone snugly in place, allow ventilation, offer access to the feet for massage, and can be released easily when you need to remove or replace the stones that have cooled.

Stones that are placed on angles or precarious parts of the body that won't allow for easy use of straps (i.e., the elbow, shoulder, ankle, knee, side of the leg, neck) can be held in place by the weight of a sand/grain bag (see Fig. 3-13). Stones can also be placed inside of a long tube sock or a pillowcase that is rolled into a tube and then wrapped around an area (like a hot pack) with its ends tucked under either side of the precarious body part to hold it in place.

STATIC PLACEMENTS FOR INDIVIDUAL BODY PARTS

Subtle variations in stone size, shape, and temperature can make a big difference in the effectiveness of static placements of individual stones. These variations are discussed below for each body region. As you read, bear in mind that each of these individual placements can be added to any of the more complex stone layouts discussed later in this chapter.

Face Placement

Stones can be placed over the third eye, eyes, and cheeks, as shown in Figure 6-1. Tiny flat stones, no larger than approximately 1 to 1.5 inches, are the best size to use for face placement.

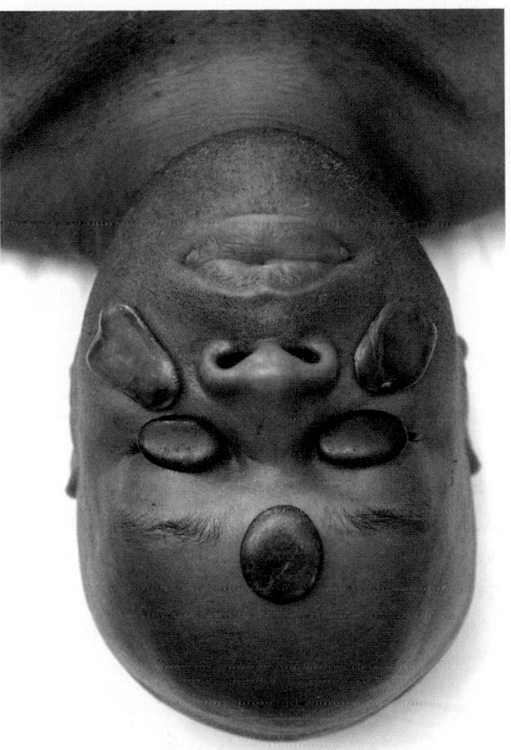

Figure 6-1 **Face Placement.** A face placement is soothing whether it is with warm or cold stones.

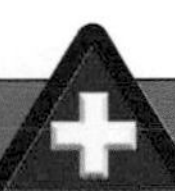

CAUTION

Before placing stones on the face, especially over the eyes, you must be sure that they are not too hot. To avoid burning or shocking your client, carefully test the stone temperature on your own eyes before placing the stones on your client.

As soon as the stones contact the eyelids, ask the client if the temperature is okay. It is important that both stones be the same temperature for the eyes or cheeks. Because the face cannot tolerate very much heat, these stones will begin with less heat and, therefore, will cool off rapidly. Nevertheless, stones feel soothing on the face whether they are warm or cold.

Instead of placing the whole stone down at once over the eyes, enter with the edge of the stone. Begin at the inside corner of the eye and slowly and gently lower the stone over the eye, without pressing.

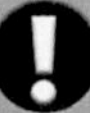

TIP

Eye stones with a slight curve to them are less likely to roll off or put pressure on the eyes; unfortunately, curved, thin, flat, tiny stones are hard to find! If you are lucky enough to have some, take good care not to lose them!

Once the eye and third eye stones are in place, it is helpful to cover them with an eye mask to hold them in place and help preserve their warmth. An eye mask with a thick lining on the bottom (see Fig. 3-12), can also serve to catch the top edges of the cheek stones and help to stabilize them as well. An eye mask also serves to relax the muscles of the eyes and help the client get out of their head, which will help to enhance the relaxing effects of the stones.

Armpit Placement

Warm stones in the armpits help to soften some of the muscles of the shoulder girdle and thereby make massage of the armpit and shoulder region less painful for your client and easier for you. (Fig. 6-2) Cold stones

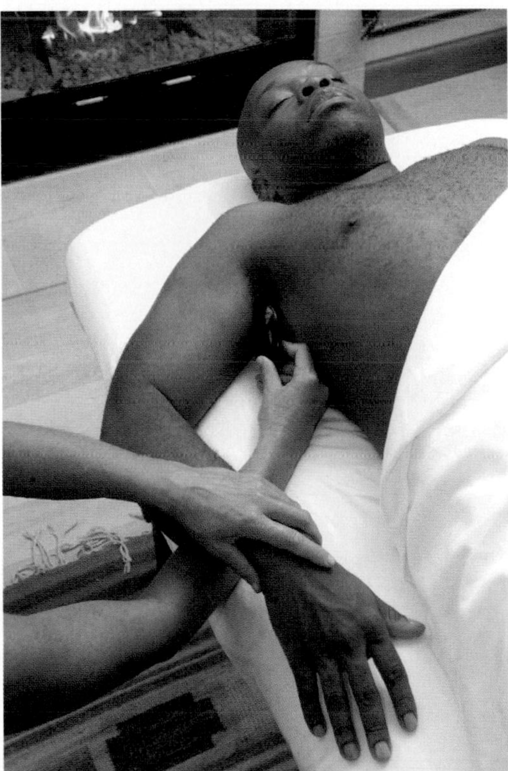

Figure 6-2 **Armpit Placement.** Stones placed in the armpit soften the muscles of the shoulder girdle.

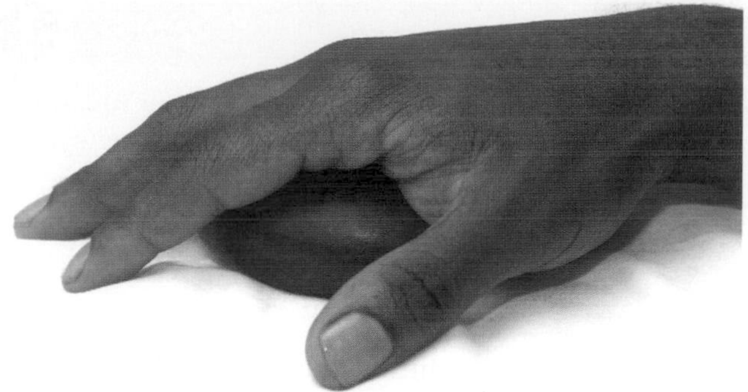

Figure 6-3 Palm Placement. Stones placed beneath the supine hand need to be thick so the palm can reach them without having to push the hand down.

are useful in the armpits when the client is overheating from the warmth of the stones, as they cool the body rapidly. Simply lift the arm up and out, place the stone into the armpit cup, and gently lay the arm back down along the body so that it holds the stone in place. This can be done with static or flowing placement.

Palm Placement

Stones can be placed beneath the palm of the hand when the client is supine or on the flat of the palm when the client is prone. The stones that are placed beneath the hands need to be round and thick so that the client's palm will naturally make contact with the stone, without having to reach or push the hand down (Fig. 6-3). Because of the lift that happens at the wrist when an arm is lying supine, the palm also has a natural lift, and if the stone is not thick enough, the hand will not make contact with it. When the client is lying prone, the stone is placed directly on the palm of the upright hand, so it does not need to be as thick.

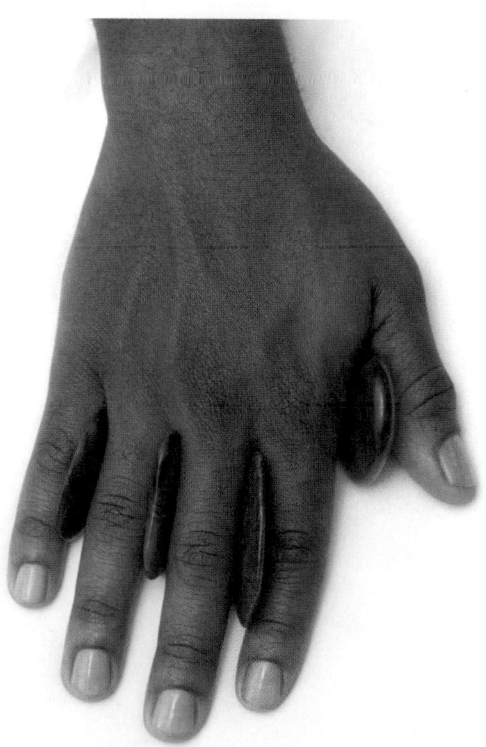

Figure 6-4 Finger Placement. Stones placed between the fingers feel pleasant whether warm or cool.

Finger Placement

When clients are supine, you can place small, flat stones between the fingers. Simply slide the stones between the fingers, as shown in Figure 6-4. Like the face stones, finger stones will lose their heat rapidly. However, both warm and cool stones feel pleasant between the fingers. It is best to use stones that are slightly longer than the toe stones for the fingers.

Foot Placement

Stones can be placed on the bottom of the feet and strapped in place, as discussed previously and shown in Figure 6-5. This often prompts clients to remark,

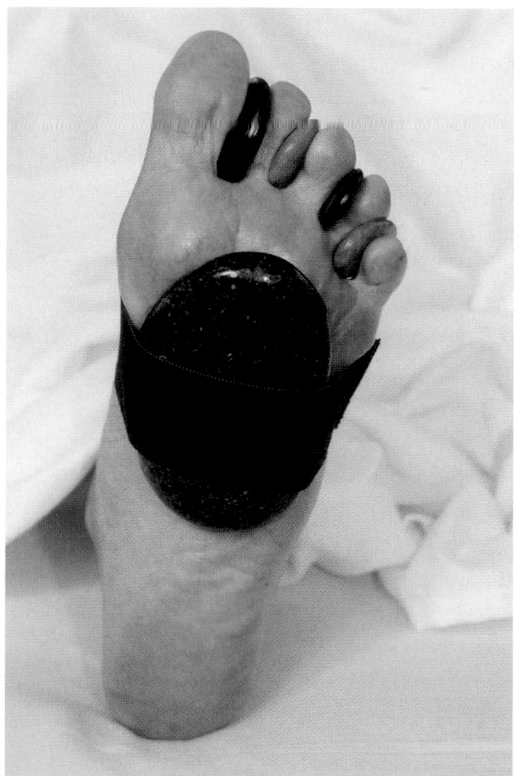

Figure 6-5 Foot Placement. An oblong stone placed on the ball of the foot and held in place with a stone wrapper feels like the client is wearing a stone bootee. Tiny stones placed between each of the toes enhance the experience.

"It feels as if I'm wearing a stone bootee!" The ideal stones to use for foot placement are thin and oblong with a slight curve. Place the stone over the ball of the foot with the curved side facing in. Be sure to enter slowly with the edge of stone, checking with the client for temperature approval as the stone is being placed. Many feet are surprisingly sensitive and can take less heat than you might assume.

Once the stone is in place, it is time to attach it to the foot with the stone wrapper. While holding the stone in place with the fingers, tuck the middle of the strap between the fingers and the center of the stone. Use the thumb on this same hand to hold the end of the strap with the bristly side of the Velcro face up along the top of the foot. This ensures that the rough side of the Velcro is never felt against the skin. With your other hand, gently tug the loose end of the strap and attach the Velcro along the top of the client's foot. Practice this on yourself until you are sure you can use the wrap without allowing the bristly side of the Velcro to scratch the client's skin. The stone wrapper allows you to slide one stone out as the replacement stone is slid in, as shown in Figure 6-6.

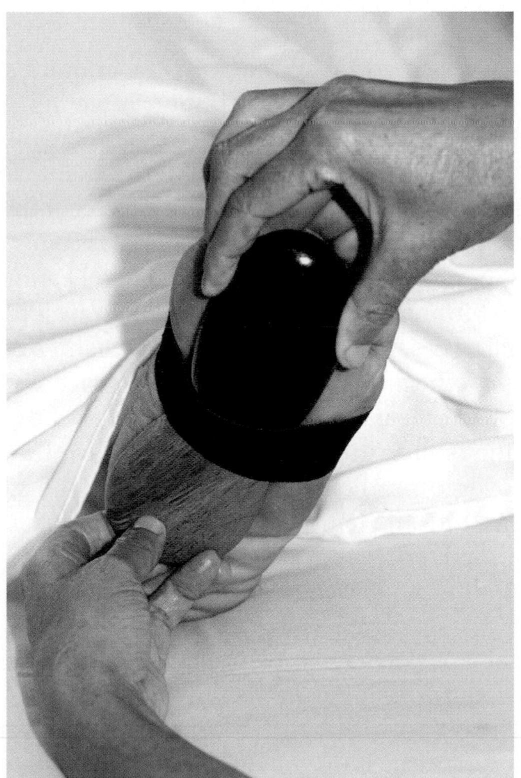

Figure 6-6 Replacing Foot Stone. Stone wrappers allow you to slide one stone out as the next one comes in.

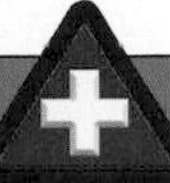

CAUTION

Be sure to check in with the client again concerning the temperature of the stone after the strap has been on for <1 minute. Sometimes a client thinks a stone temperature is okay, but shortly thereafter realizes it is intolerable. If this is the case, you need to remove the stone immediately.

Tiny stones, the same size as the face stones, can be slid in between the toes. Be sure the toe stones are flat, as thick ones can overstretch the toes and cause discomfort to the client. Like the eyelids, the skin between the toes is very tender and cannot tolerate much heat.

TIP

Therapists can carefully use their own eyes or toes to check the temperature of a toe stone.

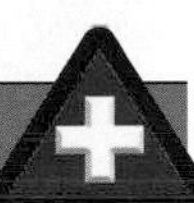

CAUTION

Each toe stone should be placed between the toes gradually rather than the whole stone at once, while checking in with the client to see if the temperature is okay.

It is an incredible feeling to have the toe stones placed while the foot stone is strapped on. Toe stones do not retain their heat for more than 5 minutes, but they can be left in longer, as the cool stones still feel good and also serve to stretch the toes. However, it's best not to leave them in longer than approximately 15 minutes or the toes can start to feel achy and overstretched.

STATIC STONE PLACEMENT LAYOUTS

Stone layouts are more complex than individual placements and require a little time and forethought. It is most effective to create the stone placement layouts that go beneath clients just before they lie down on the table, eliminating the need to ask them to sit up for you to make the placement. After clients have settled into the temperature of the stone layout beneath them, you can then make the placement layout on top of them. While the client enjoys the warmth and relaxing effect of the stones above and below them, you can begin the massage by working on the head, neck, shoulders, feet, or hands. By the time you are ready to begin the more dynamic three-dimensional massage strokes, the stone layouts will have lost most of their heat and can be removed (see the subsequent text in this chapter for stone removal techniques). After the initial layouts of stones have been removed, the rest of the placements throughout the massage will typically be flowing placements, as it is difficult to do a three-dimensional massage with complex stone layouts present. Complex static stone layouts can be reintroduced once again toward the end of the massage.

TESTIMONIAL

Sometimes, I end a massage with a static placement layout, especially if the client is in a deep state of relaxation and has time to rest for a while after the massage is over. I can only do this when I have a break between clients, something I highly recommend. I tell my clients not to worry about putting the stones away, and just to leave them where they fall when they get up. And yet, I almost always return to find the stones laid out to make a beautiful shape on the massage table as a thank you for the massage.

My students sometimes ask me if it is better to begin a hot stone massage with the client supine or prone. My personal preference is supine, because most of my moves are three-dimensional, requiring reaching under and moving the body, and are much easier to do when the client is face-up. Starting supine also gives the client's back time to soften from the hot stone placement beneath it. And lastly, starting supine allows me to work the head, face, and neck first. This is beneficial because it tends to quiet the client's mind early on in the massage, helping the client to be present with his or her body sooner. However, initial client positioning is a personal decision, and starting in either position will suffice.

The following static placement layouts are examples of what can be created with the stones for both supine and prone positions. You are invited to use these stone layouts in your practice, but you need not memorize them or follow them by rote. There is no wrong layout as long as it feels good to the client.

Supine Layouts

If you choose to begin the massage with the client supine, place a stone layout on the massage table just before the arrival of the client. Depending on the complexity of the stone layout you choose, this could take from 5 to 15 minutes. After the placement is laid on the table, cover the stones with a narrow towel or folded pillowcase to keep them warm while waiting for the client. The sheet then rests on top of the covered stone layout. If the client is on time, the folded pillowcase should be left over the stones and the client asked to lie down on top of the covered stones and beneath the sheet. As mentioned previously, using a cover for the stones optimizes the amount of time the heat from the layout will last. Later, when the stones have cooled down, the pillowcase should be removed. The stones then lie against the skin, giving off their remaining heat. If the client is late, however, the pillowcase will most likely need to be removed before the client lies on the stones, or otherwise they will not be warm enough.

When the client arrives, explain how to lie on the stones and give them permission to move any stone that is not comfortable. Then, leave while the client undresses and lies down.

As soon as you walk back in the room, ask the client how the stone temperature is feeling. If the client reports that the warmth of the stones cannot be felt at all, remove the pillowcase. If the client can feel the heat, but only slightly, wait a bit to see if the heat begins to penetrate over time. Begin massaging without stones in your hands. If the client still cannot feel the heat from the stones after a few minutes, remove the pillowcase. In contrast, if the client says the stones are beginning to feel too hot, place an additional narrow layer of cloth over the stones. If, however, the temperature feels just right, leave the original cover over the stones as is. After the client's comfort with the temperature of the stones has been established, you can then proceed to place a frontal layout, after which you can return to massaging the client.

After approximately 10 to 15 minutes (or check with client), remove the pillowcase and lower the client back onto the bare layout for more warmth. Depending on how much heat remains, stones should be removed approximately 5 to 10 minutes after the pillowcase has been taken off them.

Stone Layouts for Beneath the Supine Client's Body

The following photographs show how the stones are laid out on the massage table just prior to the arrival of the client. (As noted previously, the stones are normally covered with a pillowcase and then topped with a sheet for the client to climb under.) If you have an idea of the size of the client, try and lay out the stones accordingly.

> **TIP**
>
> Try lying on the stone layout before your client arrives so that you can make adjustments for temperature and for where the stones should be positioned, keeping in mind the client's height in relationship to yours. The stones will also relax and ground you in preparation for the session.

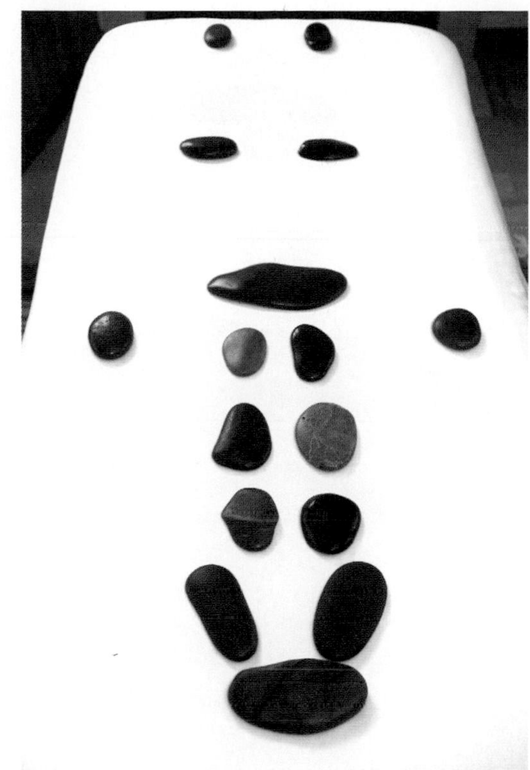

Figure 6-7 The Super Double Spinal Run. This placement has stones on either side of spine, a stone beneath the neck, sacrum, hands, knees, and feet. Client lies face up on top of stones.

CONCAVE RAVE

The "concave rave" is a very simple stone layout that accommodates all the indentations on the back of the body and takes approximately 5 to 10 minutes to arrange. The stones used for such a layout should be rounded rather than flat to fill in the empty spaces and reach the body. Arrange the stones for placement beneath the neck, low back, palms, behind the knees, and strapped to the feet.

SUPER DOUBLE SPINAL RUN

The "super double spinal run" is a bit more complex than the "concave rave," but it is the layout I most commonly use for beneath the back, as it is very comforting to the client and effective in releasing tension along either side of the spinal column (Fig. 6-7). Allow approximately 10 to 15 minutes to set it up. The stones on either side of the spine should be of similar size, height, shape, and temperature; otherwise, one will stand out and mask the others. Place the stones so that they are beneath the erector spinalis muscles, not the ribs, as that would be uncomfortable for the client. Avoid placing the columns of stones too far apart—the spinal column is narrower than you might think. Do not make just one line of stones down the spine when the client is going to be lying on top of them, because the pressure of the spinous processes over the stones would be painful. One line of stones can be used over the spine when the client is face down, as there is no pressure from the body.

Notice that the neck stone is oblong and thick, the scapula stones are wide and long, the spinal stones are smaller ovals, and the lumbar stone is shaped like the lumbar region. The hand stones are thick, the knee stones are oval and slightly thick, and the foot stones are oval and flat. Once the client lies down on this layout, wrap the foot stones onto the feet.

Stone Layouts for the Top of the Supine Client's Body

Use the following layouts on the top of the body after the client is comfortable with the temperature of the stones beneath. If time is short or the client does not enjoy having several stones placed on top of the body, use one of the lighter layouts. If the client enjoys having the full complement of stones, and time permits, then you can use more stones.

SIMPLE PLEASURE

"Simple pleasure" is a quick and simple placement that can help a client relax in a very short time. It

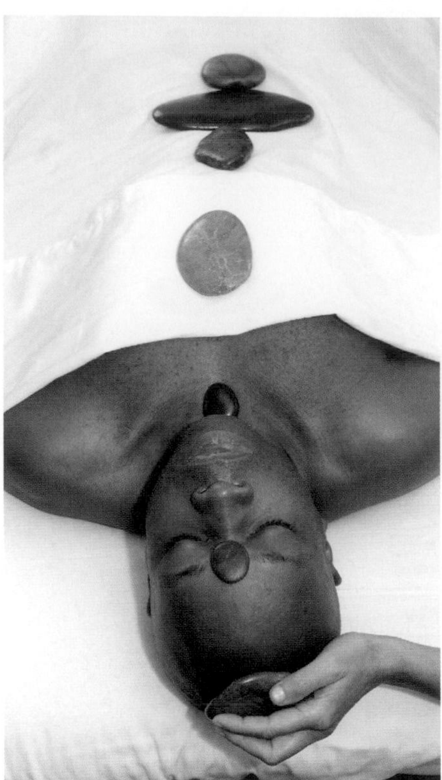

Figure 6-8 The Chakra Dance. This placement positions a stone on all the chakras but the crown.

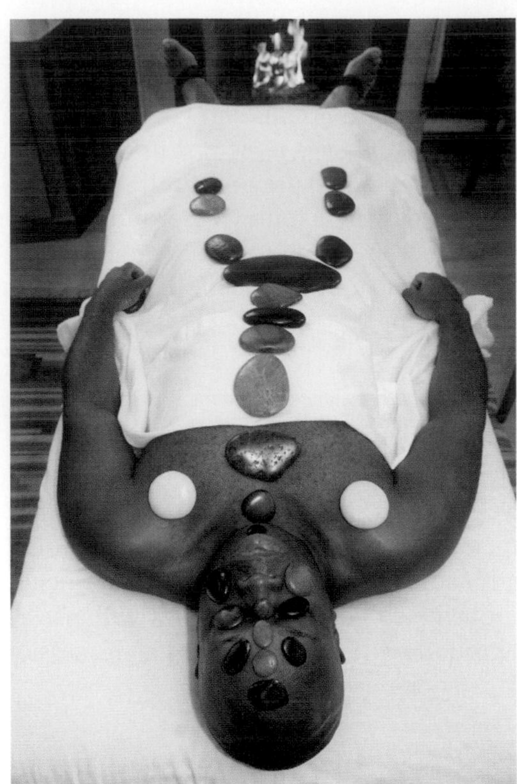

Figure 6-9 The Frontal Shebang. This placement positions stones just about everywhere they will stay.

includes just five stones: a small one on the third eye, a medium-to-large one on the heart area, a large one on the belly (doubles for hand warming as well), and two stones on the feet.

CHAKRA DANCE

The "chakra dance" layout is also quick and easy to do (Fig. 6-8). Place stones on each of the chakras: Begin with the third eye, then the throat, heart, solar plexus, belly, and pelvic bone. Exclude the crown chakra, as a stone would not stay on the top of the head! You can, however, hold a stone on the crown chakra for a few moments. This is a very balancing layout and helpful to open and realign these energy vortices.

FRONTAL SHEBANG

The "frontal shebang" layout uses a stone on just about every location on the front of the body where it won't easily fall off (Fig. 6-9). This is a good placement for starting a massage while you are working on the head and neck. Stones can be left on the face while you gently massage the neck. When you are ready to massage the face, remove the face stones. The rest of the stones can be removed as they cool off or when you are ready to work on that part of the body. If the "super double spinal run" accompanies this layout, take care to ventilate the room so that the client does not overheat.

Prone Layouts

If you plan to begin the massage with the client prone, very little preparation is needed for the stone layout on the massage table, as only a few stones are placed beneath the front of the body. After the client is lying face down on the few preplaced stones, you can place your stone layout for the back of the body on top of the client over the sheet or directly on the skin, depending on the temperature of the stones.

Stone Layouts for Beneath the Prone Client's Body

Avoid placing too many stones beneath the front of the body, as comfort is a concern whenever the client is face down.

ILLY-BELLY-PECKI-POO

The "illy-belly-pecki-poo" is a fanciful name for a modest placement that most clients find comfortable.

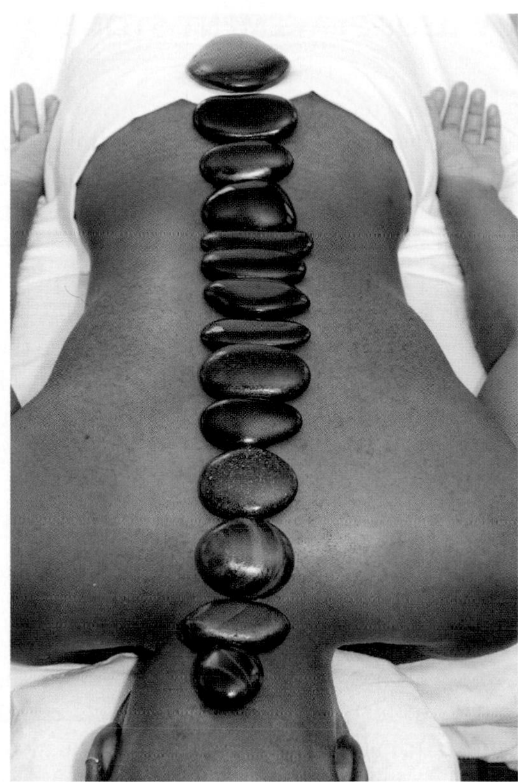

Figure 6-10 Warm Single Spinal Run Out. Warm stones placed over the spine.

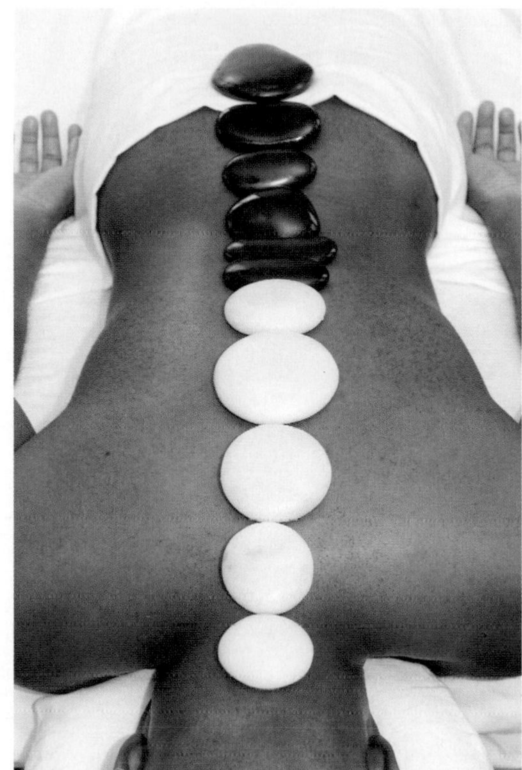

Figure 6-11 Cold/Warm Single Spinal Run Out. Cold and then warm stones placed over the spine.

It is composed of a large belly stone, two small stones for the iliacus muscles, and two round stones for the pectoral muscles. This layout takes only a minute to set up. It is enhanced, however, by the stone layouts on the back of the body.

Stone Layouts for the Top of the Prone Client's Body

The following are three possible layouts for the client's back in prone position. Remember, however, that these are only suggestions. Any number of arrangements can be made on the back of the body. Feel free to experiment.

EXTREMITY LAYOUT

The "extremity layout" is a quick and simple layout that includes a stone placed in the palm of both hands and on the sole of both feet. It is very grounding and cleansing to the client, pulling energy out of each "exit" path of the body. This is a good layout to use when time is short or you are doing long, flowing connecting strokes that encompass the whole length of the body. It is also a wonderful way to end a massage, because it is comforting and grounding without being overly intoxicating to the client who is attempting to "come back!"

SINGLE SPINAL RUN OUT

The "single spinal run out" runs a long line of stones directly on top of the spine (Fig. 6-10). Because there is no pressure or body weight pushing on the stones, it does not hurt the spine. Instead, it sends a deep, penetrating warmth directly into the spine, increasing its limberness. This is a nice layout to have on the back when you are working the client's legs. It can be done with all warm stones, relieving the muscles along and between the spinous processes, or you can place cold stones at one end of the line-up and warm stones at the other end, as shown in Figure 6-11. You can also try alternating warm stones with cold stones to invigorate the client's back and spine. You can create the "single spinal run out" by bringing the working stones to a rest, one at a time, along the spine as the massage on the back comes to an end. Or you can place fresh stones along the spine before you work the back, pre-softening the back muscles while you massage the legs.

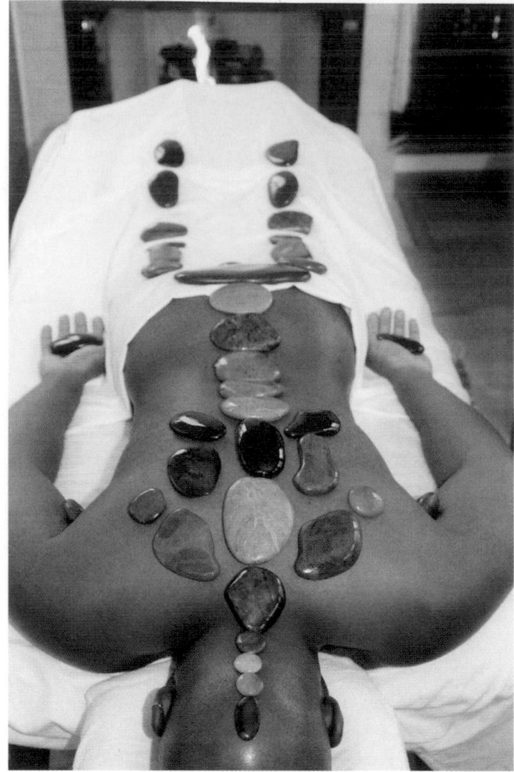

Figure 6-12 The Backside Shazam. This placement covers much of the back of the body and is a wonderful way to end the massage.

BACKSIDE SHAZAM

The "backside shazam" covers most of the backside of the body (including armpits), and it is especially soothing at the end of a massage (Fig. 6-12). Leave clients with this layout when they have time to luxuriate. Clients who are treated to a "backside shazam" at the end of a massage should wait for a few minutes before attempting to drive home.

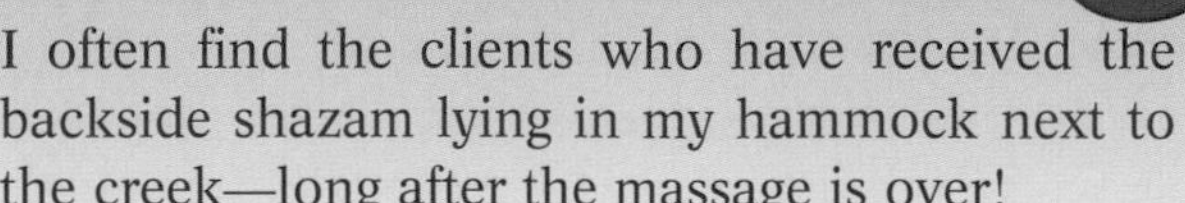

TESTIMONIAL

I often find the clients who have received the backside shazam lying in my hammock next to the creek—long after the massage is over!

CREATIVE PLACEMENTS

Any number of variations to the suggested placement layouts can be made. Have fun playing with the stones, making layouts that suit the individual client in that given moment. Experiment! Clients will likely find your inventiveness refreshing.

REMOVAL OF PLACEMENT STONES

How a stone is removed from the body is as important as how it is placed. If you lift a stone off the top of the body rapidly and carelessly, the client will likely experience your removal as jolting. If you ask your clients to sit up so that you can remove the stones from beneath their back, your clients will have to exert attention and effort during a deeply relaxing experience. This is not a good idea, and clients do not appreciate it. Use the following techniques to avoid interrupting the client's experience and achieve a seamless, flowing massage.

Stone Removal from the Top of the Client's Body

Remove each stone slowly and with consciousness, just as you would initiate contact with a stone. This does not have to be a long, drawn-out process. As long as there is awareness and presence with each removal, clients will not feel that the stone (and its energy) is being ripped from them. This type of removal also alleviates the chance of dropping a stone on the client, the floor, or your own foot! Rather than lifting the whole stone off the body at once, lift the stone to its side and turn it over as you take it away. This creates a sense of gradual departure and promotes a settling, rather than anxious, feeling. If the stone being removed is large, it can be twisted in a circle as it is lifted and taken off the body. This creates a slight spin of the energy and feels pleasant to the clients.

Stone Removal from Beneath the Client's Body

When stones need to be removed from beneath the client's body, do not ask your clients to sit up! The three-dimensional approach allows for easy and flowing stone removal and does not require you to employ the help of your clients. With this approach, you'll learn to weave the stone removal into the flow of the massage. Your clients never need to know that the stones are being removed.

The same technique that is used for removing the stones from beneath the client's back is also used for removing the strip of material that was previously placed over the stones. As mentioned previously, depending on the temperature of the stones and the lateness of the client, there may not be a strip of material over the stones, but if there is, this removal technique will need to happen twice during the massage—once for removing the material and then later

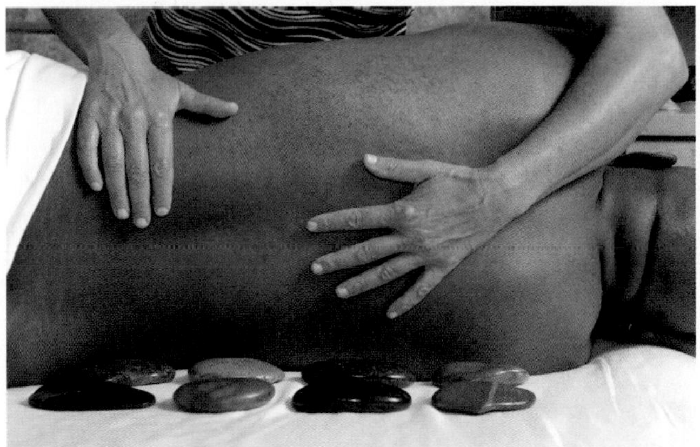

Figure 6-13 Lifting Client for Stone Removal from Below. The client is rolled to the side as part of the massage instead of being asked to sit up.

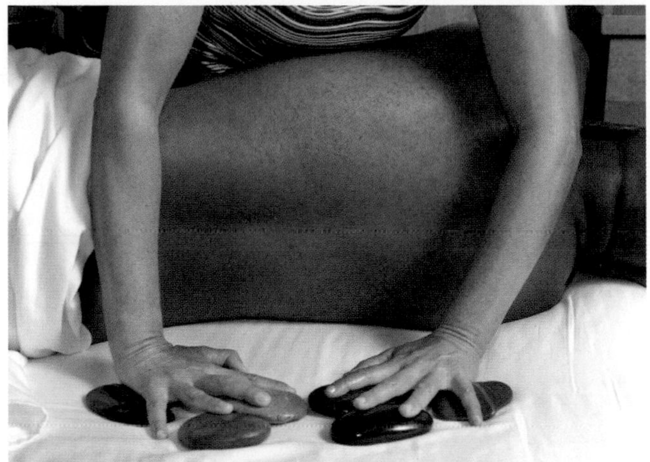

Figure 6-14 Moving Stones Out of the Way. Contact is kept with the client while pushing stones to the side of the table closest to the skillet.

for removing the stones. To avoid redundancy, stand on different sides of the body for each time you use this removal technique. Always stand on the side of the table that is closest to the skillet to remove the strip of material. Always stand on the side of the table that is furthest from the skillet to remove the stones. The reason for this will become apparent in a moment.

After you are at the appropriate side of the body, depending on whether or not you are removing the material or the stones, lift the client's far shoulder from the elbow upward, gently opening the shoulder girdle and avoiding undue stress that could wrench the shoulder joint. Once lifted, pull that shoulder toward you with one hand while you simultaneously reach behind with the other hand and push it toward you, allowing the client's body to roll to its side and against your body, as shown in Figure 6-13. Now that you have the client's body lifted up and off of the stones, you can remove either the strip of material or the stones, depending on what is called for in that moment.

When you remove the strip of material, the reason for its narrowness becomes apparent. If the material is too wide, the side of the client's body will be rolled on top of the material and it will be very challenging and disruptive to remove it. A narrow strip allows you to roll the client's body to its side without it being on top of the material. After you remove the strip of material, lie the client back down on top of the stones, which will now feel much warmer to the client. Do this slowly so that the new heat of the uncovered stones does not surprise the client.

When you are ready to remove the stones, do this same technique from the other side of the client's body. But before you begin, place two hot stones by the side of the torso closest to the skillet. Then, walk to the side of the body that is furthest from the skillet. Lift the shoulder and roll the body toward you so the client's back is facing the skillet. Before removing the stones, however, massage the back briefly. This helps to eclipse any thought the client may have had of the stones being removed.

When you are ready to remove the stones, keep both of your forearms in contact with the back so the client still feels connected to you as you push the stones away from the back and toward the side of the massage table that is closest to the skillet, as shown in Figure 6-14. This makes returning the stones to the skillet much easier and smoother, with no need to walk all the way around the table to retrieve the stones. Immediately after the stones are pushed out of the way, pick up the two new hot stones that you had previously placed by the client's torso and use them to massage the client's back some more. After the new stones you are using to massage the back have lost enough heat to become placement stones, place them strategically under the low back and slowly lower the client back down on top them. While you return the cold stones to the skillet, the client is enjoying the warmth from the new stones.

STATIC PLACEMENT OF STONES ON THE THERAPIST

Hot stones do not have to be reserved entirely for the clients! While massaging others, therapists can also be caring for themselves with the heated stones. When sitting and working the client's head and neck, for instance, hot stones can be placed beneath the therapist's buttocks or feet. This is very calming, grounding, and centering for therapists. While standing, if a stretch tank top with wide elastic shoulder straps is worn, medium-sized stones can be placed on top of the shoulders and secured in place beneath the therapist's straps. If pants are worn that have some resistance to them, large flat stones can be placed on the abdomen or lower back while working. The warmth from these stones helps to keep the shoulders dropped and the abdomen and sacral area very relaxed.

CAUTION

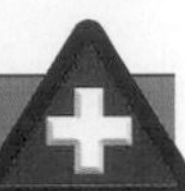

Care is required with these placements to avoid falling stones. This can be corrected by simple attention to the placements made.

At the end of a long day, hot stones can be placed on the massage table and therapists can lie on them, placing a few on their abdomen and chest as well. This is an easy way to warm and relax their tired muscles and a glorious gift to themselves.

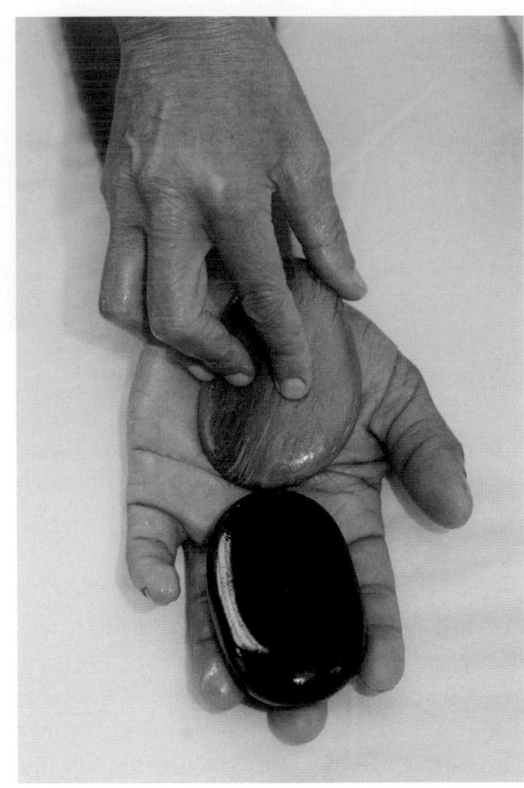

Figure 6-15 Switching Stones. As one placement stone cools off, slide a working stone that has lost too much heat to massage with into the palm by pushing the cool one off with the new stone. Every working stone can become a placement stone.

FLOWING PLACEMENT OF WORKING STONES

Every working stone becomes a possible placement stone. As a working stone loses its heat, it becomes the perfect temperature for use as a placement stone against the client's skin. It is a waste to return a warm stone to the skillet unless you already have enough stones in place and they are not needed. As explained in Chapter 5, if the working stones are too cool to be used as placement stones, then you are using them too long for massage and most likely feel boring to the client. Convert your working stones to placement stones before they lose their warmth.

Flowing placement is fun and does not require a great deal of forethought, as static placement does. However, keep in mind that the stones will cool off fairly quickly at this point, so be careful not to get carried away with placing stones, as you could end up with too many stones to replace at once.

TIP

Keep track of the stones that you place throughout the massage so that you'll know when to replace them with new ones.

When you are ready to convert a working stone into a placement stone, simply glide into an area of choice with the stone and leave it there. If a cooled off placement stone is already there, simply push it out of the way with the new one (Fig. 6-15). Presto! You've just made a flowing placement. If the old placement stone can be returned to the skillet without interrupting the flow, do so immediately. If this is not possible, then leave the stone in an organized pile to avoid confusion with the hot ones. Return these cooled stones to the skillet when there is a natural break in the massage. Flowing placements are a smart and effective way to make use of all of the stone's warmth. They are also pleasant surprises for your clients.

SUMMARY

Stone placements can be done in either a static or flowing fashion. Static stone placements are stones that are used specifically for placements and not for massage. They can be done on individual parts of the body as well as in complex layouts. Complex static stone placements are useful for the beginning and end of a massage, but not as much during the dynamic three-dimensional strokes. There are many different layouts for both the front and back of the body; however, none of them need to be adhered to like a science. Creativity is encouraged. Static placements can also be made on the therapists' bodies as well, in locations such as low back and shoulders, using their own clothing to hold the stones in place.

Flowing placements are individual stone placements that are made throughout the flow of a massage. As a working stone cools off too much to be used for massage strokes, it can be placed on or beneath the body, as the warmth of the stone is sufficient when it is stationary, but no longer when it is moving. Every working stone can become a placement stone; however, it is important not to make too many flowing placements, as they cool off rapidly and create extra work as far as removing all of them before they become too cool to be useful.

Removing a placement stone needs to be done with the same care and attention as when placing the stone. Pulling too many stones away at once and in a rapid fashion can feel jarring to the client. Remove a stone slowly, with a slide turn and with reverence.

Stone placement increases the client's experience of relaxation and creates the sensation of feeling as if additional hands were on the body throughout the massage. It is a wonderful adjunct to the hot stones that are being used to massage the body.

REVIEW QUESTIONS

TRUE/FALSE

1. A static placement layout must be followed exactly with no improvising.

   Circle: True False

2. A flowing placement happens during the flow of the massage and is the end result of a working stone losing its heat.

   Circle: True False

3. An armpit is an awful place to put a stone.

   Circle: True False

4. A hand placement stone should be thick when it is placed under a hand while the body is in the supine position.

   Circle: True False

5. When a client is prone, no stones should be placed beneath them.

   Circle: True False

MULTIPLE CHOICE

6. A device that is used to help hold stones in place is:
   a. Stone wrapper
   b. Oven pocket
   c. Sand bag
   d. Only a and c
   e. a, b, and c
7. Face placement should be comprised of:
   a. Warm stones
   b. Cold stones
   c. Either warm or cold or both at the same time
   d. Large stones
   e. Black stones
8. Static placement stones are to be used:
   a. Instead of massaging with stones
   b. Constantly throughout the massage
   c. In addition to massaging with the stones
   d. When you are too tired to massage
   e. None of the above
9. Supine layouts can only be done:
   a. With heavy clients
   b. With light clients
   c. When no injuries are present
   d. When the client is lying face down
   e. None of the above
10. When making a layout for the client's back to lie on, you want to first cover it with:
    a. A narrow thick towel
    b. A narrow thin strip of material or pillowcase
    c. A wide thin towel
    d. A wide thick towel
    e. The sheet

SHORT ANSWER

11. Complex static stone layouts are best done at the ____________ and __________ of a massage.
12. Every ________________ stone becomes a _________________ stone.

13. A stone should be removed ______________ if it is too hot for a client and ______________ when it is ready to be returned to the skillet.
14. Flowing placements are more ______________ than static layouts; however, they __________ __________ more quickly.
15. Therapists can also place stones on _______ ______ during a massage.

MATCHING

16. Concave Rave
17. Super Double Spinal Run
18. Chakra Dance
19. Frontal Shebang
20. Single Spinal Run Out

a. Should be used only in prone position
b. Covers most everywhere on the front of the body
c. Is most commonly used in supine position
d. Fills the spaces beneath the back of the body
e. Stones are left in place over all but one chakra

Answers to Review Questions can be found in Appendix D.

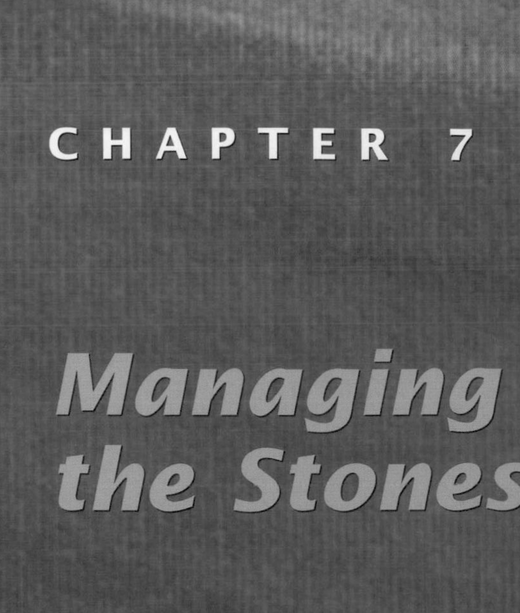

CHAPTER 7

Managing the Stones

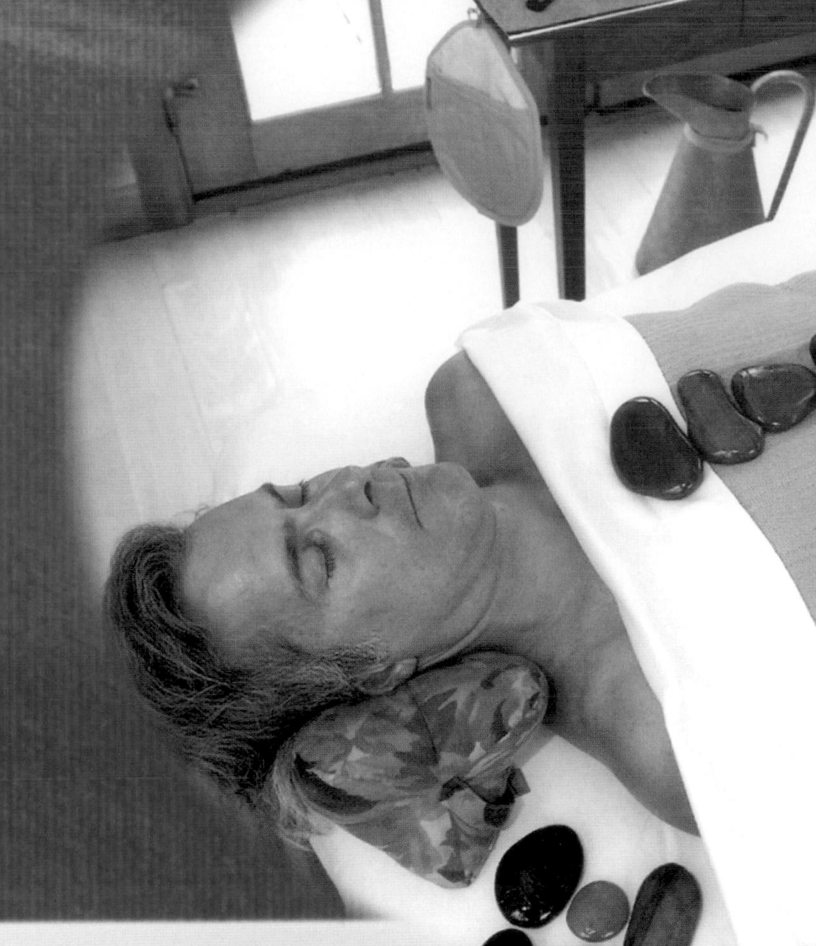

Outline

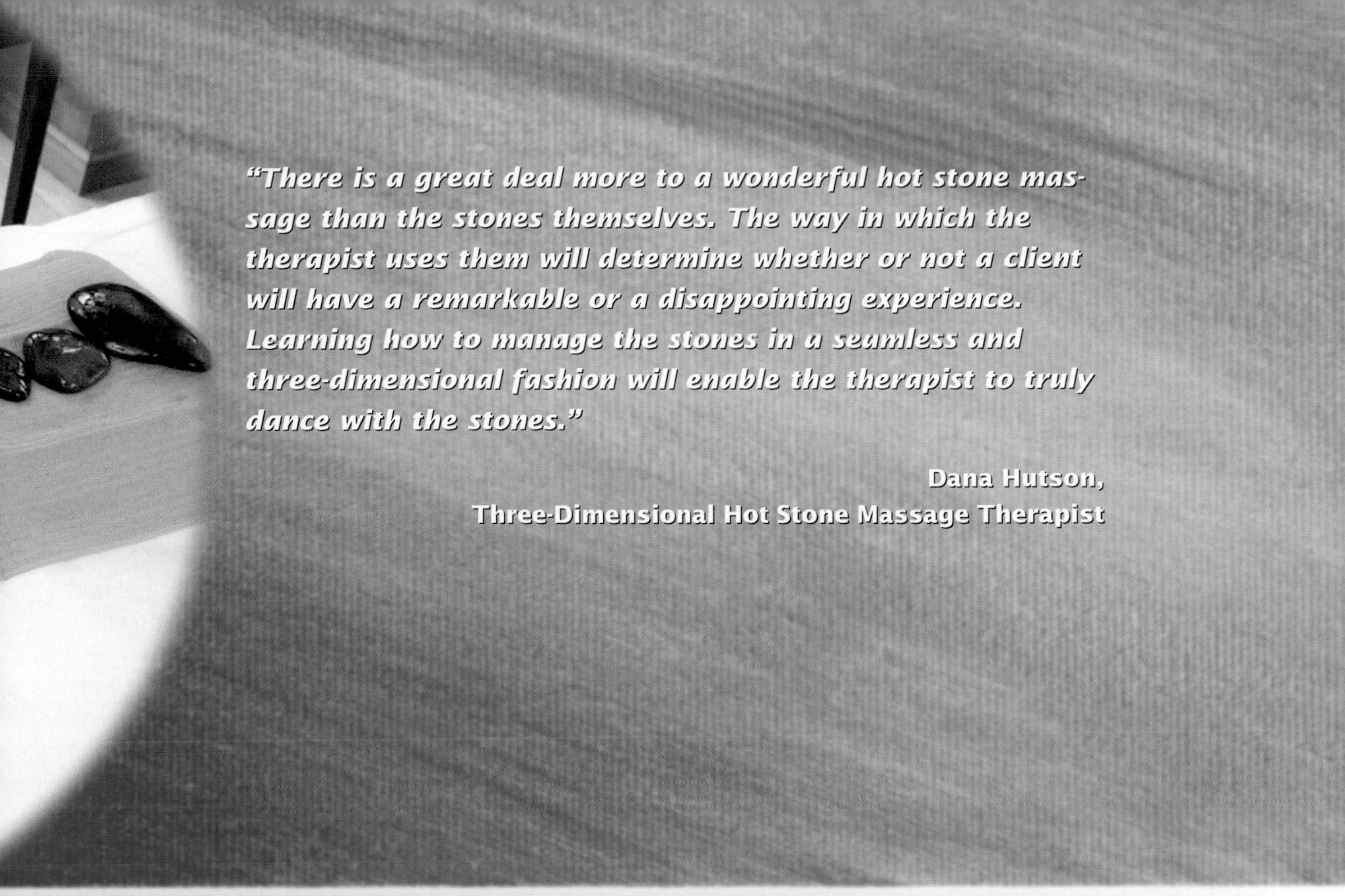

"There is a great deal more to a wonderful hot stone massage than the stones themselves. The way in which the therapist uses them will determine whether or not a client will have a remarkable or a disappointing experience. Learning how to manage the stones in a seamless and three-dimensional fashion will enable the therapist to truly dance with the stones."

Dana Hutson,
Three-Dimensional Hot Stone Massage Therapist

Objectives

After reading this chapter, you should be able to:

- Explain the purpose and benefits of an organized system of stone management.
- Describe the four-pile system of stone management.
- Identify the advantages of using oil versus cream in a hot stone massage.
- Explain when to introduce the stones into the massage and how many to use.
- Describe the approach, timing, temperature, stone size, speed, and pressure for effective contact of stone to body.
- Explain the safety guidelines for preventing injury to both the therapist and client.

Key Terms

Four-pile system: A system of stone management created by the author to reduce the amount of interruption necessary during a hot stone massage.

Stone entrance: The way in which a stone is brought into the massage and first makes contact with the skin.

Stone flipping: A technique used with a very hot stone to prevent burning or discomfort for both the client and the therapist.

The stones themselves—even with their beauty, earth energy, and capacity for holding heat and cold—are only part of the equation for giving an exquisite hot stone massage. Just as important as the stones is the way in which the therapist uses them. Many people have shared with me their negative experiences of hot stone massage. I, too, have been disappointed as a hot stone massage client. These stories and experiences helped me recognize the need for a new approach. This chapter, in particular, is a result of the experimentation and creativity that ensued. As such, it is one of the most important chapters in the book.

This chapter describes many managing techniques that, although may appear trivial, are critical for helping to make hot stone massage satisfying to clients.

TIP 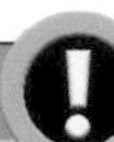

It is often not the obvious things that make a difference in a massage, but rather the attention that is paid to the subtle details.

If a hot stone massage is riddled with interruptions; if you introduce the stones to the body abruptly instead of gradually; if you hold the stones by your fingers only and not with the rest of your hand; if you use the stones too quickly, too slowly, too lightly, or too roughly; or if you use too many stones and do not perform enough massage with your hands alone, clients will not have a positive experience. It is not enough simply to heat the stones and apply them to the body. Adhering to the guidelines in this chapter will make all the difference in your clients' experience of hot stone massage.

SYSTEM FOR OPTIMAL STONE FLOW

When first attempting to give a hot stone massage, many students say how challenging it is for them to retrieve and replace the stones throughout the massage. Deciding which stones to use, which ones are no longer hot, which ones are too hot, and so forth takes a great deal of time and energy away from the massage. Unfortunately, most hot stone massage classes and videos fail to teach stone management. Instead, they have the therapist taking one or two stones at a time out of the skillet and returning them to the skillet randomly when they are no longer hot. This method has three disadvantages: First, it requires constant interruption, forcing the therapist to leave the client's body every minute or so to select appropriately heated stones from the skillet. Second, it requires the therapist to hunt around in the skillet for a stone heated to just the right temperature, and this takes the therapist away from the massage for too long. Third, it forewarns the client every time stones are about to be used. That is why I developed the four-pile stone management system.

The Four-Pile System

At first, you might find the **four-pile system** cumbersome, but once you've mastered it, you'll find that the amount of time you spend managing your stones is greatly reduced. As the system becomes second nature, your clients will barely notice the few brief interruptions you make. In addition, because you will not have to leave your client each time you need a stone, your client will have no idea when the stones are coming. This creates an invisible flow that gives the client the impression that the stones appeared out of nowhere.

The four-pile system allows you to work with three piles of stones over a period of approximately 10 minutes before having to retrieve more stones from the fourth pile that is in the skillet. This means that in a 90-minute massage, you'll have to leave the client only 9 or 10 times to retrieve stones!

The Four Piles

The number of stones suggested for each pile is appropriate for therapists who have developed some experience with the system.

TIP 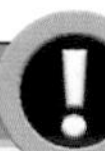

When you're starting out, use fewer stones in each pile, except for the one in the skillet. Eventually, as the system becomes more natural to you, increase the number of stones you use until you can manage the numbers recommended below.

1. **Pile One** is placed on the massage table and is comprised of 6 to 8 stones that are the least hot of all the piles (Fig. 7-1). Their temperature should be appropriate for almost immediate use (within 5 minutes). For this pile, choose

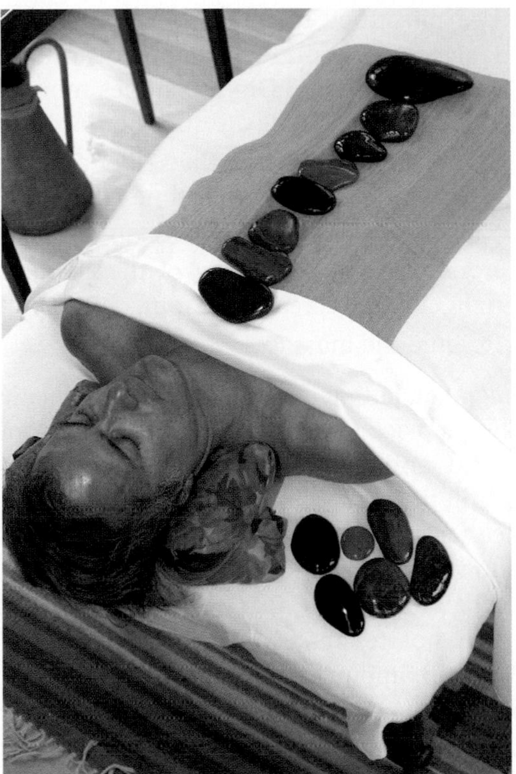

Figure 7-1 Piles One and Two. Pile one is laid on the massage table, while pile two is laid on top of the client over the sheet and possibly a narrow strip of material.

stones that are sized and shaped according to the area of the body where the massage is to begin. Place the stones on the massage table near the place you intend to begin the massage, but not so close to the client that they could touch the client's skin.

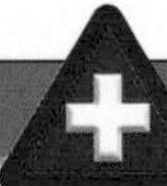

CAUTION

Clients should be advised on the location of the stones so they don't inadvertently move their body and contact them. You could also place a pillowcase between the stones and the client's body to prevent accidental skin contact.

2. **Pile Two** is placed directly on the client over the sheet or a strip of fabric and is comprised of 6 to 8 stones, as shown in Figure 7-1. This is the second set of stones you will use in the massage, so their temperature should be a bit hotter than those in pile one. They also should be of the appropriate size and shape for the area of body where you intend to use them.

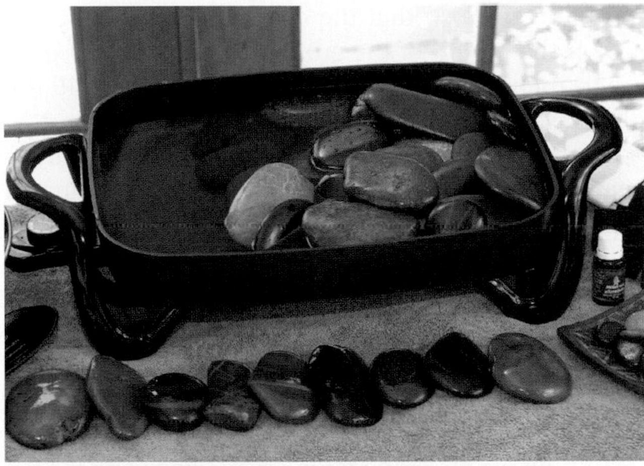

Figure 7-2 Piles Three and Pile Four. Pile three is "waiting in the wings" on the stone table in front of the cooker. Pile four is comprised of the remainder of stones that are pushed to the right side of the cooker.

3. **Pile Three** (otherwise known as "waiting in the wings") is placed over a towel on the stone table, directly in front of the skillet, and is comprised of 12 to 16 stones, as shown in Figure 7-2. This pile should be considerably hotter than pile two, as it will be approximately 10 minutes before the stones will be used. This pile will be used to replace both pile one and pile two, and thus more stones are required.
4. **Pile Four** is comprised of all the stones that remain in the skillet after the first three piles have been made. These stones should always be pushed to the far right side of the skillet, as shown in Figure 7-2. These 16 to 20 stones are the hottest of all the piles, as they are left in the skillet and kept at an approximate temperature of 160°F. You will eventually use these stones to replace pile three.

Creating the Piles

When first generating the piles, you'll need to create the temperature variations of each. Before the client arrives and after making a stone placement on the massage table (see Chapter 6), remove 24 to 32 stones from the skillet (depending on the size of your piles) and place them on the stone table in front of the skillet. Dip about half of them in the cold water, preparing them for piles one and two, as follows: Dip the stones that you'll use for pile one for approximately 5 to 10 seconds, and then dip the ones for pile two for approximately 3 seconds. Then, arrange the stones on the stone table from left to right according to temperature so that the coolest of the hot stones are on the far left of the group, the next hottest ones are to their right, and the hottest (which you did not dip in water) are all the way to the right.

After the client is on the table and you are ready to begin the massage, place the piles in their designated locations. The stones on the far left of the stone table will be used for pile one. Place them directly on the massage table closest to the area of the body where you will begin the massage. The next hottest group of stones on the stone table will be used for pile two. Place them on a fabric strip on top of the client's body near the area where you will be working. The stones remaining on the stone table are pushed towards the left and will be used for pile three. If there is a cool breeze in the room, it is advisable to cover pile three with a pillowcase to preserve their warmth while they wait to be used. Push the stones in pile four all the way to the right side of the skillet so that there is room for returning the cold stones to the left side of the skillet without having to stop to make room for them during the massage. Now the massage can begin.

Order of Stone Flow

The same stones are continuously reused and reheated throughout the massage. The stone piles automatically keep their variation in temperature as you move them systematically from one pile into another. The time that elapses between these transitions allows for each pile to cool or heat to its appropriate temperature. As long as you adhere to the recommended flow and amount of time to use each stone, you should not experience any problem with the temperature of the piles. However, an extended delay in the use of any of the piles will result in stones that are either too cold or too hot to use. If this happens, simply replace the cool stones in the skillet or cool off the heated ones by dipping them in cold water and begin the pile system over. However, even with brief interruptions such as these, the four-pile system is still more efficient than the alternative method of constant retrieval.

Here is the ideal order in which the piles should be used for the most efficient management.

1. Use pile one first and then return it to the left side of skillet (or move it out of the way on the massage table until it is easy to return to skillet).
2. Next, use pile two and then return it to the left side of the skillet.
3. Use pile three to replace piles one and two. Place pile two on the client for warmth before creating pile one. Dip the stones momentarily in cold water if they are still too hot for use.
4. Remove pile four from the skillet and use it to replace pile three on the stone table.
5. Now that there is room to do so, push the stones from the left side of the skillet to the right side to recreate pile four.
6. Resume the massage.

Remember, left means cooler and right means hotter. Always place stones so that the coolest ones are to the left and the hottest ones are to the right, whether in the skillet or on the stone table.

Once mastered, adhering to the four-pile method will allow you to spend more time tending to your clients than tending to your stones. Therefore, it is as important not to make adherence to the four-pile method more important than the individual needs of the clients.

TIP 

If a client needs your attention in a way that requires you to alter the flow of the four-pile system, do so. After you have taken care of the client's needs, you can then start the system over.

OILING OF STONES

Although the benefits, order, and method of using massage oil during a hot stone massage may appear trivial, the cumulative effect of lubricating the stones hundreds of times throughout a massage has a significant impact on the overall flow, safety, and ease of a hot stone massage and is thus worthy of discussion. The following section will discuss: the advantages of using oil versus cream or other types of lubricants, when to apply oil to the stones, and the most efficient way to oil your hands.

Benefits of Using Oil Versus Cream with Stones

Hot stones need to be well lubricated on all sides in order to be safe for use. Thus, adding the element of hot stones into a massage necessitates the use of oil rather than other forms of lubricants. Although the use of cream, lotion, or gel is not impossible, they take more time to apply and spread out evenly over the stone, thus impeding the seamless flow of the massage and increasing the chance of a stone sticking and burning the client. Oil spreads out quickly and evenly over a stone, allowing it to be used rapidly. Although the time difference between applying oil versus cream is small, the accumulation of many applications add up to become a large difference by the end of the massage.

High-quality almond oil seems to have the perfect viscosity for hot stone massage—not too thin and not too thick. Oils that are scented with essential oils are nice to use because the heat of the stones brings out the pleasant aroma of the oil. However, because some clients are sensitive to certain fragrances, it is important to have an unscented almond oil on hand as well.

CAUTION

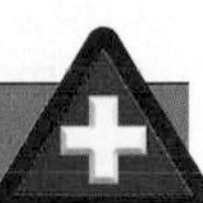

If you are drawn to a scented oil, ask clients whether or not they are sensitive to fragrances before using it. If so, use your unscented oil for them.

Dipping Method for Rapid Oiling of Stones

To achieve optimal flow during a hot stone massage, it is vital to have a quick and easy system for accessing oil. Stopping to pick up and squeeze oil out of a bottle each time you need to re-oil your hands and stones will significantly slow down the flow of your massage. Using a pump bottle on a holster strapped around your waist is one solution, but it is much faster and more effective to dip hands into a small oil-filled bowl (Fig. 7-3).

TIP

A small hot stone can even be dropped into a bowl of oil to warm it.

You can place several small oil-filled bowls on tables or shelves around your massage table for easy access. Only put as much oil as you might need for each massage so that you are not reusing the same oil for each client.

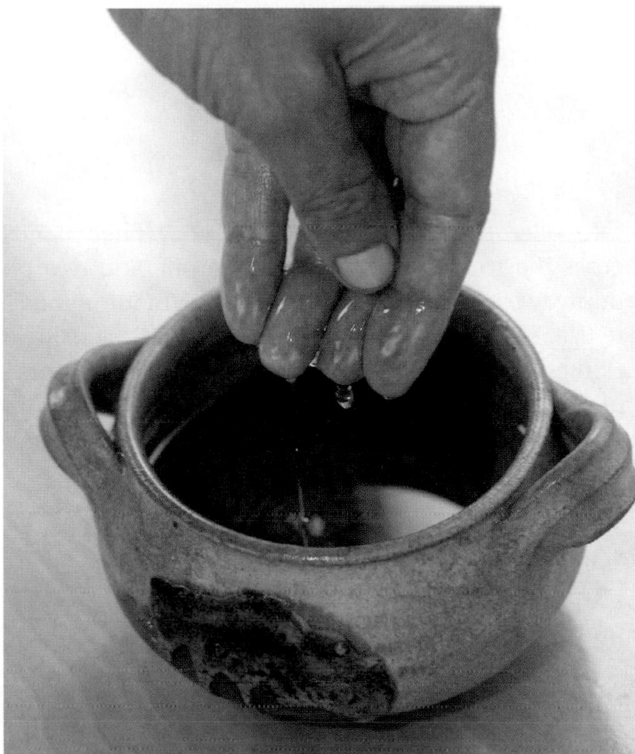

Figure 7-3 Dipping Hand in Oil Bowl. Dipping your hand in a bowl of oil is a very fast and efficient way of bringing oil to the stones.

Order of Oiling

Even though I recommend that you begin the session massaging with the hands rather than the stones (next section), it is important to pass your oiled hands across the face of the stones as you approach the client's body, as shown in Figure 7-4. If you do this consistently, you'll then be able to introduce the stones seamlessly, without having to stop and oil

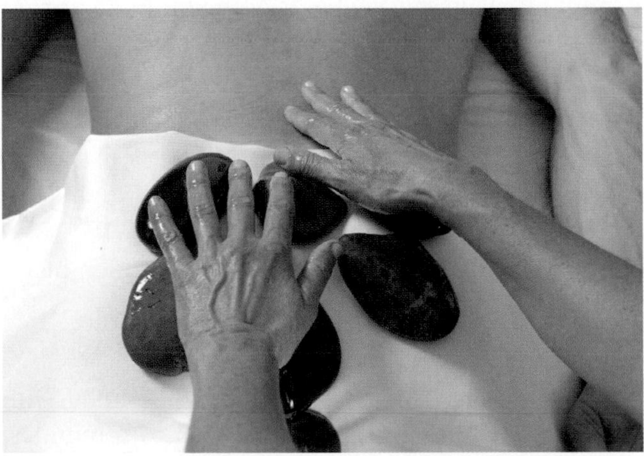

Figure 7-4 Order of Oiling Stones. Slide oiled hand across the face of the stones on your way to massage the body.

them each time they are about to be used. Use the following sequence:

1. Oil your hands.
2. Oil the stones.
3. Oil the client's body.

To oil the stones, simply slide your oiled hands across the top of the stones in pile one and two on your way to the body. This prepares them for immediate use. This easy yet important step helps to ensure a seamless flow. When you are ready to use the stone, you no longer need to stop and oil it first—simply lift the stone and roll it once in your hand to oil the other side and begin massaging with it.

MASSAGING WITH STONES

How you handle the stones, at which point you bring them into the massage, the ratio of stones you use to hands-on massage, the way you make your initial contact of each stone against the skin, the size of the stones in relationship to your hand, the speed at which you move the stones, and the amount of pressure you create with the stones against the client's body all have an impact on the quality of the hot stone massage you will give.

Order and Ratio of Using Stones

Always begin a hot stone massage with your hands alone (no stones). This allows you and your clients to connect. Stones are not replacements for your hands; they are tools to be used in conjunction with them. Although their warmth can soften a muscle with amazing speed and power, when you use stones, you cannot as easily sense what is going on in an area of the body. The hands perceive what stones cannot.

TIP 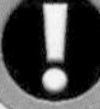

Use your hands to palpate and explore the tension, density, temperature, and configuration of a muscle.

Once you have massaged the client's body with your hands alone for approximately 3 to 5 minutes, you can then incorporate stones into the massage. Because the body is always pre-oiled with this hands-first method, less oil is required for using the stones.

It is important to find the right balance between using stones and hands. In general, if you use too many stones and do not make enough contact with your hands, the client is going to miss your touch. And yet, if there is too much hand contact and not enough stones, the client will be fixated on when the next stone might appear. Finding the perfect balance takes time, experience, and communication with the client. Each person's unique needs will alter this balance slightly.

Proper Stone Size for Optimal Contact with Body

The size of stone you use and the way in which you hold it in your hand will dramatically affect the quality of the contact that it makes. The proper size of stone is one that allows for optimal contact of stone and hand together; thus, you should choose working stones that fit nicely in your particular palm with some of the palm still showing, as shown in Figure 7-5. Your fingers should be able to curl around the outer third of the stone. If the stone takes up the entire surface of the palm (Fig. 7-6), then the fingers will not be able to curl around the stone enough to make skin contact with the body. However, if the stone is so small that there is too much hand and not enough stone, the effect and power of the warm stone will be lost. Finding the perfect ratio of stone to hand will allow for optimal contact and set the stage for giving the best hot stone massage possible.

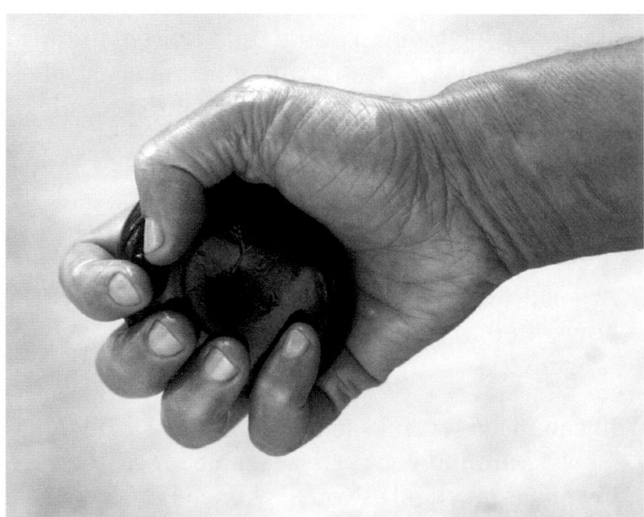

Figure 7-5 Proper Size of Working Stone. The perfect ratio of stone to hand for a general working stone is when the fingers are able to curl around its outer one third.

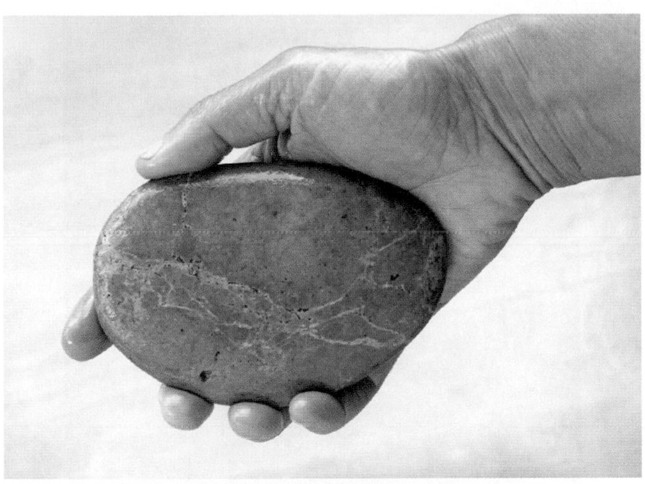

Figure 7-6 Improper Size of Working Stone. This stone is too large to be a good general working stone, because the fingers are not able to curl around the outer one third of the stone.

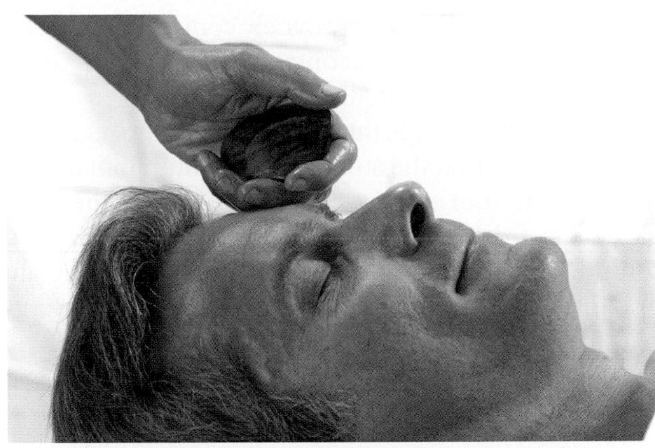

Figure 7-7 Stone Entrance Part 1. Ease in with stone making initial contact with fingertips.

Stone Entrance

Introducing an object such as a hard and hot stone into a massage requires care and skill. An effective **stone entrance** is imperceptible, causing a deepening of relaxation for the client. It may elicit a deep sigh or moan from the client and generally enhances the client's relationship to the stones. In contrast, a poor entrance is abrupt and sudden and may cause the client to jump, gasp, or exclaim "Oh!" It can close a client off to what might otherwise have been a pleasant and possibly healing experience. An abrupt entrance can even discourage a client from ever considering a hot stone massage again.

Proper stone entrance consists of three main elements: approach, timing, and temperature. The key to all three is being gradual.

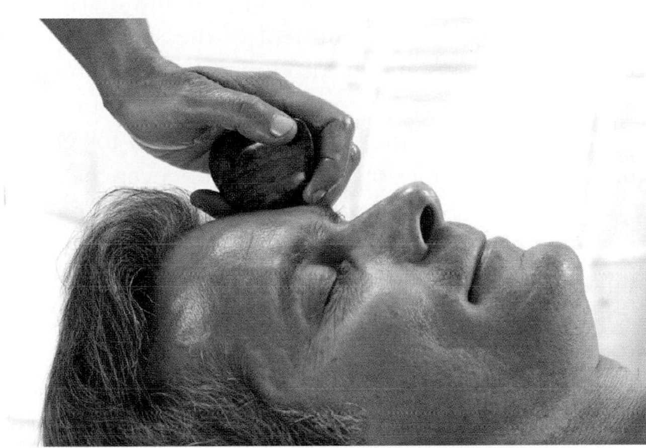

Figure 7-8 Stone Entrance Part 2. Continue entering by letting the edge of the stone make contact with the client's skin.

Approach

A stone needs to be introduced to the skin gradually. In other words, never apply an entire stone against the skin at once. Begin by placing your fingers on the edge of the stone. Contact the client's body with only your fingers to the skin, as shown in Figure 7-7. Next, let your fingers quickly slide out of the way so that the edge of the stone is in contact with the skin, as shown in Figure 7-8. Finally, allow the stone to make full contact with the skin by following it from its edge to its center and then to its entire length, as shown in Figure 7-9. This entire procedure happens in a matter of microseconds; nonetheless, the quick but gradual unfolding of the stone onto the skin makes a major difference in its reception. This kind of entrance allows the stone to enter the massage almost invisibly.

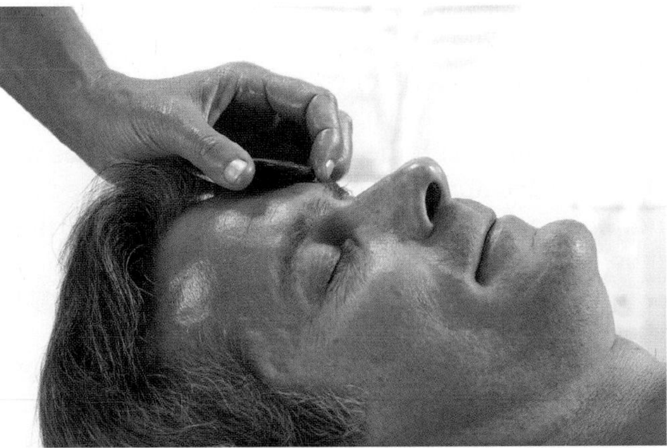

Figure 7-9 Stone Entrance Part 3. Complete stone entrance by allowing the full surface of the stone to make contact with the skin.

The opposite, and unfortunately common, approach to stone entry is to make contact with the entire stone against the client's skin all at once. This is shocking to the system and reduces the client's capacity to relax, feel safe, and trust that the stones will not burn him or her. With this kind of entrance, the client spends the massage on guard waiting for the next abrupt stone arrival. On the other hand, when entrance is made gradually and invisibly, the client is able to leave the mind behind and fully take in the effect of the massage.

Timing

Using a stone immediately after it has been brought to the massage table will ensure its arrival is predictable. The clients will start to associate every break you make to retrieve a stone with the arrival of one. Not only does this predictability remove the "magical" experience of not knowing when a stone will appear, but it also creates an unconscious resentment of the stones, which begin to be seen as an interruption rather than an addition to the massage. Even the best hot stone massage must include some interruptions in the flow to accommodate the dynamics of the stones. However, the more you separate these interruptions from the introduction of stones, the less your clients will associate interruptions with the experience of hot stone massage.

Here is one way you can creatively and seamlessly weave the stones into the massage: Before recreating your piles of stones, first lay some new warm placement stones on or beneath your client to soothe the client while you refresh your piles. Once your piles of stones have been recreated, resume the massage with your hands alone. This way, the client does not associate the break with the arrival of a stone. After massaging for a few minutes with stoneless hands, pick up a stone in each hand midstroke. Continue to massage, but use your forearms instead of your hands, as shown in Figure 7-10. The client will have no idea that you have a stone in each hand. Then, when the timing is right, allow your stone-filled hands to make proper contact with the client's body. The stones will seem to have appeared out of nowhere, but they will not be shocking to the client's body because of their incremental entrance onto the skin.

TESTIMONIAL

A client recently remarked during her massage, "It feels as if you're pulling the stones out of midair!"

"In a certain sense, I am," I said.

Even in jest, we were acknowledging the mysterious quality of this method of stone entrance.

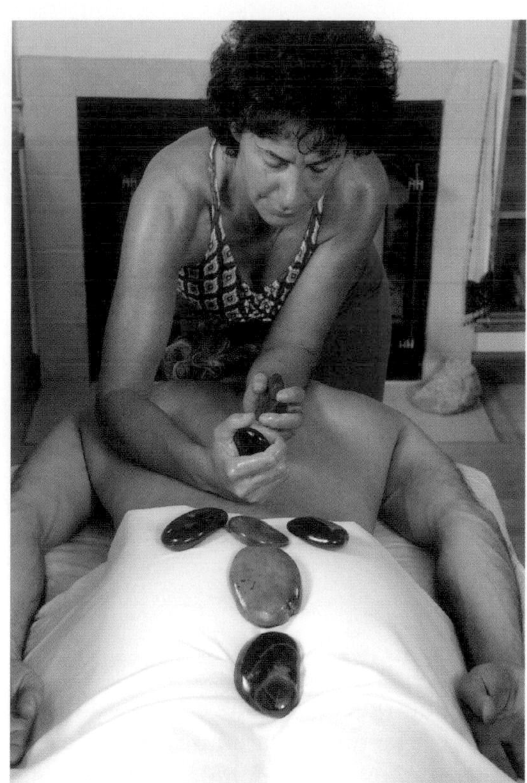

Figure 7-10 Timing of Stone Entrance. Holding stones in your hands as you massage with your forearms allows the stones to seem to appear out of nowhere when you begin to massage with them.

Temperature

The temperature of the first few stones that make contact with the client's skin will determine, to a great extent, the temperatures that clients will be able to tolerate for the rest of the massage. At the beginning of a massage, the client's body is unaccustomed to heat. If you begin with hot stones, you are likely to provoke a hypersensitive reaction that will reduce the amount of heat the client feels he or she can tolerate throughout the entire massage. The client will continually report that the stones are too hot when, had they been properly introduced, their temperature would probably have been considered just right. This response is largely psychological and could be avoided simply by giving the client enough time to adjust to gradual increases of temperature.

TIP

When a client resists even minimal heat, try reintroducing the stones gradually, beginning with stones that are body temperature. From there, gradually increase the temperature. Eventually, you might discover that the exact same temperature of a stone the client had perceived as too hot is now perfect.

For a comfortable stone entrance, begin the massage with a stone that is tepid. Use the tepid stone for a few seconds, and then switch to the next stone, which should be a bit warmer than the first one. Use this stone for approximately 5 seconds, and then bring in a third stone, which should be even warmer than the last one. This gradual increase in temperature allows the client's body the time it needs to adjust so that you can eventually employ a level of heat that is optimally soothing and healing. Once the client's desired stone temperature has been established at the beginning of the massage, you can use this temperature throughout the remainder of the massage without having to reintroduce the temperature gradually each time you use a stone. However, when you have two or three stones to choose from in pile one, it is always advisable to begin with the stone of the coolest temperature of the group. This not only abides by the gradual temperature entrance guideline, but it also extends the length of time your stone pile will retain its heat.

Because stone entrance is so pervasive throughout the massage, it can and will make or break the entire experience for the client. When you pay attention to approach, timing, and temperature, you enable clients to find a level of relaxation with the stones that they might not otherwise be able to experience.

Making Body Contact with Stone and Hand Together

When massaging with the stone, make sure that the client is able to feel your hand, as well as the stone, against his or her skin (Fig. 7-11). When you hold a stone in such a way that it is the only thing making contact with the skin, a client can feel cut off from the human element of touch (Fig. 7-12). Clients report that the feeling of a hand caressing the body along with the warm stone is more soothing than the

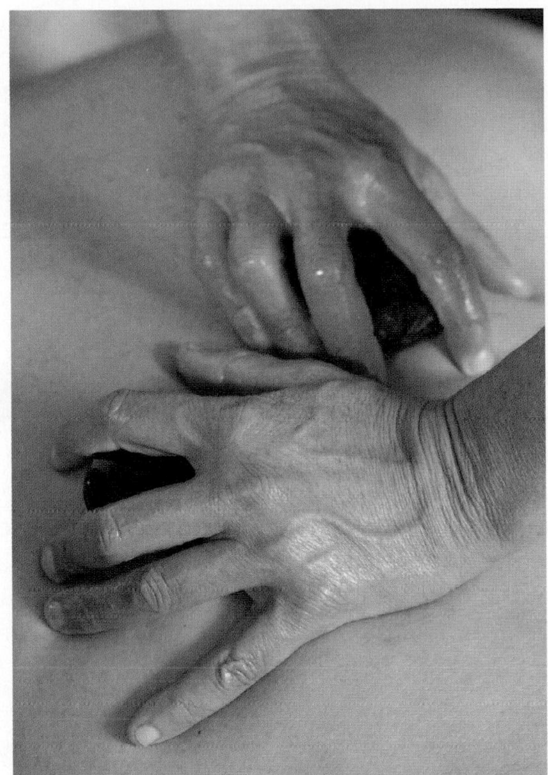

Figure 7-11 Proper Working Stone Contact. With proper contact, the hand makes contact with the body as well as the stone.

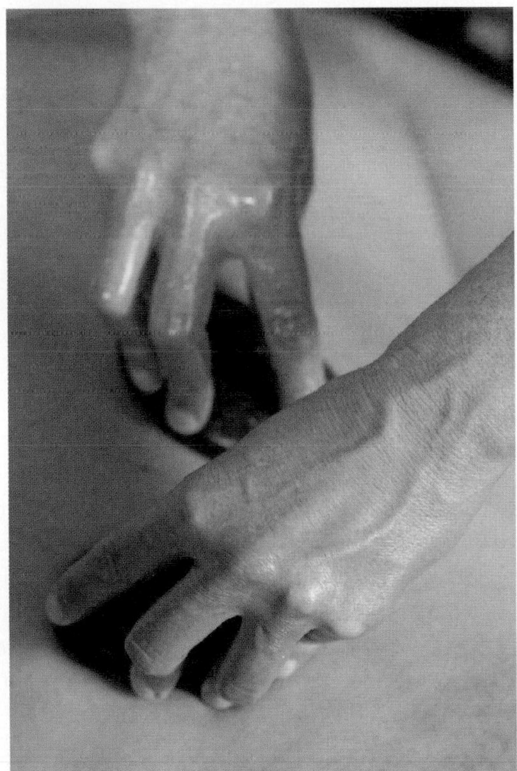

Figure 7-12 Improper Working Stone Contact. With improper contact, the stone makes contact with the body without any hand contact at all.

feeling of a stone by itself. In addition, the sensation of the therapist's hand keeps the client feeling connected to the therapist. Part of the power of a massage stems from that connection. Stones are powerful tools, but stones and touch combined are a richer combination. When your hand can make contact with the skin while maneuvering the stone against the muscle and your client can feel both hand and stone at the same time, you are using the stone correctly.

TIP

One way for you to tell if you have reached this perfect balance is if your client responds by saying, "I can't tell if that's your hand or the stone" or "Boy, your hand feels so warm." This indicates that the client is noticing the *effect* of the stone, rather than the stone itself, and you can feel confident that you're using the stone well.

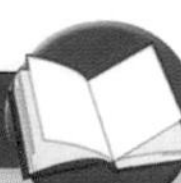

TESTIMONIAL

A client told me of a disconcerting experience she had with a hot stone massage that led her to not want one again, until she experienced the three-dimensional approach. She was at a very high-end spa and the stone therapist walked into the room wearing rubber gloves. She began setting the stones up for the massage wearing the gloves. My client said she was expecting her to remove the gloves, but instead she began massaging with the stones still wearing them! Finally, she asked the therapist if she was planning on removing the gloves and, to her amazement and horror, the therapist said that she always wears gloves throughout a hot stone massage to prevent burning her hands, but there was no reason for concern because her hands would never be making contact with the client's skin, only the stones would. She apparently stated this with enthusiasm, as if having contact with the stones alone was preferable to hands or any combination of the two. Needless to say, this was a very sterile experience for my client, turning her off to hot stone massage—for good reason!

There are a few times when it is appropriate to use a stone by itself, for instance, as a tool to work a trigger point or to accomplish a particular technique, as shown in Figure 7-13 (explained in detail in Chapter 8). As noted previously, you should use hands alone at the beginning of and during the massage to accurately diagnose and treat a muscle, as well as to provide the full human contact that is so essential. But the majority of the time, the stone and hand will be working together as a team, relying on the perfect fit for their optimal contact. This approach of making contact with the hand and stone together ensures that the benefits and pleasures of both a regular and hot stone massage are achieved.

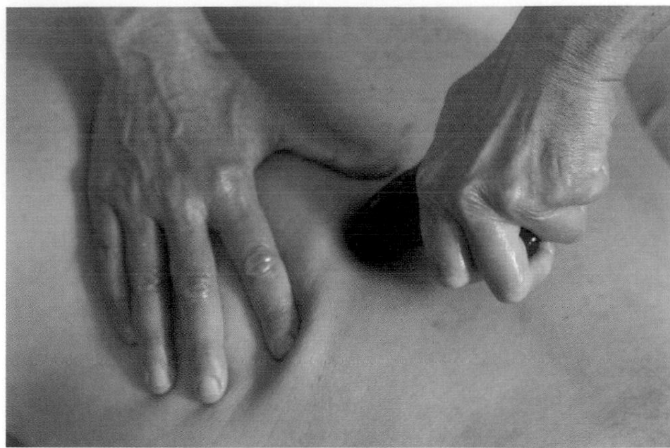

Figure 7-13 Proper Tool Stone Contact. With a tool stone, it's appropriate to have only the stone touch the body.

TESTIMONIAL

When clients tell me they're not interested in a hot stone massage, I ask them why. Often they tell me, "I want hands, not stones, to massage me." After I explain that my particular style of hot stone massage provides for contact with both hands and stones, they are usually willing to try one session, after which they almost always become happy converts.

Speed with Which to Move Stones

The speed with which you move a stone along the client's body depends on the temperature of the stone, the quality and size of the area of the body being massaged, and the purpose and intention of the stroke. Moving a stone either too slow or too fast could disturb or even injure the client. Here are some guidelines for using stones at the most effective speed.

Based on Temperature

When a stone is extremely hot, you need to move it swiftly along the skin to spread out its heat. When you move a hot stone quickly along a muscle, it remains in contact with each particular area for less than a second; thus, the heat is more widely distributed and less concentrated. If you move it too slowly, too much heat will penetrate a given area, and the sensation will quickly become intolerable to the client.

As the stone begins to cool, you need to slow down the speed at which you move it so that the client can still perceive the heat from the stone. At a slower speed, the heat remains longer in each given area; thus, the client experiences the stone as hotter than if it were to be moved more quickly. If a stone that has lost much of its heat is moved too rapidly over an area, the client will not perceive it as warm. This is why it is very important to move at the speed that matches the particular temperature of each stone.

After gradually introducing the stones at increasing temperatures, use the hottest stone you feel the client and your own hands can tolerate, moving it swiftly in long strokes to allow the heat to dissipate. Then, as it begins to cool, slow down your pace until, eventually, you are almost holding the stone still over the area. This progression allows for a longer period of uninterrupted stone use than is possible by using a stone of a lesser temperature from the start.

Based on Quality and Size of Area

Generally speaking, the tighter the area of the body, the slower you should work with the stones. When working on a tight, tense muscle, slow down the speed of stone movement to give the tissue a chance to soften. If an area feels loose and very open, you can speed up the movement of the stones.

That said, the size of the body part should also influence the speed at which you work. Over larger areas of the body, such as the back, arms, and legs, you can move the stone more quickly. Over smaller areas, such as the face, neck, and feet, you should move more slowly. This makes common sense: When there is less room, you have to slow down. It also means that you can use hotter stones on larger areas of the body where you're able to move the stones quickly and cooler stones on smaller areas of the body where speed of movement is limited.

As an example, if a large body part has a lot of tension in it, I will work quickly at first, gliding a hot stone in long broad strokes. As the stone cools down, I will hone in on the smaller, more specific areas of tension within the large body part. This method takes into account the size of the area, the temperature of the stone, and the tension in the muscle, which are all important factors involved in determining the speed at which a stone should be moved.

Based on Purpose and Intention

Your intention for your work in a particular area should also influence the speed at which you move the stones. If your intention with a particular stroke is to lengthen, invigorate, break up, or bring new blood and oxygen to a muscle, use quick strokes, either short or long. If your intention is to soften tissues, coax a muscle into opening, relax the client, or be sensitive to a client's tender emotions, slow down your stone movement. Varying speeds appropriately makes for a fulfilling massage, one in which the rhythm is tailored to the needs of the client's body and soul.

Flipping the Stones

Because it is desirable to get as much heat, thus time, out of each stone as possible, it is more advantageous to use a stone as hot as possible (once you've worked up to a high temperature) rather than simply waiting for it to cool down before using it. When a stone is too hot for you to hold it in your hand for more than a few seconds, but not too hot for you to pick it up, you can begin to use it by employing a technique called **stone flipping.**

Before learning the technique, it might be helpful to understand the principle behind it. The client's body absorbs the heat from the underside of the stone as it glides along. This quickly makes the underside of the stone cooler than the side facing your hand. You can take advantage of this variation in the rate of cooling by flipping the stone. Start by making one long, quick glide down the client's body with the hot stone. Within seconds, the stone will be too hot for you to hold. At this moment, flip it over so that the cooler side is now facing up against your hand and the warmer side is against the client's body. Again, glide the new side of the stone quickly along the surface of the body, cooling it off slightly before flipping it again. Use this flipping technique as many times as necessary until you can work with the stone comfortably held in your hand.

Remember that as the stone cools off, you'll need to slow down its movement so that the client can feel its heat as it passes over the muscles. However, you can still flip the stone as it begins to cool down. Applying the principle that the side of the stone that is away from the body is always a bit warmer, flip the stone to extend the amount of time the client can feel its heat.

Using Pressure with Stones

One of the chief complaints I hear from clients who have had negative experiences with hot stone massage is that they feel they had to sacrifice depth for heat. That is, their massage therapist, perhaps afraid of injuring them with the stones, backed off on the amount of pressure and depth used. Although many therapists apparently assume that because the stones are hard they should not drop in as much, the exact opposite is true.

When a stone is appropriately hot, its hardness is not perceptible. In fact, its heat enables you to drop quite deeply into a muscle without causing the client pain. If you avoid pressure when using stones, your clients will have a very superficial and boring experience.

TIP

When using hot stones, think of them as extensions of your hands and give the same amount of pressure, depth, and specificity as you would if you were massaging with hands alone. Before doing so, however, make sure that the stones are truly hot: Stones that have cooled off are experienced as hard, so you should avoid deep pressure with them.

CAUTION

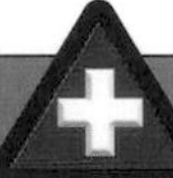

Never use deep pressure with stones in situations that call for avoiding deep pressure with hands.

CAUTION

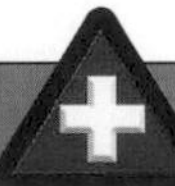

A hot stone does not feel hard, but a cool stone does. When applying pressure with stones, be sure that the pressure is suitable for the temperature of the stone. Also remember that even though a hot stone does not feel hard to the client, it is in reality much harder than the hand, so use it with caution, especially around bony protuberances. While it is important to give depth in a hot stone massage, it is just as important to avoid injuring your client by overdoing it!

SAFETY GUIDELINES

As wonderful as the application of hot stones is when done properly, there are pitfalls to avoid. Some of them are inevitable and some will occur in the process of learning how to perform a hot stone massage. But over time, it is possible to avoid most of these potential problems. Until that happens, however, there is an important rule of thumb that must be followed: When therapists hurt themselves by either picking up a stone that is too hot or dropping a stone on their feet, it is imperative that they do not yell "Ow!" out loud. I know this may sound silly, but imagine how much confidence it instills in clients receiving a hot stone massage when their therapists are hurting themselves! I learned this the hard way when after exclaiming "Ouch, I burned myself!", my client said "You know, I think I'll just have a regular massage after all." I didn't blame her, and after that, I withheld all of my exclamations until eventually there was no more need to exclaim as my proficiency level had improved. Common errors to avoid are described in the following sections.

Burning Self or Client

It is rare for a therapist or a client to experience burns during a professional hot stone massage, but it can happen, especially in the learning phase. Precautions must be taken to avoid burns from happening. Over time, as therapists gain experience in their techniques and greater familiarity with the way in which stones receive and release heat, there will be little chance of burning.

While learning how to give a hot stone massage, these are the ways a burn might occur. Using a stone that is too hot can burn a client's skin as well as the hands of the therapist. Not using enough oil on the stone or on the body part will keep the stone from gliding and thus increase the chances of producing a burn. Leaving hot stones in place on clients' bodies after they have indicated that it is too hot, forgetting to keep a hot stone moving while talking, or leaving a stone on the massage table too close to the clients' bare skin can all create a burn. Reaching into the hot water with a hand rather than a spoon can cause burns for the therapists. Dropping a stone into the cooker and splashing hot water can also cause burns for both the clients and therapists.

It is critical that therapists learn proper stone temperatures and stone handling to avoid these problems. Although the "learning" burns tend to be minor, they have a major impact on clients' experience. It is best to begin professional use of hot stones only after enough practice has taken place to eliminate these possible burns.

There are many easy ways to avoid burns. Therapists need to get very familiar with the proper temperatures to use with both the working and placement stones (discussed in Chapter 6). If a stone is too hot for the therapist to hold for 3 seconds, it is too hot to use without flipping. Practicing using different stone temperatures on people with different tolerances to heat will help therapists get a good sense of what is too hot to use on the average person. Working up to higher temperatures rather than starting with the hottest stone and checking in with clients every time a higher level of temperature is introduced will also minimize the chance of burning clients.

Therapists need to avoid picking up stones with their hands from the cooker or immediately after they have come out of the cooker. Therapists need to use enough oil so the hot stones will glide properly, attend to the clients' needs immediately when they say a stone is too hot, pay attention to the stones in their hands when they are talking to the clients, place the hot stones that are on the massage table away from the clients' skin, and return the stones gently into the cooker to avoid splashing. If all of these details are attended to, no one will get burned.

Hurting Self or Client

Both client and therapist can incur injuries when therapists drop stones. To avoid such occurrences, therapists should work slowly, carry only one stone at a time in each hand, always walk around the client to return stones to the skillet, and never reach over a client's face with a stone. Stones may still fall to the ground from time to time, and therapists need to be prepared for this eventuality and learn to avoid being hit by them as they fall. But there is a big difference between dropping a stone on the ground and dropping a stone on a client's face! Stones are hard, and care must be taken not to drop them on clients or therapists.

Because of their warmth, the hardness of the stones gets masked when massaging with them. Working too long with a stone as it cools can feel uncomfortable for the client and also may produce abrasions a therapist may not immediately recognize. The best way to avoid this is to stop working with a stone as soon as its temperature has dropped significantly. It is better to get a new stone than to work too long with a tepid one. A hot stone loses its soothing, relaxing effect as it cools, becoming increasingly boring, hard, and annoying. When stones are used too long after their heat has subsided, it is no longer a hot stone massage but a hard stone massage! Therapists need to remember that stones are hard and they should not go too deep or hit bony protuberances with them.

Shocking Client

The sudden abrupt application of a hot stone can be shocking for clients. To avoid this, therapists should introduce stones in a gradual fashion, beginning with the edge of the stone and moving into the full surface of it. It is important that the hands make contact with the skin at the same time as the stone. Finally, therapists should begin with stones that are not quite as hot as the others being used and then gradually introduce increasingly hotter stones, giving the body time to adjust. Therapists should always be sure that they precede the introduction of a cold stone with a warm one, weaving the cold stone in on the heels of the warm stone, while simultaneously warning the client. Shocking the system with a stone that is too hot, too abruptly placed, or too cold will ruin the experience of the massage, and it may even have medical consequences depending on the state of the client's health.

Overheating Client

Because the stones are warm, the massage room can tend to get a bit hot or stuffy. The amount of heat experienced from the combination of both placement and working stones accumulates over time, and it may require cooling off the client and the room. Sometimes a client will suddenly feel flush and realize that they are overheating. Other times, a woman may have a "hot flash," making the heat from the stones suddenly intolerable. Should either of these situations happen, the placement stones should be removed immediately, and the room should be ventilated with either a fan or an open window. If more cooling is required, the sheet should be replaced with a small towel over the pelvic and chest region. If more action is still required, use some cold stones to help cool off the client even further. Checking with the client periodically throughout the session about comfort and keeping some ventilation in the room can remedy such complications before they can occur.

Creating Lightheadedness

After a hot stone massage, especially if the client already has low blood pressure, a feeling of wooziness or lightheadedness can be experienced when getting up. Activities such as walking and driving should be delayed until the therapist is convinced that the client is able to safely drive or walk. If dizziness occurs, the therapist can help alleviate the situation by using cold stones on the face. Breathing and eye contact exercises along with a cold drink of water can help undo some of the feelings of lightheadedness. If it is necessary to delay the departure of a client, the therapist should never hesitate to insist upon it.

SUMMARY

Proper management of the stones transforms a mediocre hot stone massage into a superb one. The four-pile system makes it possible for optimal stone flow and allows you to spend more time with your client than your stones. Pile one goes on the massage table closest to where you will begin the massage, pile two goes on top of the client, pile three goes in front of the skillet on the stone table, and pile four remains in the skillet on the right side. The piles are made in increasing gradients of temperature so that they will still have heat in them by the time you reach the last pile. Always push the remaining stones in the skillet to the right and return cool stones to the left side of the skillet so you can know where the hottest and coolest stones are to be found. This system of stone management makes it so you do not have to leave the client every few minutes to retrieve a new stone from the skillet.

Hot stone massage necessitates the use of oil versus cream or other lubricants as oil spreads quickly and evenly over the stones and does not interfere with the seamless flow. Place several small bowls of oil around the massage room so that you can easily dip your fingers in for oiling your hands. This is a much faster and fluid way to retrieve oil. Once your hands are oiled, slide them across the top of the hot stones in piles one and two on the way to the client's body. This easy step does not interrupt the flow of the massage and makes it so the stones are ready for use. Not having to stop and oil each stone just before you use it adds to the seamless flow of the massage.

Always massage without stones for a few minutes before introducing them so that you can make a connection with the client and assess the state of the muscles. Find the correct ratio of stones to hands that is appropriate for each client. When ready to introduce the stones into the massage, do so gradually, making initial contact with your finger tips, then the edge of the stone, and then the entire stone. Begin with a tepid stone and gradually increase the temperature of the stones until you find the appropriate temperature for each client. After replenishing the piles, massage once again with hands rather than stones so that the arrival of the stones is unpredictable and not related to their retrieval.

The stone should fit in the center of your palm so that your fingers can curl slightly around its edges. When making contact with the client's body, your fingers should be able to massage the skin along with the stone. Move the stone quickly along the skin when a stone is hot or when the area you are working on is large or supple. On the contrary, move the stone slowly along the skin when the stone is not as hot or when the area you are working on is small or tense. Move the stone with quick strokes when your purpose is to create invigoration or break up a stagnant area of the body. Use slow strokes when your intention is to relax a muscle, open a muscle, or connect with the client on a deeper level. Flip the stone if it is too hot to comfortably hold in your hand. Don't let the hardness of the stone fool you into thinking you should forgo deep pressure. Work as deeply with the stones as you would normally with your hands.

Take care not to burn or hurt yourself or your client by splashing hot water, reaching into the skillet with your fingers, dropping a stone on your client or self, or not using enough oil to make a stone glide properly. Be careful not to shock a client with improper entrance or temperature, or by forgetting to warn the client before the arrival of a cold stone. Do not overheat a client by using too many hot stones or not enough ventilation. Be sure that your client is not too lightheaded by the end of the massage and is completely ready to drive before leaving the massage.

REVIEW QUESTIONS

TRUE/FALSE

1. Adding a stone management system takes no practice and will be easy to incorporate right away.

   Circle: True False

2. The stone management system includes a three-pile system.

   Circle: True False

3. Pile two is located on the massage table and is the second pile to use.

   Circle: True False

4. Pile one is the hottest pile of all.

   Circle: True False

5. Pile three is also called "waiting in the wings" and is the third hottest.

   Circle: True False

6. Pile four always gets pushed to the left side of the skillet before resuming the massage.

   Circle: True False

7. It's key to put stones from pile number two on the client before placing pile number one on the massage table.

   Circle: True False

8. After pile one is used, therapists should immediately get more stones from the skillet.

   Circle: True False

9. After pile one is used, therapists should use stones from pile two.

   Circle: True False

10. Stones are always laid out with hottest ones on the left and coolest ones on the right.

    Circle: True False

MULTIPLE CHOICE

11. The order of oiling is:
    a. Hands / stones / body
    b. Hands / body / stones
    c. Body / hands / stones
    d. Feet / hands / stones
    e. None of the above
12. For effective stone entrance one needs to:
    a. Enter with whole stone
    b. Buffer edge with fingers
    c. Enter with edge of stone
    d. Both b and c
    e. None of the above
13. The first stone that is introduced to the skin should be:
    a. Equally as hot as the others
    b. Hotter than the others
    c. Cool
    d. Tepid
    c. None of the above
14. Therapists need to be careful not to:
    a. Say "ouch" if they burn themselves
    b. Splash hot water on client or self
    c. Use a slotted spoon to remove the stones from skillet
    d. Both a and b
    e. All of the above
15. If a client is feeling lightheaded during or after the massage, therapists should:
    a. Use ice cold stones all over client's body
    b. Stop the massage
    c. Use less stones and less temperature
    d. Be sure client is safe to drive before leaving
    e. Both c and d

SHORT ANSWER

16. Once the therapist becomes adept at the pile system, the recommended amounts for each pile are: Pile One ______ Pile Two ______ Pile Three ______ Pile Four ______.
17. Stone should always be returned to the __________ side of the skillet.
18. The last thing therapist needs to do after creating piles but before resuming the massage is to ____ ______.
19. If a client requires tending to in a way that would interrupt the flow of the stone management system, a therapist should ________________________.
20. Therapist should massage the client with _________ first before using ___________.

Answers to Review Questions can be found in Appendix D.

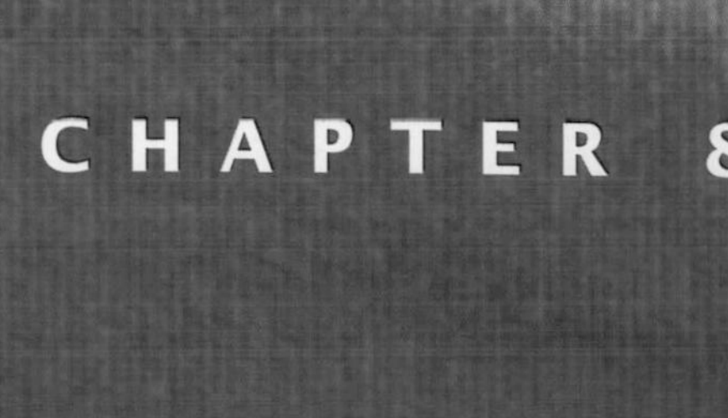

CHAPTER 8

Principles of Three-Dimensional Hot Stone Massage

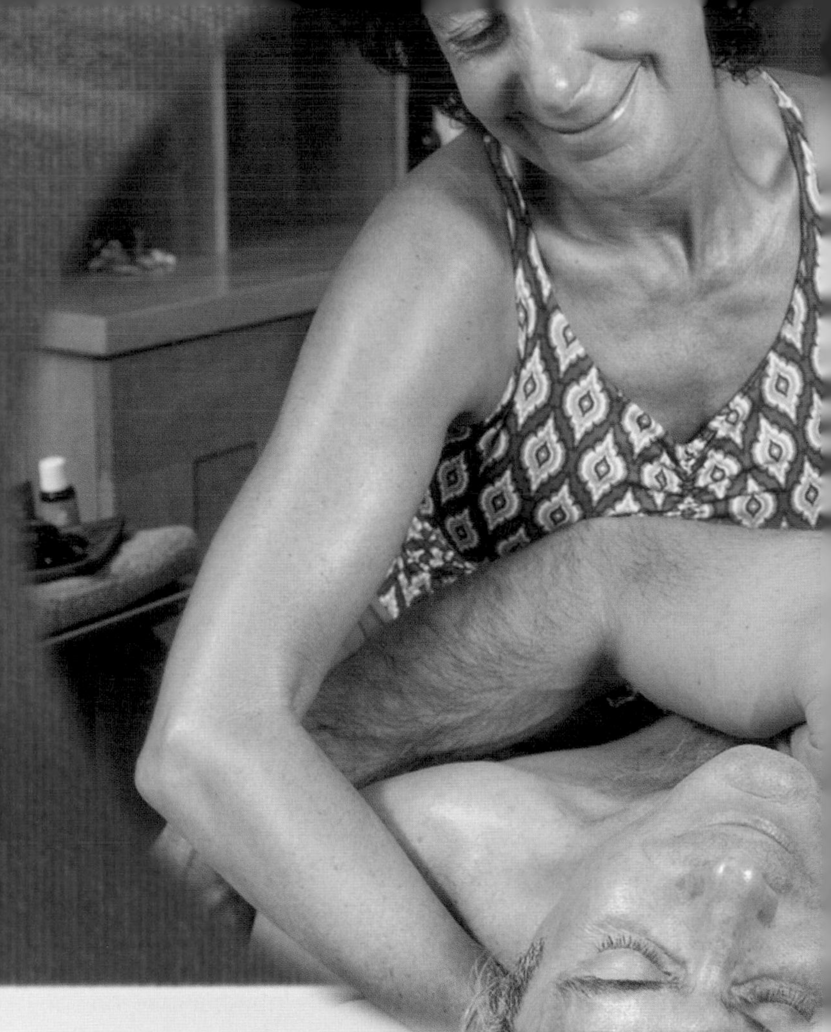

Outline

Be Fully Present

Create a Constant Flow
- Overlap Hands and Stones
- Make Seamless Transitions between Body Parts

Touch in Specific Ways That Encourage the Tissues to Soften
- Work with Shortened Muscles
  - *Anatomical Shortening*
  - *Manual Shortening*
- Honor the "Speed Limit" of Every Part of the Body
- Utilize Opposition and Resistance
  - *Opposition*
  - *Resistance*

Work Three-Dimensionally
- Embrace
- Move the Body in Space
- Undulate
- Be the Wave

Utilize Effective Body Mechanics
- Use a Staggered Stance
- Make Feet Mimic Hands
- Lean against the Massage Table
- Use Gravity
- Lift from the Joints
- Use Body Levers and Fulcrums
- Stay with Your Move
- Use Your Momentum
- Apply Pressure Effectively
  - *Use Your Weight*
  - *Drop in Vertically*
  - *Use Client's Weight*
- Protect Your Joints

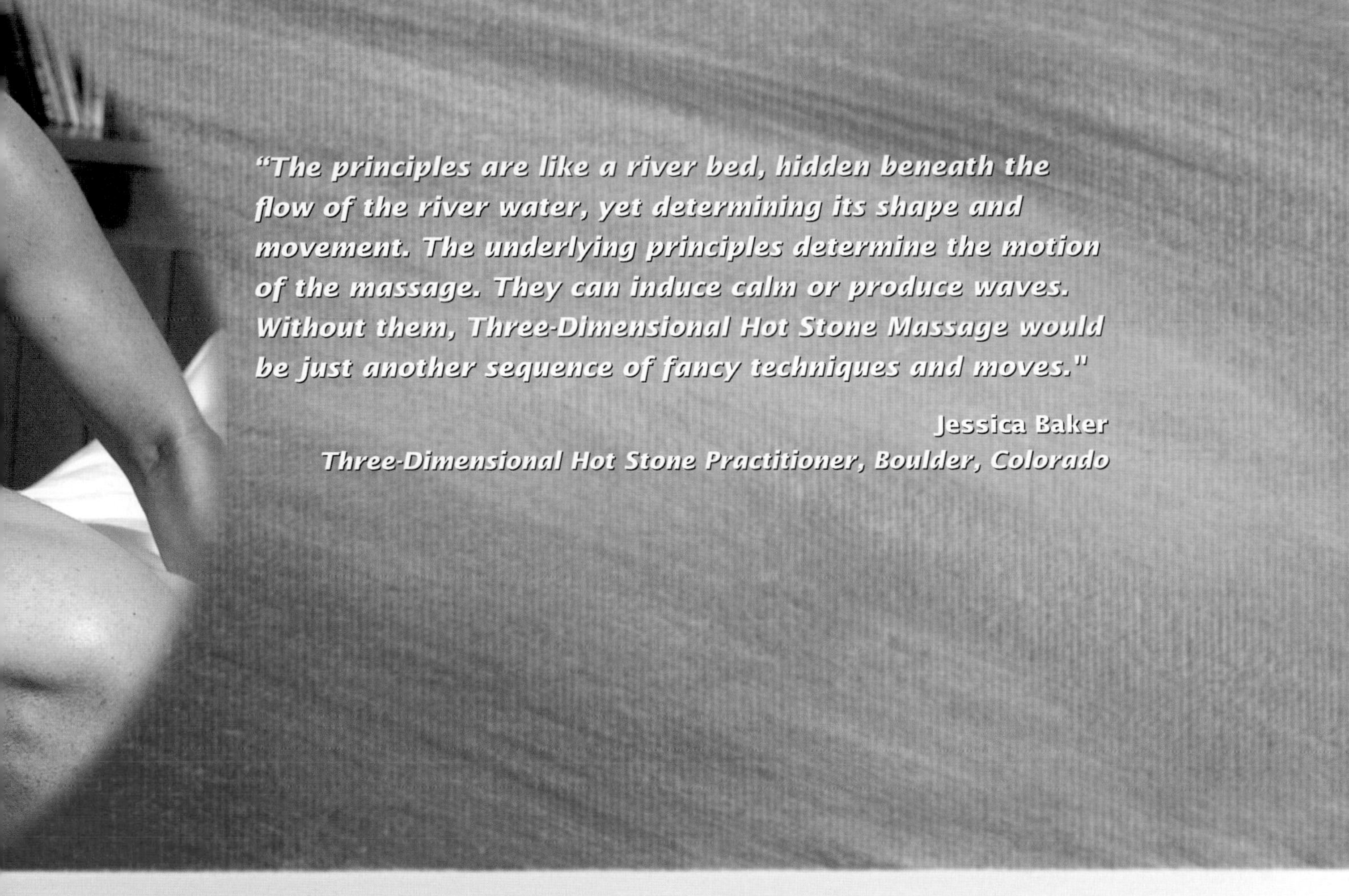

Objectives

After reading this chapter, you should be able to:

- Explain the importance of being fully present in a hot stone massage.
- Identify several principles discussed in this chapter that help tissues to soften.
- Compare and contrast active and passive resistance.
- Demonstrate three aspects of three-dimensional massage: embracing, moving the body in space, and being the wave.
- Demonstrate healthful and efficient body mechanics for providing hot stone massage.
- Describe ways for applying pressure without hurting yourself or your client.

Key Terms

Carpal tunnel syndrome: A type of entrapment neuropathy in which the median nerve, which runs through a narrow tunnel formed by ligament and carpal bones at the base of the hand, is compressed by inflammation of the nearby tendons and surrounding tendon sheath. This inflammation is typically due to chronic repetitive stress, such as working with the wrist in a bent position.

Embracing: Technique for encompassing and massaging both sides of the client's body simultaneously.

Fulcrum: The point at which a lever's force is transmitted to a weight.

Lever: A rigid object, such as a metal bar or long bone, fixed to a stationary fulcrum and used to lift a weight.

Mother–father technique: Massage technique used to shorten muscle fibers in an area of the body that cannot be anatomically moved into its short position. The "father" hand uses the thumb or a stone to penetrate the muscle while the "mother" hand pushes the tissue towards the father hand. The term originated with massage therapist Grant Freeman of Crestone, Colorado.

(Continued)

Key Terms

Opposition: The movement of opposite ends of a muscle or body part further away from each other, which lengthens and (when released) softens the tissue.

Phenomenal Touch Massage: Massage modality created by the author from which the three-dimensional principles and moves (used in this book) are derived.

Resistance: Tension created when a muscle opposes pressure. This tires and thereby relaxes the muscle.

Undulation: A wavelike rippling motion created by moving the client's body in a gravitational dance.

This chapter covers some of the essential principles that underlie an extraordinary hot stone massage. No matter how wonderful stones are or how expertly you handle them, if you don't adhere to these foundational principles of touch, the overall quality of the hot stone massages you give will be greatly diminished. The principles include the following:

- Be fully present
- Create a constant flow
- Touch in specific ways that encourage the tissues to soften
- Work three-dimensionally
- Utilize effective body mechanics

If you were to learn the moves and techniques covered in Chapter 9 without these underlying principles, they would not unfold from their source, but rather from rote directions and memory. In contrast, if you were to learn only these principles, and worked from them consistently, a set of effective moves and techniques would be born from them. In short, these principles are the basis of artful touch. They contribute to the extraordinary nature of this work.

BE FULLY PRESENT

Presence encompasses and underlies all the principles included in this book. Without presence, the rest of the principles are rendered virtually ineffective. Without presence, you cannot authentically meet your client. You cannot know the type of contact, pressure, speed, and direction of movement that the client requires. Most importantly, without presence, you cannot transmit the most essential ingredient for healing and transformation, which is love.

Being present means bringing all of your self to the massage, clearing your mind of clutter and your own agenda, staying completely focused, paying full attention, and bringing your entire (selfless) awareness to your client.

Being fully present with your client requires some preparation. Before your client arrives, begin clearing your mind. As thoughts arise, acknowledge them, and then set them aside until your mind is calm and there is space within it. From the moment the client arrives, pay attention. Notice any changes in the client from the last time you worked with him or her, or if this is a new client, try to sense his or her expectations and any unspoken needs. Watch the way in which the client moves and holds his or her body.

Maintain this same attention throughout the massage. When you notice that your mind has strayed, bring it gently back to the present moment. Watch the way the client breathes, notice the direction the tissue wants to be moved, tune in to the speed at which a muscle wants to be touched, and feel the way your body needs to move to best support the area where you are working. Notice the effect your words have on a client. If what you say causes the client's body to tighten, change your words or intonation. Value the client's body language more than the client's words. If a client says your pressure is fine, yet the body withdraws or tightens, pay attention to that. The body never lies.

Listen deeply and follow the client's unspoken needs. Attend to or revisit an area that may be asking for work, even if it is not "next in line." Find the rhythm of each massage. Is the body asking for long strokes, deep specific point work, or stillness? While it is essential to check in with your client from time to time, don't rely on that for all your information. If you have to ask, you may not be paying enough attention. Being fully present allows you to truly meet the client. Presence invites all of the other principles to emerge organically. Where there is presence, there is the possibility for reverence and love.

CREATE A CONSTANT FLOW

Not only do you want to create a seamless flow with the integration of the stones, but you also want to do the same with your hands and with the transitions between each stroke. Proper entrance with your hands is just as important as it is with the stones. Rather than placing your hand down all at once, as with a stone, you enter gradually, with the edge of your hand or your fingers first and then allow the rest of your hand and body weight to follow. Even though this "gradual" entrance occurs very quickly and thus might appear to be trivial, it is imperative to follow this procedure, or otherwise your hand entrance will feel very abrupt to the client.

As important as hand entrance is, there are also additional aspects required for creating a flow. Overlapping your hands and making a seamless transition from one body part to the next are imperative for creating the integrative dancelike quality of the massage.

> **TIP**
>
> It is important to note that to create a constant flow, it does not mean that you must keep your hands in contact with the client's body at all times. As explained previously, to manage the stones, you must break physical contact with the client throughout the massage. However, when you are in physical contact with the client, it is critical to overlap your hands and make seamless transitions to create a constant dancelike flow throughout the time that you are massaging.

Overlap Hands and Stones

To overlap hands and stones, you need to introduce the next hand or stone before removing the hand or stone that is presently on the body (Fig. 8-1). In other words, begin the next movement within a stroke before finishing the previous one. This overlapping of hands and stones creates a continuity of touch that makes it feel like one long movement within each stroke instead of a multitude of breaks. This continuity of touch magnifies the calming effect and helps the client drop into an even deeper state of relaxation.

Make Seamless Transitions between Body Parts

In addition to overlapping your hands within each stroke, you also want to overlap each part of the client's body throughout the massage. This is accomplished by using transition strokes that tie the last body part you worked on into the next. For example, when you are done massaging the head and neck, rather than walking over to the arm and beginning again with the arm, instead, from the head, you can slide your arm under the client's neck and move your body to the client's arm while you are still under the neck. Then, allow your arm to slide from the neck to the shoulder and then down the arm. Another possibility for seamless transition could happen while moving from the leg to the abdomen. Before your arm leaves the upper thigh, bring your other hand onto the abdomen and begin massaging there while still working on the leg, as shown in Figure 8-2. Then, slowly let your hand on the leg slide up to join the other hand on the abdomen.

Contact is never broken during the transition between the two body parts. Seamless transitions can be made between every two parts of the body, both as you move sequentially along the body and when you move out of order revisiting areas requiring more attention. Seamless transitions create such a sense of continuity and integration of the body parts that the client tends to lose track of what part you're working on. Indeed, clients have told me, "It feels as if you are massaging everywhere all the time!" This principle truly helps to calm the controlling mind and create a

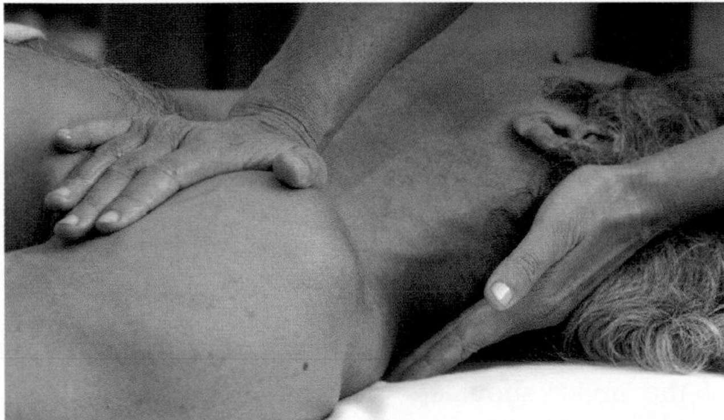

Figure 8-1 Overlapping. Before one hand or stone is removed from the body, the next one slides in creating a sense of overlapping.

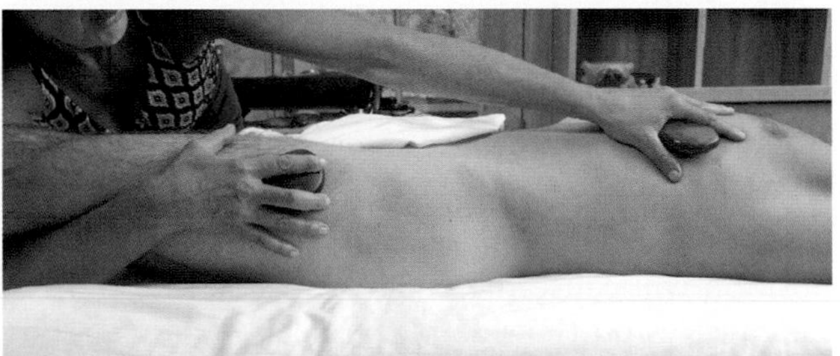

Figure 8-2 Seamless Transition. One hand transitions to the next body part before the first hand has left the body part it is working on, creating an uninterrupted flow.

sensation of one long flowing stroke throughout the massage.

TOUCH IN SPECIFIC WAYS THAT ENCOURAGE THE TISSUES TO SOFTEN

The way in which you touch will affect your client more than the actual strokes or stones that you use. The type of touch described here encourages the body's tissues to soften and allows the client to let go. When you follow these principles of touch, the client will be able to receive deep pressure comfortably and relax into the pressure rather than resist it. These are some of the secrets that allow the tissue to welcome deep penetration and release with ease.

Work with Shortened Muscles

It is much easier to enter and soften a muscle when it is in its shortened state, rather than its elongated state. The shortened position provides more space and thus access to the tissue, whereas the elongated position lengthens a muscle that is already tight increasing the challenge of penetration into the tissue. If instead you move the muscle, either anatomically or manually, into its shortened position, you'll be able to soften the tissue and achieve deep penetration without creating pain or resistance for the client.

Anatomical Shortening

You can shorten most muscles anatomically by bringing the associated joint into its flexed position. This makes the muscle shorter and softer. For instance, when the client is prone, you can bring the calf towards the buttocks to shorten and thus loosen the hamstring muscle. With the client supine, you can bring the hand toward the shoulder, shortening and thus softening the bicep muscles for easier and less painful penetration.

A common mistake many therapists make when working the neck is to work it in the open, outstretched, elongated position. Although this position offers better access to the muscles, it also elongates them, making them too taut to enter. This position is acceptable for broad, gentle, caressing strokes, but working with any kind of specificity or depth in this position will cause the client pain. Instead, shorten the muscles on the side of the neck by bringing the head toward the shoulder (on the side you are working), as shown in Figure 8-3. This creates more space in the muscle. Now, with the neck in this position, you can easily create deep specific pressure in the neck. When this is done properly, clients are pleasantly surprised to discover that deep pressure does not have to induce pain to be effective. In fact, it's more effective when it is painless.

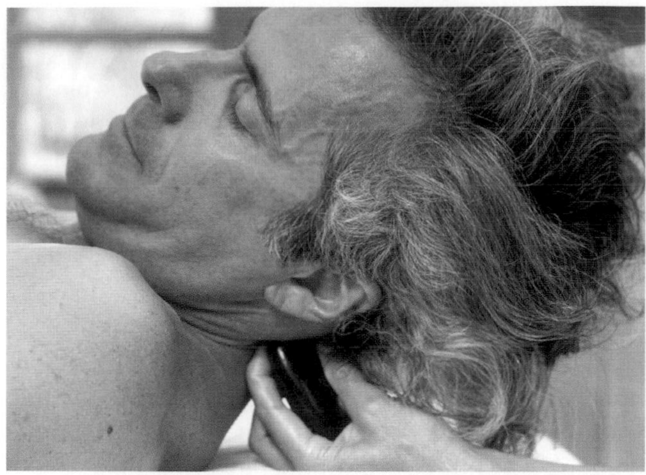

Figure 8-3 Anatomical Shortening. Shorten the neck by bringing it toward the shoulder on the side you are working. This softens the neck muscles and makes penetration much more easy and painless to accomplish.

TIP 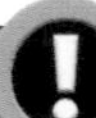

Try this yourself! First try the ineffective way. Turn your neck all the way to the right and then with your left hand, using either fingers or thumb, locate a spot (on the left side of the neck) that is tight. Now, with your neck in this extended position, begin massaging specific spots as deeply as you can. Notice how much pain is involved and how difficult it is to find an entrance into the taut muscles. Now, try the new way. Hold a spot on the left side of your neck and allow your neck to fall slowly over your hand towards the left side. Try massaging your neck in this position. Notice how much more space there is to deeply penetrate your neck muscles and how much less pain is involved. This is true for every part of the body.

Manual Shortening

You cannot easily move certain muscles, such as those of the upper shoulders, forearm, buttocks, iliotibial band, or back, into an anatomically shortened position. Instead, shorten these muscles manually by using the

mother–father technique. The father hand is the one that works specifically and deeply, whereas the mother hand pushes the tissue towards the father, creating a shortening effect ("snowdrift") around the area of penetration. The mother hand is used in a broad fashion, offering support to the father hand. The mother–father technique shortens the muscle very specifically in one area, softening the once taut tissue and allowing the stone or thumb to penetrate with ease.

To perform the mother–father technique, begin with your two hands approximately 3 inches apart from each other. To accomplish this without stones, spread the fingers of the father hand out on the client's body for support, set the knuckle of the thumb (by drawing it in) and plant the thumb on the spot you intend to penetrate. To perform this technique with a stone, wrap the fingers of the father hand around the stone. Place the mother hand (either with or without a stone) in a palm-down, outstretched, but slightly cupped pose a few inches away from the father hand. Use the outside edge or the heel of the mother hand to create your pressure. Next, while keeping the hands planted on the client's skin, move them slowly towards each other with the emphasis on the mother hand "pouring" the snowdrift of muscle towards and over the father hand, as shown in Figure 8-4. Do not just slide the hands along the skin. Instead, allow them to first push vertically into the muscle and then move the muscle itself horizontally.

Check the following aspects of your technique:

- Place the father thumb or stone in a 45-degree angle to the area of penetration.
- Use the mother hand to move the tissue toward the father hand, creating a mound of muscle that pours onto and slightly over the father hand.
- On the client's exhale, move both hands slowly toward one another (with depth) until they are approximately 1 inch apart from each other.
- On the client's inhale, release the pressure and allow the hands to slowly move away from one another (while remaining in contact with the skin).

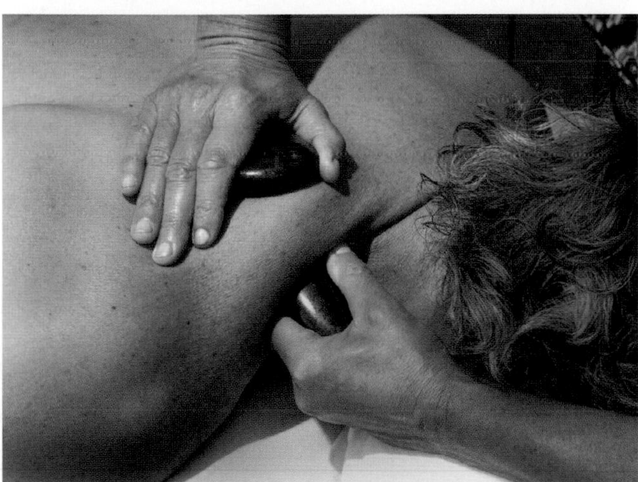

Figure 8-4 Manual Shortening. The "mother-father" technique shortens the muscle so there is more space and thus softens it to penetrate the tissue without causing pain.

CAUTION

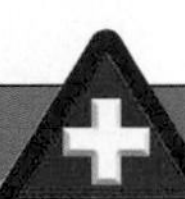

Be careful not to pinch the skin or muscle when coming close together. Be sure that your mother hand has a slight lift to it and drops the mound of muscle onto and over rather than directly into the father thumb.

Apply the accordion motion once or twice in a given spot, and then, during the client's inhale, slide the hands slightly (0.25 inches) up or down to a new spot nearby. Keep performing the technique, moving as needed, until a muscle or a particular segment of a muscle is softened.

TIP

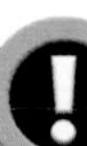

The mother and father hands can be interchangeable when you are working an area that is level; however, when the body surface is uneven, it is easier to have the mother hand higher up than the father. This allows for a larger "snowdrift."

The amount of depth and pressure you can achieve with the mother–father technique would be intolerable for a lengthened muscle. It would not permit such penetration. This extremely useful technique can be done on any part of the body that is tight, especially in areas that cannot be shortened anatomically. If a tight muscle flips out from under your fingers, or jumps into spasm when you apply deep pressure, the mother–father technique is needed. It will not only soothe the intensity of deep pressure by creating more room in the muscle, but also simultaneously "trick" the client's mind into relaxing.

TIP

Try the mother–father technique on yourself. Find a spot on your thigh or calf and press your thumb deeply and directly into an area of tension. Now, staying in that same exact spot, bring the mother hand into the equation. Create a snowdrift of muscle by pushing the surrounding muscle towards and over the place of penetration. Notice how much deeper you can go without it feeling painful or invasive. Now, while holding the same depth of penetration with your father hand, release the mother hand and see how much more painful that level of penetration is without the mother hand shortening the tissue.

Honor the "Speed Limit" of Every Part of the Body

Muscles vary in their ability to withstand work at different speeds and still remain relaxed. It is crucial to find and honor the "speed limit" of every part of the body you are working on. If you work too quickly on a tight muscle, it will jump, spasm, or flip out from beneath your hands. When this happens, avoid the temptation to continue working at the same speed and depth, or to lighten up, or go away. Instead, slow down. A tight muscle can handle deep pressure when it is given slowly. Once you slow down, if a muscle still resists, then it is appropriate to lighten up, but not until after you have first tried slowing down.

TESTIMONIAL

In workshops, I have heard many students tell the person working on them that their pressure was too deep, but after I had the student slow down, they said the pressure was perfect, even though the student had not reduced the pressure at all. I have also had clients say that the pressure and speed were perfect, but their bodies were tightening up. If this happens to you, slow down regardless of what the client says, as it is common for people to expect that they can receive more pressure than they are actually capable of.

To find the proper speed, you must pay attention to the subtle reactions of the client's body. If you are working too fast, the body will contract, but if you are working too slowly, the body will ask for faster movement. Muscles need to be met; they need to be worked in a particular direction, at a particular depth and a particular speed in order to release. It is your job as a practitioner to pay close attention to your clients' bodies and adjust your speed, depth, and direction accordingly. You need to rely on asking with words only if you are not listening carefully enough with your hands. The body will tell you all you need to know.

Utilize Opposition and Resistance

Another principle for softening tissues is to utilize opposition and resistance whenever the opportunity presents itself. There are endless creative ways to weave this principle into the massage without breaking the flow. Once you set the intention to create opposition or resistance in the client's body, opportunities will present themselves often.

Opposition

Opposition is the movement of opposite ends of a muscle or body part further away from each other. This gently stretches and lengthens the muscle, releasing tension. Opposition can be done is a subtle fashion; for example, when you hold the wrist while you effleurage up the arm to prevent jamming at the shoulder. Or it can be done in a more grandiose fashion utilizing the weight of the client's body, employing fulcrums to gain leverage, using your own body weight by leaning back (Fig. 8-5), or allowing gravity to do the work for you by lifting the client's body and letting it

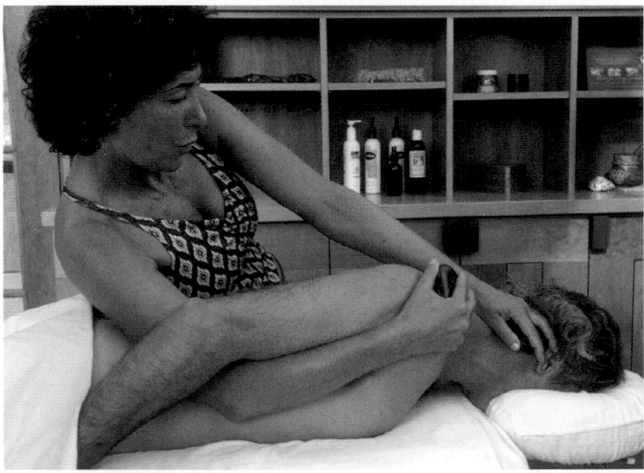

Figure 8-5 Opposition. The therapist uses her weight, rather than strength, to lean back against her hand placements and create an oppositional pull in the neck area.

hang and fall away from itself. Opposition is a gentle way to invite a muscle to let go and open up in its own time. It can be incorporated into the massage seamlessly, wherever the opportunity presents itself.

Resistance

You can also soften tissues by producing **resistance**; that is, by applying pressure that the muscle actively or passively resists. This tires and thereby relaxes the muscle. You can apply passive resistance to the client without the client's participation, or you can create active resistance by eliciting the assistance of the client.

With active resistance, you move the joint in a specific direction, and the client resists it. Active resistance works by tiring out the muscle enough that it releases its spasms or holding patterns. It is more effective than passive resistance because the movement is initiated from within the client's body, but if the client is too relaxed or simply prefers not to be interrupted during the session, passive resistance is a great alternative for certain areas of the body.

Active resistance can be applied on every part of the body that involves a joint. For instance, to loosen the hip joint push into the client's lateral thigh while the client resists you by pushing back. To release muscles around the ankle, pull down on the foot while the client pulls the toes up toward the head. To release the muscles of the forearm, have the client twist the forearm in one direction while you twist the client's hand in the other direction, and simultaneously slide your hand up the forearm. To soften the tissues of the neck, push on one side of the head while the client pushes into and against your hand. To release the muscles of the chest, push down on the client's chest on the exhale, then have the client push your hands up with the breath as you resist against it. There is no end to the openings that can be created in the body when utilizing the effective principle of active resistance.

Passive resistance is a bit more limited because, without the client's participation, you are restricted to particular parts of the body. For instance, you can't push the client's leg into your resisting hands, or the client's breath against your hands, or the client's head against your hands. On the other hand, without the participation of the client, you still can pull the forearm down with one hand as you push up on the bicep with the other, you can push down on the foot while using your other hand to push up on the front of the ankle, and you can push the client's wrist forward with one hand while you slide down the top of the forearm with the other, as shown in Figure 8-6. And you can do the opposite resistance by pushing back on the client's hand while you push down the underside of the forearm. There are also many other places that will allow for passive resistance for the client who does not want to participate in resistance activities. Use passive resistance in any way that you can. Although it may not have as dramatic an effect as active resistance does, it will still soften the tissue.

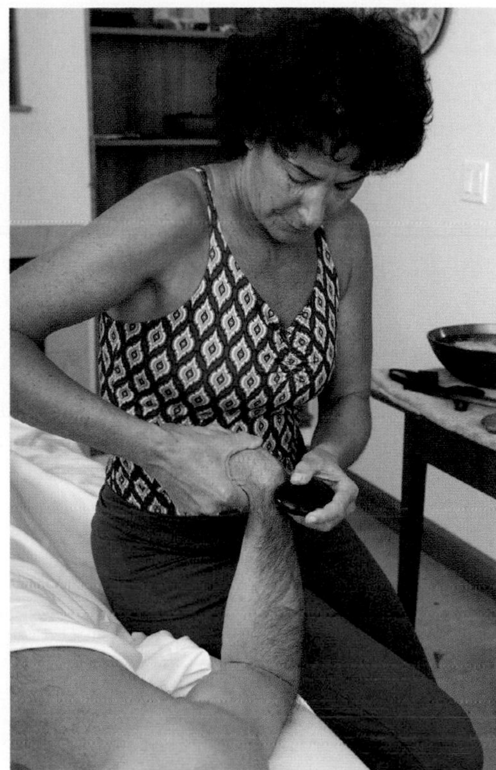

Figure 8-6 Resistance. The therapist slides her hand down the top of the client's wrist/forearm while creating passive resistance with her other hand by pushing down and away with the client's hand.

WORK THREE-DIMENSIONALLY

In a broad sense, to give a three-dimensional massage means to incorporate every principle that is stated in this chapter. But in this particular section of this chapter, we focus on a more limited aspect of three-dimensionality; that is, working both sides of the body at once and enveloping the body as the three-dimensional organism that it is. So, there is a principle of working three-dimensionally within the modality I call three-dimensional hot stone massage.

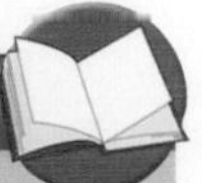

TESTIMONIAL

A 76-year-old Scandinavian client began to cry after being touched three-dimensionally for the first time. "This is the way I always dreamed of being touched," she said, "but no one ever did it, so I thought I was crazy for wanting it. Now I have finally found the massage I have been waiting for my whole life. Thank you so much." Sadly, this reaction is common. So many people long to be touched three-dimensionally, yet the technique is missing from so many massages. Follow the principles below, and it will no longer be missing from yours.

This section describes four techniques for working three-dimensionally: embracing, moving the body in space, undulating, and using your own body movement to move the client.

Embrace

Embracing is my term for massaging both sides of the client's body at once. It can be done on any and every part of the body and makes each part being worked on feel as if it is getting double the massage. When you massage the body on both sides at once, your touch creates a feeling of wholeness and connection front to back. When the body is massaged on only one side at a time, the tension in that area tends to move to the other side. For instance, when the abdomen is worked alone, its tension often flows backward, away from your hands, and lodges in the lower back. When the lower back is worked by itself, the tension often moves forward and hides in the psoas or rectus abdominus muscles. However, when the lower back is massaged at the same time as the abdomen, as shown in Figure 8-7, the tension has nowhere to go and simply dissolves.

When only one side of the body is worked at a time, the client can fixate on the tension in that area and sometimes tighten even more against the massage. Working both sides of the body part at once helps the client's mind to relax because it is too challenging to fixate on both sides of the body at the same time. The focus then becomes more internal and the area of tension rapidly melts. And even if there is no significant tension in an area, the client's body still feels more complete and met when it is embraced on both sides at once.

Embracing can be accomplished by using one hand on either side of a body part, but it is not limited to the use of your hands. You can also use your forearm, or even your leg, to achieve the effect. Or you can reach both hands around the body and embrace with your hands and forearms at the same time. No matter what part of your body you are using to embrace the client's body, it is imperative that your two body parts massage in relationship to one another and do not do their own individual dance—when one hand squeezes, the other hand releases; when one lifts the other one lifts or when one goes forward, the other may need to go backward. The two body parts you are using to embrace must listen to one another and create a synchronized dance between them, or otherwise they could create a feeling of chaos.

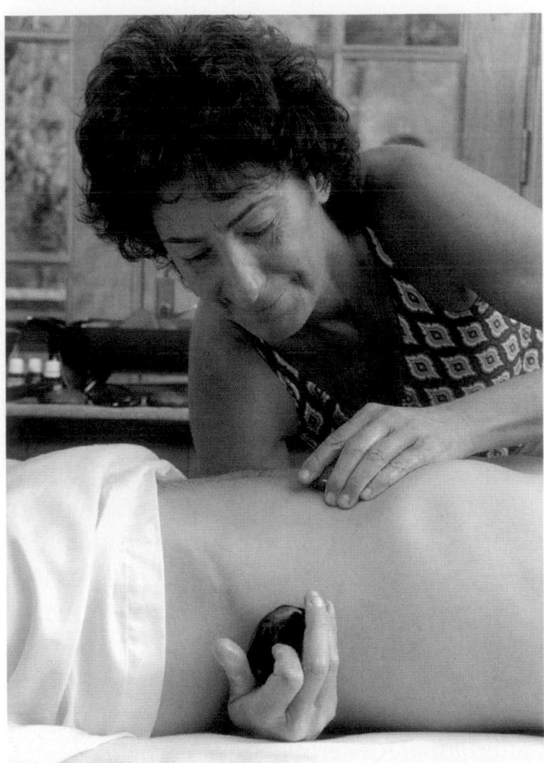

Figure 8-7 Embracing. The therapist embraces the client's torso by massaging the abdomen and low back at the same time.

TIP

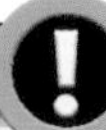

Try it on yourself. Reach down to your thigh and massage just the top of it. Now, reach one hand beneath your thigh and work both sides at the same time. Try this on your calf, your foot, and your belly with your lower back. Notice the difference when you work each area one-sided versus two-sided. Notice what it feels like when your hands are in synch with one another and when they are not. Experiment on your friends to discover all the ways you can creatively embrace both sides of their body. Then, do the same body parts one-sided. Let them report the difference to you. You will never want to work one side at a time again. It not only feels better to receive three-dimensional touch, but it is also more fun to do. Neither you nor your clients will ever get bored when you embrace their bodies.

TIP

If the images in the photographs appear to call for more intimacy than you are comfortable with, don't worry. Embracing looks much more intimate than it actually feels. When clients receive this kind of encompassing touch, they are in such a deep state that they don't realize what is occurring. Usually, they are not focusing on how close your body is to them as much as they are enthralled by the sensation of the experience. However, you must always honor both your client's and your own level of comfort with this kind of contact and if it feels too intimate for either of you, then minimize the extent of the embrace.

Move the Body in Space

The power and healing potential of your massage increases even more when you lift the embraced body part and move it in space. As three-dimensional as embracing is, it can still be done in a flat fashion. In contrast, raising the body part off the table while you embrace it frees the body's tissues deeply and assures that it is not done in a flat fashion.

Lifting the body off the table and moving it in space gives the client a sensation of freedom and vitality. Some clients get bored or fidgety lying still on a massage table for 60 or 90 minutes. Many will begin to plan their day, worry, run through their taxes, write letters, or "go to work" while being massaged in a flat fashion. But when clients' bodies are lifted off the table and moved, they suddenly get more involved in the session and return to the present moment. And yet, because they do not have to initiate any movement and are encouraged to just fall into the gravitational pull, they can remain completely relaxed, like a rag doll.

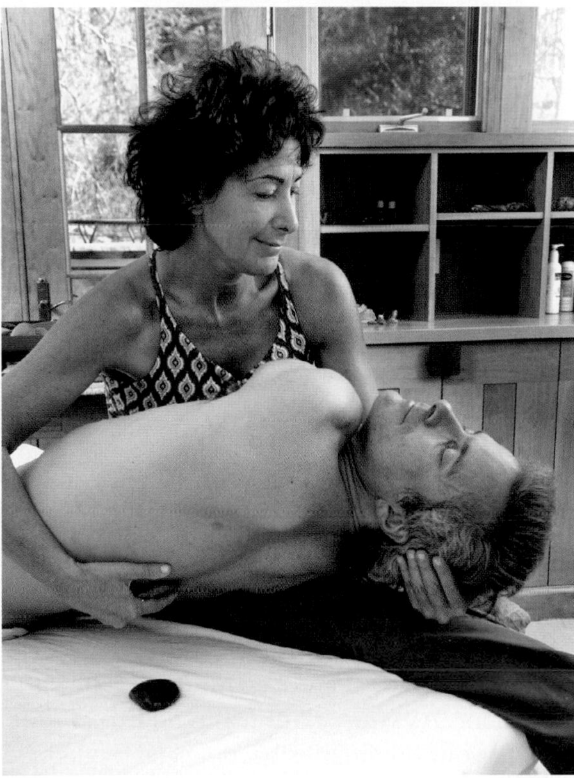

Figure 8-8 Moving the Body in Space. The therapist lifts and moves the client's body in space adding a whole other dimension of freedom to the massage.

There are a variety of ways in which you can move your client in space. The movements can be very small and simple, such as lifting the neck off the table, or they can be large and grandiose, such as lifting the entire upper torso off the table (Fig. 8-8). Your clients will appreciate whichever way you choose to lift their bodies and move them in space, whether subtle or grandiose, as long as you are checking in and listening to what their bodies want.

TESTIMONIAL

I have used this principle with young, athletic clients as well as bed-ridden and paralyzed people. It is not for you as a therapist to decide what is best for each client, but it is your job to listen to what is appropriate for the body you are working on. Sometimes, when we get our own limited concepts out of the way, we are surprised by how much more a client can move than we might expect, and we can offer our clients a whole new way of liberating their bodies.

TIP

Because new clients are unaccustomed to being moved in this way, they may need a little coaching and/or permission to fall into your arms before they will let themselves do it. Saying something like, "It's okay to let your head fall into my hands," or, "Go ahead, give me all your weight!" is very useful in helping clients to give themselves permission to be held and moved in this new way.

CAUTION

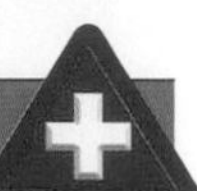

When experimenting with these principles, be sure to match the degree of lifting and undulation with the level of comfort and trust you have previously developed with this particular client. Generally, I recommend beginning slowly with a new client. As your relationship and trust deepens and your boundaries become clearly defined, you can increase the amount of lift and embrace. Some clients, however, are ready to take this principle to its fullest extent immediately. As usual, it is your responsibility as a therapist to recognize what is happening with the body of the person you are working on in the present moment, rather than base your decisions solely on rote rules.

Undulate

Embracing and lifting the body in space are brought to an even more phenomenal level when **undulation** is added to the equation. Undulation is a wavelike rippling motion that is created by allowing the body to fall (in a controlled fashion) and then be caught and lifted over and over again in a rhythmical dance. The fall happens by allowing the head or torso to give way to its natural gravitational pull. The catch of the fall occurs in a rubbery fluid fashion. When the client's spine is undulated, it creates a snakelike motion that opens and releases deep tension held around the vertebral column. A forward and backward undulation is simulated in Figures 8-9 and 8-10. The motion of your own body, which simulates the motion of the client's body, enhances the undulation. Similar to both embracing and moving the body in space, undulation can be done in a gentle subtle fashion or in large rippling motions, and in a variety of speeds, all which can be determined by listening to the client's body.

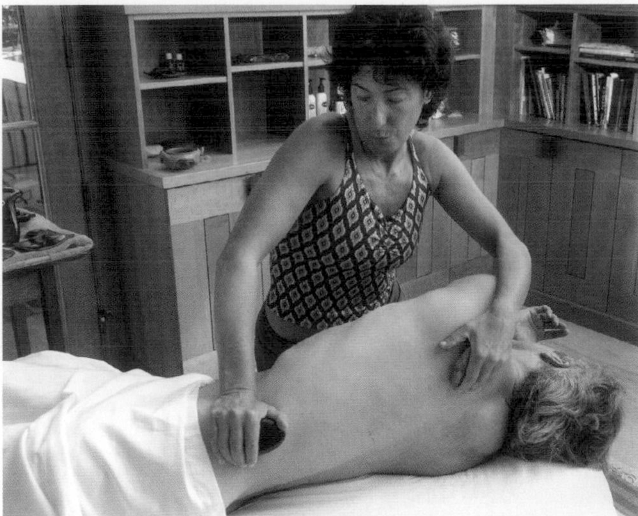

Figure 8-9 Forward Undulation. In undulation, the therapist moves the spine forward and backward with a dynamic rhythmical fluid rippling motion. This photo shows the forward movement aspect of the undulation.

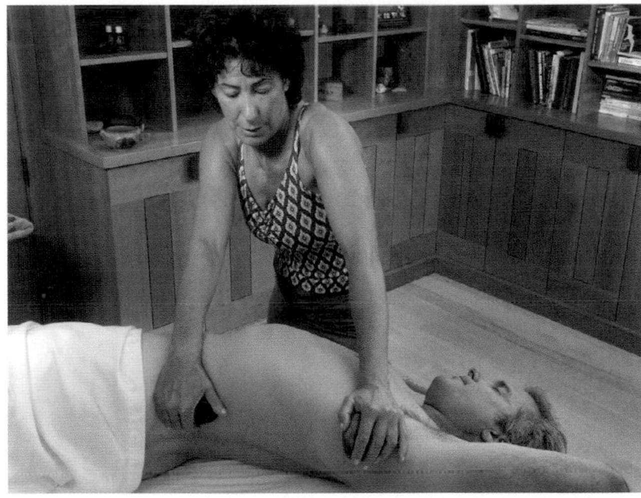

Figure 8-10 Backward Undulation. This photo shows the backward movement aspect of the undulation; however, the movements are never stagnant, but instead done in a continuous wavelike motion.

Be the Wave

"Be the wave" is my fanciful name for the principle of allowing the client's body to be moved by your own body's movement. This principle is easier to demonstrate than it is to describe and is virtually impossible to capture through photographs, so you will have to use your imagination and be willing to experiment.

Imagine a piece of seaweed floating on a wave. The seaweed moves in accordance with the movement of the wave. The wave moves and the seaweed is lifted. In applying the analogy to you and your client, you are the wave, and the client is the seaweed. Rather than manipulate the client's body with your strength, let it be moved by your body's motion. You move your body and the client's body moves as an end result of your movement, not the other way around. When the movement of your own body initiates all of the movement that you create in your client's body, you will not get tired or sore, and the massage will feel more fluid and relaxing to the client.

Here are some examples of "being the wave":
From the supine position:

- While holding your client's head, sway your body in a wavelike motion and allow the head to be moved by that motion rather than lifting the head and moving it with your arms and strength.
- From the side of the table, with one hand beneath the client's lower back and one hand on the top of the abdomen, make a sweeping motion with your body toward the client's feet and back toward the head, creating circles on the back and belly by your body's motion, not by the pushing of your hands.
- Place one hand beneath the client's knee and one beneath the ankle or on bottom of the foot. Bend your knees down and, as you lift your own body up, allow the client's leg to be lifted and swept up by the lifting motion of your own body, rather than by your hands.
- Sitting on the side of the table near client's head, with the client's torso embraced in your arms, allow your body to make wavelike motions, left and right, up and down, and forward and back as the client's body follows suit. Don't move the client's torso with your arms, but let it be moved by your own movement.

From the prone position:

- Sitting at the client's shoulder, reach across and place both hands beneath the opposite shoulder. Lean your body back toward the side of the table you are on, lifting the client's opposite shoulder as you lean.
- Standing at the client's foot, let your body lunge forward toward the head and your knee bend down as you let one hand slide up the top of the client's leg and the other hand slides underneath the client's thigh from the inside. No pushing is necessary when your whole body's motion initiates the movement of your hands.

TIP

Try lifting and moving your friends' bodies by being the wave and then by keeping your torso still. Notice the difference? Ask your friends how the two experiences felt for them. Being the wave can make lifting and moving the body a fun dance rather than a chore.

UTILIZE EFFECTIVE BODY MECHANICS

Injuring yourself over time is possible with any form of massage, and yet the threat of injury does not, unfortunately, force massage therapists to work ergonomically. Proper body mechanics protect your own body and enhance the flow of any type of massage; however, they are even more important when performing three-dimensional hot stone massage. Embracing, lifting, and undulating the body all require proper stance and use of gravity, fulcrums, body weight, and momentum in order to not rely on strength, which can strain the body. Fortunately, when you work three-dimensionally, you're forced to take care of your body because you simply will not be able to sustain marginal postures. Here are some important tips that will enable you to perform three-dimensional hot stone massage with ease.

Use a Staggered Stance

It is important to have your legs situated so that they give you the most support and freedom of movement possible. A staggered stance (Fig. 8-11) allows you to bend your knee, shift your weight, and move your body forward and back without losing control. In the "horse" stance, you are limited to bending your upper body forward and back but cannot move your weight or lower body forward (to any great extent) without falling. It is a limiting position that does not offer support and thus stresses the lower back. A staggered stance offers you the freedom of optimal range and comfort.

Make Feet Mimic Hands

Once in the staggered position, be sure that your arms and legs mimic one another. If your left arm is

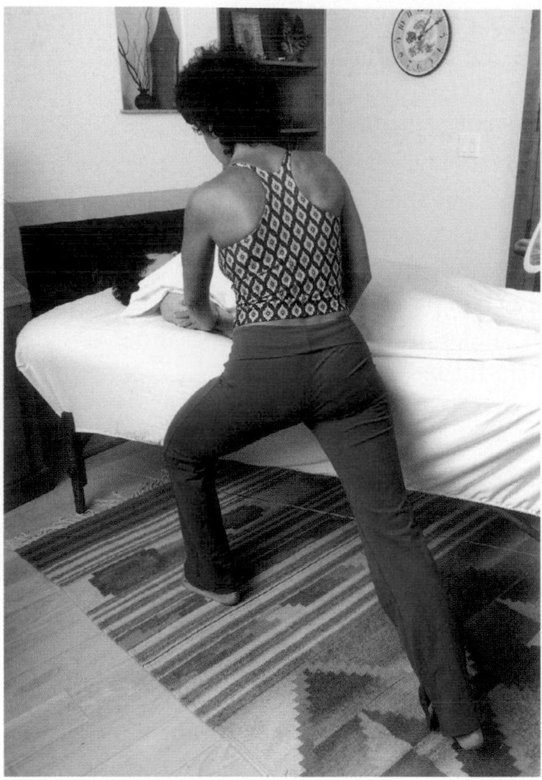

Figure 8-11 Using a Staggered Stance. Staggering the legs, one in front of the other, allows you to move forward and backwards with support. The "horse" stance limits your forward and backward mobility.

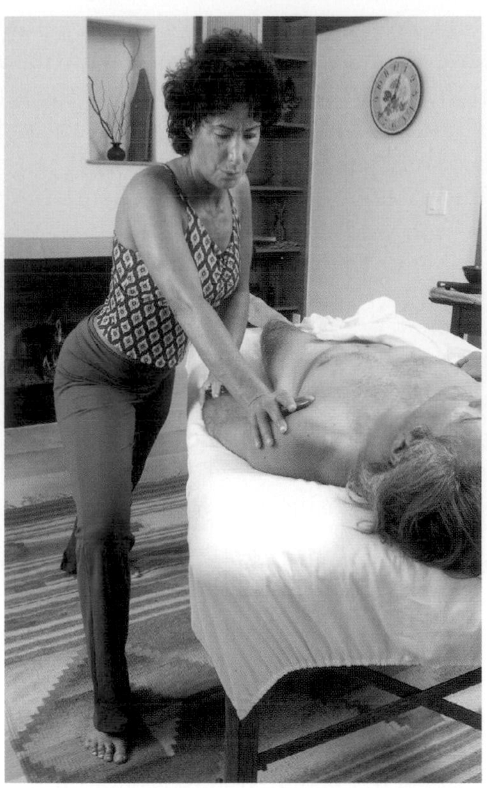

Figure 8-12 Feet Mimicking Hands. When the left arm is forward, the left leg needs to also be forward. Notice how straight the body is when proper stance is used.

forward, then your left leg should be forward, as shown in Figure 8-12, and vise versa. This position offers a greater range of movement for your body while keeping your hips and spine aligned. When your arms and legs are not mimicking each other, as shown in Figure 8-13, the spine twists. This not only limits your own body's range of motion, but it also creates an uncomfortable torque that gets translated to your client.

Lean against the Massage Table

When using the staggered position, standing perpendicular to the massage table, you can lean your forward leg against the table for extra support (Fig. 8-14). Being able to push off of the table when leaning over eliminates having to rely on your own body's strength.

While the thigh of your forward leg is pressed up against the massage table, you can put your opposite elbow into the crook of the hip of your back leg to aid you in pushing forward. Rather than relying on the strength in your hand or arm, you can push forward with your hip and derive your power from there. This is not only much easier on your body, but it also feels smoother to the client.

Use Gravity

Using gravity rather than strength allows you to gain pressure and open an area without being invasive or injuring your clients or yourself. You give clients their weight by lifting the body part and then letting it slowly fall over your hand or arm, while slightly resisting the gravitational pull, as shown in Figure 8-15. For instance, lift your client's head, hold it up from beneath the neck, and then as you slowly allow the head to fall with gravity, simultaneously lift the neck. When you lift the neck, be sure you do it slowly and low enough on the neck to allow the head to continue its controlled fall with gravity. This creates an opening in the muscles of the neck that is much deeper and more effective than had you pushed into the neck muscles with your strength.

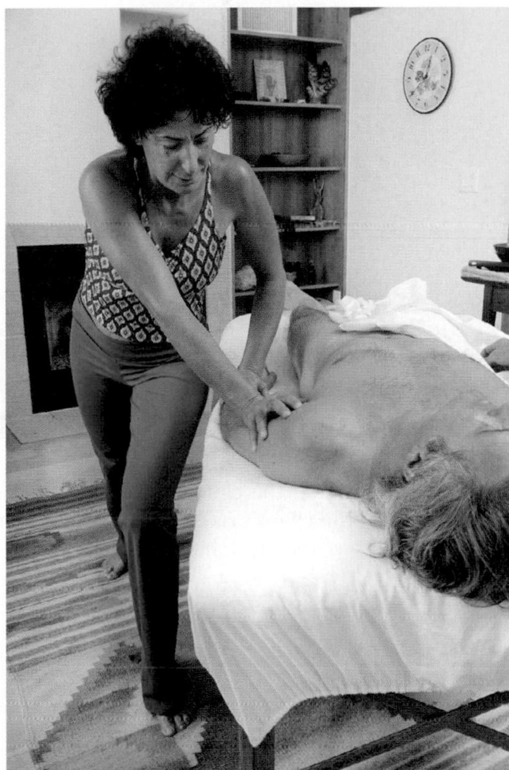

Figure 8-13 Feet Not Mimicking Hands. Notice how torqued the body is when the legs do not mimic the arms.

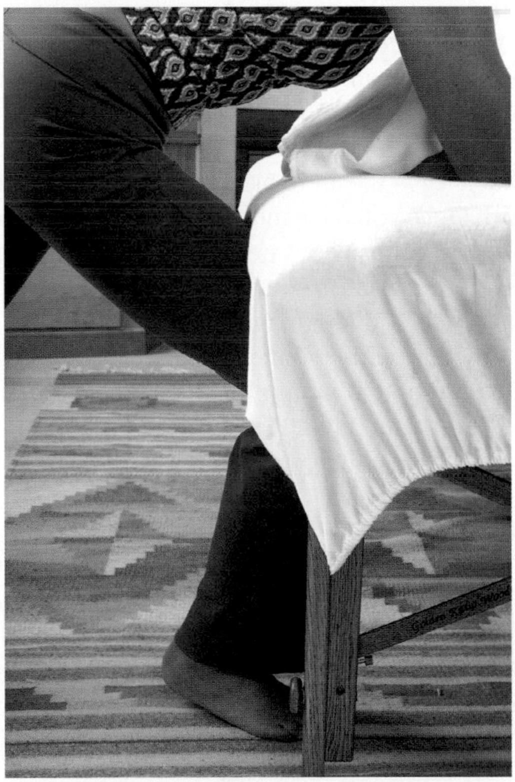

Figure 8-14 Leaning Against Massage Table. Leaning the front of your thigh against the side of the massage table offers great support to your body, especially when doing movements that require leaning across the table.

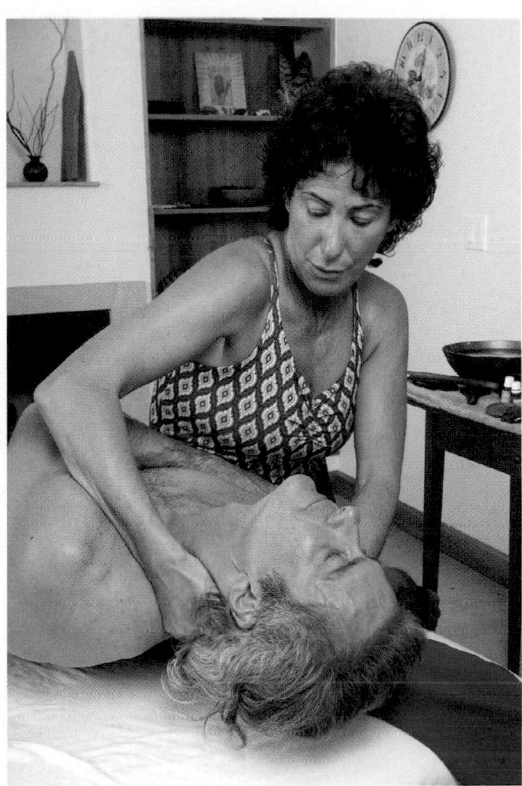

Figure 8-15 Using Gravity. Letting the client's body slowly fall back with gravity is very relaxing to the client and helps the muscles naturally release on their own. Notice how the head is allowed to gently fall with gravity as the upper torso is lifted slightly to resist the pull.

TIP

Try it on yourself. Take your right hand and bring it behind and across your neck to the left (opposite) side. Let your hand completely cover and embrace the entire left side of your neck. Then, slowly drag your hand to the right as you simultaneously let your head fall slowly down toward your left shoulder. Notice how good this feels. Now, try squeezing and pulling your hand to the right while holding your head straight up. Without the resistance of the gravitational pull, the move is stagnant, requires strength, and feels invasive. Relying on gravity rather than strength not only lessens your workload, but it also creates an exquisite sensation for the client.

Lift from the Joints

When lifting a body part, be sure that you lift from the joint rather than the middle of the muscle, as it is much lighter and easier to move limbs this way. For

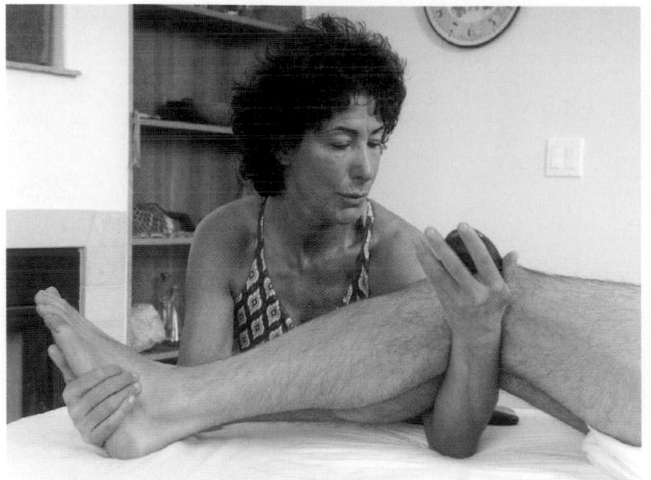

Figure 8-16 Lifting from the Joints. Lifting the legs from both the knee and ankle joints makes the leg feel much lighter and is easier to lift without injuring yourself.

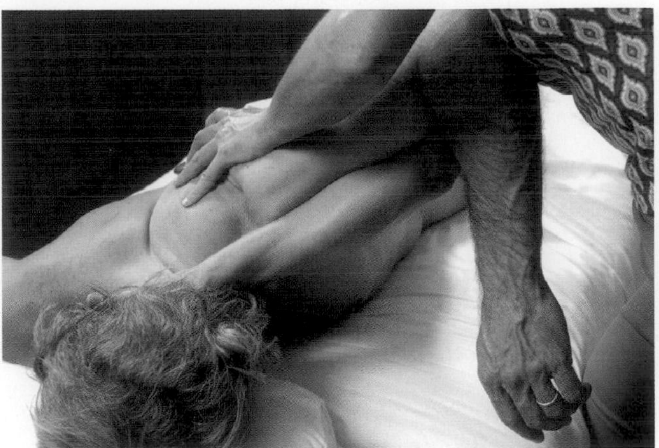

Figure 8-17 Using Fulcrums and Body Levers. The therapist weaves her hand under the client's elbow, in front of the shoulder, and behind the client's neck to create a fulcrum and lever. This makes lifting and stretching the body much easier on her body.

example, when bending the knees, lift from the bottom of the feet and behind the knee joint (Fig. 8-16), rather than from beneath the calf and thigh. When lifted from the joint areas like this, limbs become so much lighter, move with ease, and feel to the client as if they are being levitated rather than lifted. Clients are much less likely to try and help you lift when you lift in this manner.

Use Body Levers and Fulcrums

Imagine lifting a large boulder using just your body strength. Not possible. But if you were to put a large pole beneath the boulder and push off of it, the boulder would move. This pole that you put beneath the boulder and to which you applied force is called a **lever**. The fixed point on which the lever moves is the **fulcrum.**

Massage therapists injure themselves when they try to lift the client's body, like the boulder, with their bare strength. If instead you apply an understanding of levers and fulcrums to your work, you'll be able to lift the client's body without having to rely solely on strength. This will feel better and easier for you and much smoother and more supportive for your client. Figure 8-17 shows an example of the therapist creating a fulcrum with her hand in a fixed position against the back of client's neck and then straightening her elbow joint to use as a lever to lift the client's shoulder with ease. You can use your hand and elbow as a fulcrum and lever under the client's neck, shoulders, lower back, abdomen, hips, thighs, and calves to create an easy lift.

Stay with Your Move

It is imperative that you stay with each move that you do. To accomplish this, you must shift your body weight and bring it with you as you reposition your body throughout the massage. For instance, if you start moving up the client's arm but leave your body weight behind, you will not have any power behind your move. Your hands will be there, but the rest of you will not. When you cannot shift your body weight enough to stay with a move, you need to move your body forward along with your weight. You may need to raise your back leg in the air to bring your weight sufficiently forward. Once you have moved up the arm, if you continue beneath the client's neck, you need to then move your body to the side so that you can be directly behind your move, as shown in Figure 8-18.

To fully stay with a move, you also need to position your body so that it approaches the client at the proper level and angle. If you are working the upper trapezius, for instance, this would require you to drop your body down to get directly behind the upper shoulders, which are vertically positioned. But if the body part you are working on is flat, like the back, you need to get up on your toes to be able to get on top of your move. Otherwise, your client will feel your hands but not your body weight. Staying with your move engages your client's interest, takes the client to a deeper level, and is much easier on your own body.

Use Your Momentum

Working with momentum is another great principle for protecting your body from injury and for making

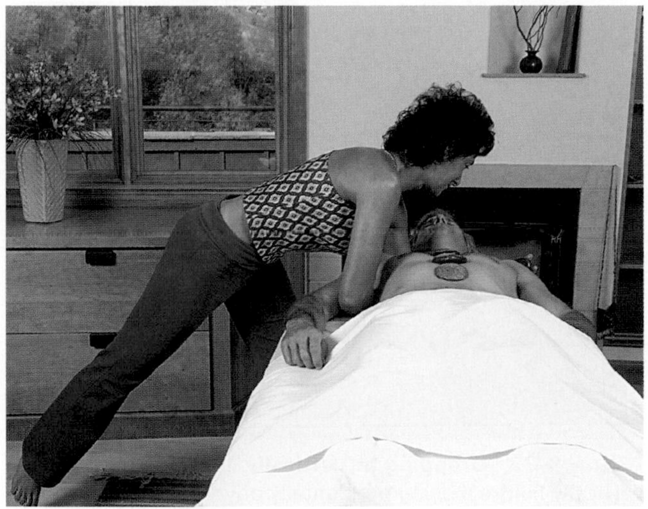

Figure 8-18 Staying with Your Move. To stay with your move, you must move your body into a new stance to reflect the new angle at which you are working.

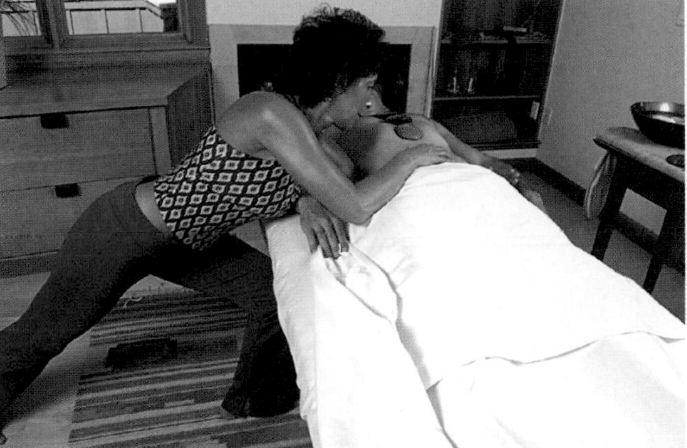

Figure 8-19 Using Your Momentum. Using momentum enables you to get beneath the client's body without straining yourself or distressing the client.

your movements smoother and easier to do. For example, to get beneath the client's lower back, step back from the side of the table, lower your stance, and come in with momentum, as indicated in Figure 8-19. This momentum will help you slide under the body without having to use your strength to push your way in. Using momentum makes moving beneath the body fun and easy rather than rigorous and awkward, and it feels much better to both the client and the therapist.

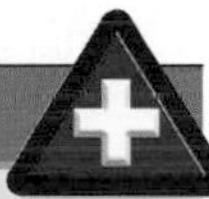

CAUTION

Even though you are entering with momentum, you still need to be gentle upon initial contact with the client's skin. Pre-oiling the forearm makes for a much easier glide on the entrance when going underneath the body.

Apply Pressure Effectively

In addition to shortening the muscle, there are other ways to give deep pressure without being invasive or injuring yourself or your client. The following principles will enable you to give effective deep pressure that fully meets your client's needs and feels good to both of you.

Use Your Weight

Going deep does not require strength, as is demonstrated by the very strong practitioner who could not go deep enough on me when relying on his strength alone, but it does require being able and willing to drop your own weight into a client. If you hold back your body's weight and try to give the massage with just your arms and strength alone, you will not only tire yourself out and not meet the client, but you will also give a massage that feels very mechanical. To avoid this, you must use your own body weight to attain pressure from above.

Going up on your toes before dropping into the body helps you to drop your weight even more, especially when using the thumbs for pressure. The forearm makes a great tool for allowing you to drop in with your weight, as shown in Figure 8-20. You can use your forearm as deeply or as lightly as each body needs, and you can be as specific (using more of the

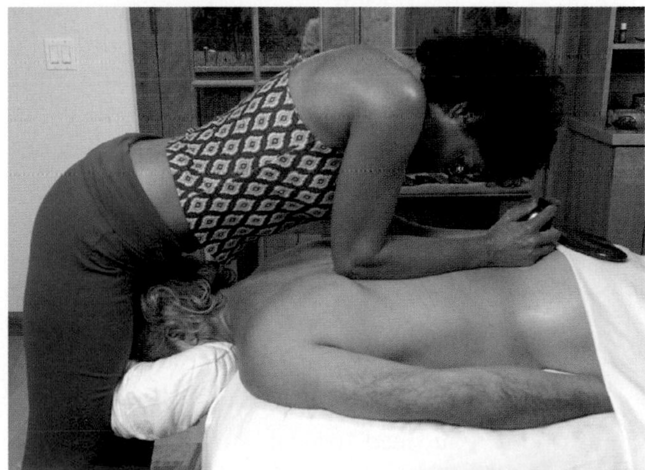

Figure 8-20 Using Your Own Weight To Gain Depth. The therapist uses her weight rather than strength to gain her depth and pressure. This is much easier on her and feels much better to the client.

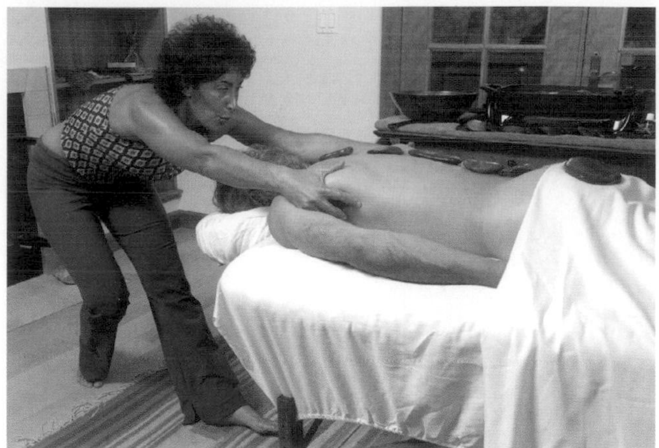

Figure 8-21 Leaning Back to Use Your Weight. The therapist uses her own weight to gain depth while pulling up the back. This creates a taffylike sensation for the client.

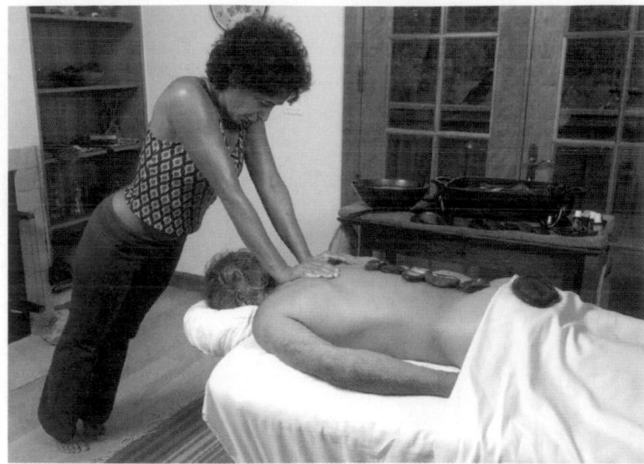

Figure 8-22 Dropping In Vertically. It is critical to drop in vertically before moving horizontally or you will lose the depth you have gained. Notice how the therapist goes up on her toes in order to increase the vertical drop.

elbow) or as broad (staying on the meatier part of the forearm) as is required.

Weight is not only useful for dropping in to a stroke, but it can also be useful for pulling out of a stroke. For instance, to create a slight feeling of traction in the client's neck, lean back with your weight and allow the head and neck to naturally unwind. When massaging down the arm, grip both sides at once and lean your body weight down toward the feet. When coming out of the back effleurage, use your weight to fall back and rake your fingers up the sides of the back, as shown in Figure 8-21. This feels deeply satisfying to the client, like warm taffy being slowly stretched out.

Always use your full weight to attain pressure whenever it is possible. You can determine if you are using all of your weight if the client were to suddenly disappear, you would fall either flat on your face or flat on your back, depending on if you were dropping forward or pulling back. But if you are only using part of your weight and holding back and the client were to disappear, you would not lose your balance or fall. You want to massage in such a way that if the client vanished you would fall. This feels the best to your client and creates the deepest pressure with the least amount of work for you.

Drop in Vertically

To gain depth when you are working from above the client's body, you need to drop straight in vertically with your weight before moving horizontally, as shown in Figure 8-22. After you've reached the desired depth, you can start to glide along the muscle, but be sure that you do not lose the vertical pressure gained previously.

CAUTION

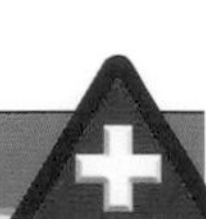

If you start gliding before you have found the amount of pressure the client desires, you will either begin too deep, causing the client's body to tighten more and pull away from you, or you will miss the beginning of each muscle by the time you drop in more. This is why it is so important to drop vertically first, wait until the body is met, and then move horizontally for the glide.

You will know if the body is met both by listening with your hands and watching with your eyes. If the body retracts, withdraws, tightens, or if the breath stops, you can be sure you are going too deep. If the body seems to reach up for more, if the client's eyes flutter, or if the client begins to talk a lot or fidget, you are not going deep enough. When clients feel met, their muscles relax, their tissue softens and opens up, they stop talking, they take a large breath, and they are right there with you.

TIP

If you do not know what this feels like, experiment with friends. Try different depths of pressure and see if you can guess what is just right without the client having to tell you. With practice, this sense will become more heightened, and you will know when you have met your client.

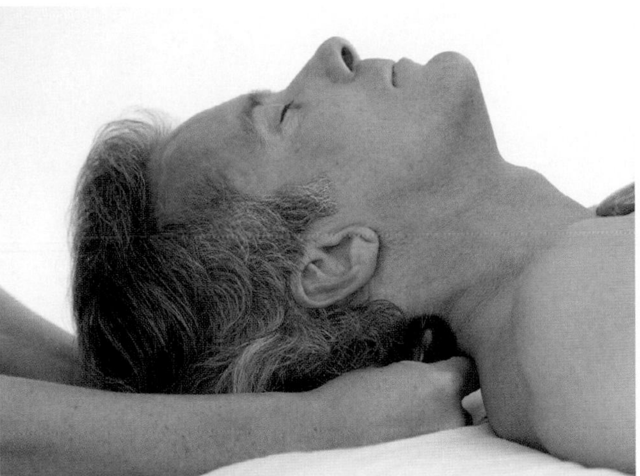

Figure 8-23 Using Client's Weight Over Stone. The therapist uses the weight of the client's head to gain pressure. This feels much less invasive to the client's muscle and is easier on the therapist as well.

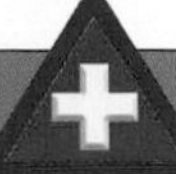

CAUTION

Pushing up with strength does not feel good to the client and will hurt your hands or wrists. Avoid it entirely.

TIP

Contact the body from beneath only when there is an easy opening such as the curve of the neck, shoulder, lumbar region, or behind the knee. Never try and force your hand underneath an area of the body where there is no space. This will feel uncomfortable and invasive to the client, who might then lift up and try to help you.

Use Client's Weight

When you are working from beneath a client, it is always essential to use the client's own weight to help attain the depth of pressure desired. Gravity and the weight of the client go hand in hand; that is, gain depth by letting the weight of the client's body fall over an "altar" that you create with either a stone, as shown in Figure 8-23, or your fingers, as shown in Figure 8-24, rather than pushing up into the muscle with your strength.

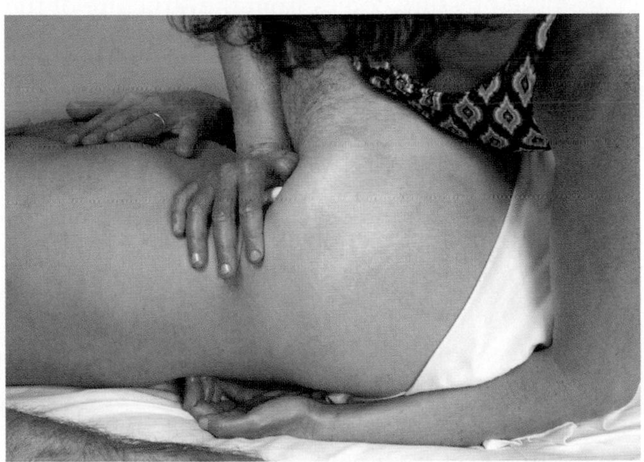

Figure 8-24 Using Client's Weight Over Fingers. It is even more imperative to use the client's weight when massaging without stones to protect your fingers. The therapist makes an "altar" and allows the client's weight to slowly drop over her hand to gain her depth.

Occasionally, clients will try and help you by lifting their weight even when you do reach under the open spaces. When this happens, I usually make a joke saying, "Oh, I forgot to tell you that I charge double when you help!" Bringing humor into it usually breaks the ice, sets them at ease, and removes any shame or judgment they might feel about their helping. This gives them permission to let go, rather than you telling them they should let go. Alternatively, you might say, "It's okay to give me your weight if you want to" or, "I can hold you up. You don't have to do anything, you can just fall back into my hands."

Sometimes clients need to be given permission from you before they will give permission to themselves to be cradled in their own weight. After you succeed in gaining the clients trust and having them give you their full weight, the massage will become much easier on you and feel much better to them.

Protect Your Joints

When dropping in with your weight, it is very important to take care of your joints (i.e., your thumbs, wrists, fingers). One way to protect your thumbs is to set the joints before dropping in with your weight. The larger joint, where the thumb meets the hand, needs to be dipped into its socket. Try it on yourself. You will see how that joint can click in to be set. This position allows the thumb joint to carry your weight as you drop in. In contrast, when the large thumb joint is allowed to come away from its socket and the next joint down is bent out, the thumb joints are no

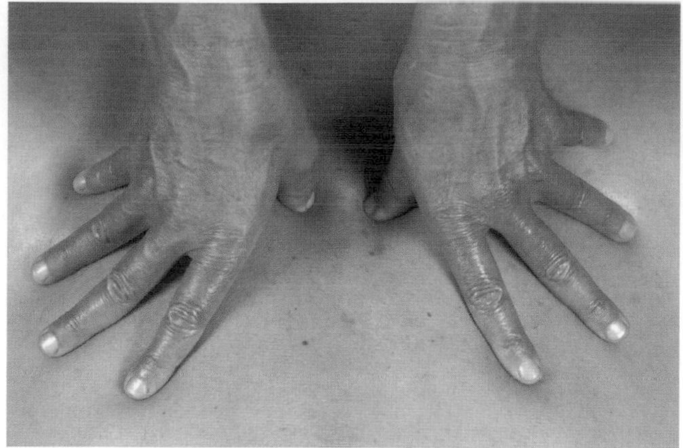

Figure 8-25 Protecting Your Thumbs. Setting the thumb joints (as indicated by the thumb on the right side of photo) will save your thumbs and allow you to go deep without pain. When the thumb joints are not set (as indicated by the thumb on the left side of photo), they offer no anatomical support and set you up for injury and painful joints.

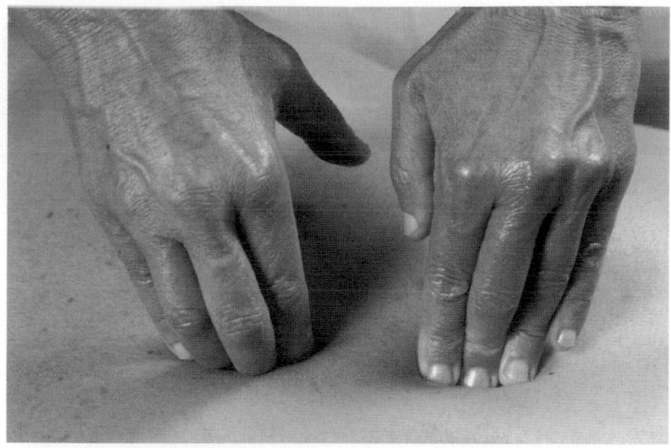

Figure 8-27 Protecting Your Fingertips. Using the finger pads (as indicated by the fingers on right side of photo) offers anatomical support to the finger joints and feels better to the client than using the fingertips (as indicated by the fingers on left side of photo), which offers no anatomical support for the finger joints and feels pokey and "finger-naily" to the client.

longer anatomically supported and will tire out and ache. In Figure 8-25, notice the thumb joint on the right side of the photo is slightly tucked in towards the body, whereas the thumb joint on the left side of the photo is not.

It is also important to keep your wrists as straight as possible, rather than cocked, when dropping in vertically to a muscle to avoid developing **carpal tunnel syndrome** over time. Cocking the wrist not only impinges the carpal tunnel nerve but also blocks the flow of energy and could eventually lead to pain in your entire arm and shoulder. In Figure 8-26, notice how the wrist on the right side of the photo is uncocked and the wrist on the left side of the photo is cocked. See which onc looks more comfortable and powerful to you.

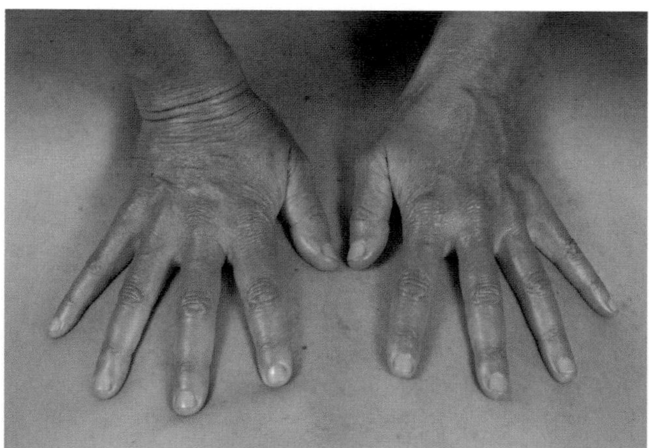

Figure 8-26 Protecting Your Wrists. Keeping your wrists at a slight angle (as indicated by the wrist on right side of photo), rather than cocked (as indicated by the wrist on left side of photo), will help to prevent carpal tunnel syndrome from developing.

You also need to take care of the distal phalanges of your hands. When using the ends of the fingers, it is tempting to rely on the fingertips rather than the finger pads; however, this is a dangerous error that not only leads to pain and wear and tear in those joints but also does not feel as pleasing to the client. If you use the pads of the fingers, as shown on the right side of Figure 8-27, the fingertips can be bent forward slightly while the first joints are bent slightly in and are set. This anatomical support relieves the need for relying on the muscles in the fingers, and instead the pressure comes from the structure of the bones. This position also avoids the pokey sensation and nail cutting of the fingertips and feels broader and more spread out to the client. When you use your fingertips, as shown on the left side of Figure 8-27, there is no anatomical support for the joints just above them, so the fingers tire out quickly. The tips also feel as if they are poking rather than kneading the client's skin. The pads are much more comfortable and effective for both client and therapist.

If you feel pain in any of your joints at any time during the massage, notice if they are not being properly supported and take immediate action: Either change the position of your joint or, if this does not alleviate the discomfort, stop the motion you are doing that is causing the pain. Without your joints, you will not be able to massage. Take the same care of yourself as you would for your client.

SUMMARY

The principles in this chapter are the keys to transforming your hot stone massage into an extraordinary experience. To set the tone and allow the other principles to organically unfold, you must be fully present with your client. Selfless awareness such as this creates a sacred temple where love and reverence can reside.

To create a constant flow in the massage, it is important for you to overlap your hands and stones within each stroke and to make seamless transitions between each body part. To encourage the tissues to open: Work them in their shortened position, either anatomically or manually, and honor their speed limit by working only as fast or as slow as the tissue will allow. Use opposition and resistance anywhere it presents itself to enhance the opening of the tissue.

Work three-dimensionally by embracing both sides of the body at once, moving the client's body in space, and undulating the head and upper torso in a rhythmic fashion. Do not move the client with your strength, but instead move your own body and let the client's body move on account of your movements.

Three-dimensional hot stone massage requires that you use effective body mechanics in order to prevent injury to yourself and your client. To accomplish this, you should use a staggered stance for your legs, have your feet mimic your hands, and lean against the massage table (when appropriate) for added support. In addition, rather than using your own effort to lift the client, allow gravity, momentum, and fulcrums with levers to do the work for you. Always stay with your move, shifting your weight each time you reposition your body.

To apply deep pressure in an effective and easy manner, use your own body weight and drop in vertically before moving horizontally. Additionally, allow your client's weight to fall over your thumb, fingers or stone, to create the pressure you desire. Last, be sure to protect your joints from injury by setting your thumbs, uncocking your wrists, and using the pads rather than the tips of your fingers when working specifically.

First and foremost, listen deeply to the needs of both your, and your client's bodies, heart and soul, and all of the other principles will unfold naturally. These principles are the foundation for the techniques and strokes you will learn in Chapters 9 and 10. Bring them with you as you travel through the next pages.

REVIEW QUESTIONS

TRUE/FALSE

1. The principles are not as important as the techniques and massage moves.

   Circle: True False

2. It is important to gracefully revisit an area of the body when it calls out.

   Circle: True False

3. It is important to remove one hand fully before entering with the next.

   Circle: True False

4. It is best to enter a muscle deeply when it is in its elongated position.

   Circle: True False

5. All muscles can be shortened anatomically.

   Circle: True False

6. The mother–father technique is used to make long full-bodied strokes.

   Circle: True False

7. The "snow-drift" effect is made by the mother hand.

   Circle: True False

8. Gravity makes more work for the therapist.

   Circle: True False

9. When using gravity, you need to offer a slight resistance in the opposite direction to feel its effect, or otherwise the body part will simply fall to the table.

   Circle: True False

10. You should massage all muscles at the same speed for consistency.

    Circle: True False

MULTIPLE CHOICE

11. If the body part being worked on is not level, the mother hand should always be:

    a. Left of the father hand
    b. Right of the father hand
    c. Higher than the father hand
    d. Lower than the father hand
    e. Doesn't matter

12. When a muscle kicks you out, you should automatically:
    a. Go away from the muscle
    b. Slow down
    c. Lighten up
    d. Go deeper
    e. Work exactly as you are
13. You only need to rely entirely on words when asking what the client needs if:
    a. You know the client well
    b. Client is new
    c. You are not listening deeply enough
    d. Client is talkative
    e. Client is not talkative
14. Using opposition in a massage has which ultimate effect on the client's muscle:
    a. Tightens it
    b. Causes inflammation
    c. Releases it
    d. Creates redness
    e. Irritates it
15. Resistance can be created in a client's muscle by:
    a. Actively engaging client
    b. Passively engaging client
    c. Irritating the muscle
    d. Penetrating deeply into the muscle
    e. Both a and b

SHORT ANSWER

16. The principle "being the wave" means to move the client's body as an end result of the ________________________________.
17. When using your body as a fulcrum and a lever, most positions you will be in have your hand serving as the ____________ and your elbow joint or forearm being used as the ____________.
18. Using ________________ makes it easier to get beneath the client's body and to protect your body from being injured or overworked.
19. Going beneath the body only where there is ______________ makes it easier and more fluid for you to enter.
20. To gain depth when you are working from above the client's body, you need to drop your own ________________ and go ____________ first before moving __________________.

Answers to Review Questions can be found in Appendix D.

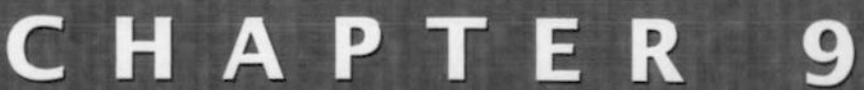

CHAPTER 9

Techniques for Working with the Stones

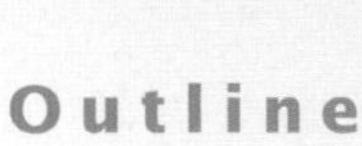

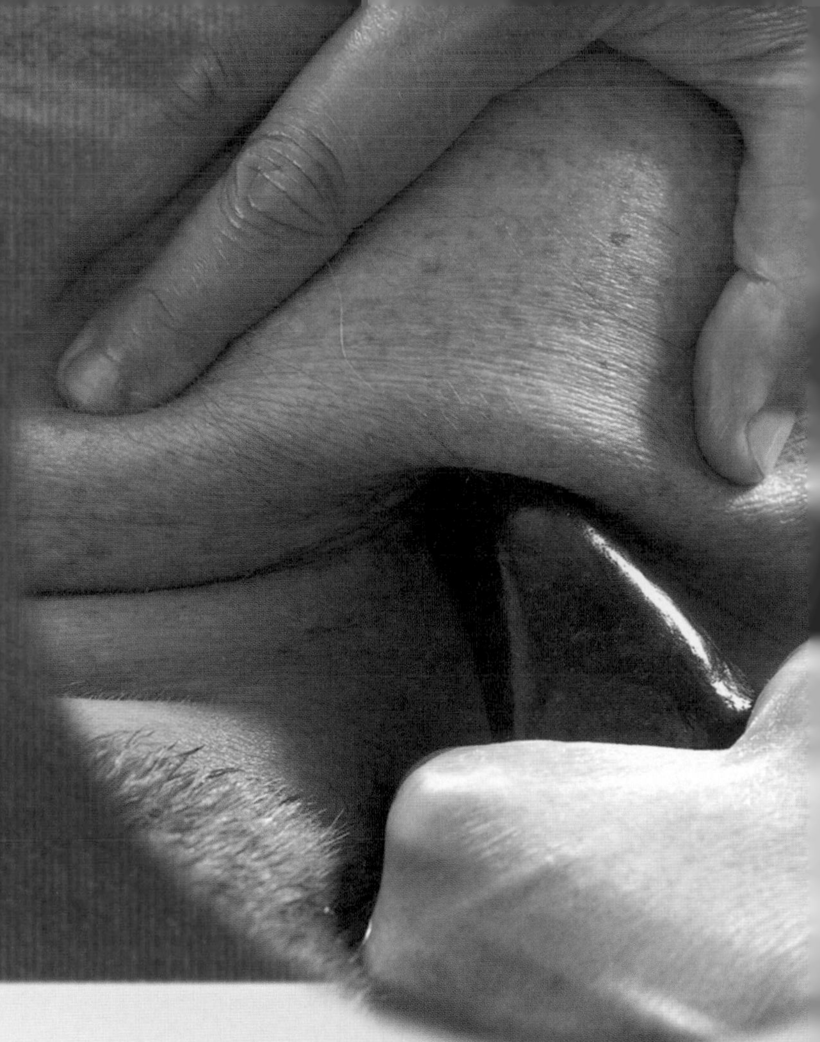

Outline

Techniques for Working with Tool Stones

- Using a Pointed Tool Stone
- Using a Concave Tool Stone
- Using a Curved Tool Stone
- Edging
- Compression
- Energetic Stone Vibration
  - *Tapping*
  - *Clanking*
  - *Rubbing*
- Friction
- Pin and Stir
- Snaking the Spine

Techniques for Using Stones above the Body

- Gliding
- Heeling
- Circling
- Paws Digging
- Crisscrossing
- Rolling
- Elephant Walking
- Flushing

Techniques for Using Stones beneath the Body

- Alternating
- Draping
- Teetering
- Squeeze, Twist, and Slide
- Sandwiching
- Lift and Drag
- Sneaking Under

"These techniques turn a hot stone practitioner into a hot stone sorcerer."

Selina Borquez,
Student of Three-Dimensional Hot Stone Massage,
Denver, Colorado

Objectives

After reading this chapter, you should be able to:

- Compare and contrast techniques for using pointed, concave, and curved tool stones.
- Explain how to use stones to generate vibrations that transmit energy into the client's body.
- Demonstrate several techniques for using stones from above the client's body.
- Demonstrate several techniques for using stones from beneath the client's body.

Key Terms

Alternating: A technique that involves alternating the stone-held hands beneath any part of the body.

Circling: A technique that involves the vertical dropping of weight through the heel of the hand to make circles with the stone.

Clanking: A technique whereby the edges of placement stones are struck against one another.

Compression: A calming technique that utilizes the weight of an additional stone or sand/grain bag, laid on top of the placement stones. Compression can be increased by adding the weight of the hand(s).

Concave tool stone: A stone with a concave or indented surface that accommodates the contours of a bony protuberance.

Crisscrossing: A technique that is similar to gliding but done in crossing patterns.

Curved tool stone: A stone with a curve, either on its side or tip, that is useful for working the various shapes and contours of the body.

Draping: A technique that allows the client's body weight to drape or fall over the stone.

(Continued)

Key Terms *(Continued)*

Edging: A technique that opens a muscle by using the edge of a stone to push or "scrape" the muscle fibers into submission.

Elephant walking: A technique similar to compression but done with alternating hands that move up and down the body slowly like an elephant's feet walking.

Energetic vibration: Using stones to create a vibration that sends energy deep into the body by means of tapping, clanking, or rubbing together.

Flushing: A technique that uses light, sweeping strokes with a large flat stone to soothe and "clean out" an area that has just received deep specific work.

Friction: A technique similar to rubbing in which stones are rubbed back and forth against the client's skin.

Gliding: A technique that involves sliding a hot oiled stone along the muscle in a long sweeping motion.

Heeling: A technique that utilizes the heel of the hand to increase the depth or specificity of gliding.

Lift and drag: A technique that involves lifting a stone against the underside of the body so that it drags rather than glides along the muscle.

Paws digging: A technique for softening tissues using stones in a motion similar to that of a dog digging in the sand with its two front paws.

Pin and stir: A technique that involves pinning the tip of a stone in place on the belly of a muscle and moving the limb in a range of motion around the pinned stone.

Pointed tool stone: A stone with a pointed tip that is used for working trigger points and very specific areas of tension.

Rolling: A simple technique accomplished by rolling a round stone back and forth or up and down the body.

Rubbing: A technique accomplished by vigorously rubbing the sides of two stones against each other.

Sandwiching: A technique that involves covering a body part with a stone on either side.

Snaking the spine: A technique that uses the point of a stone to carve an S-curve down the spine.

Sneaking under: A technique that involves bringing a stone beneath the body in a smooth and subtle fashion.

Squeeze, twist, and slide: A technique that involves squeezing a stone up from beneath a body part, and then rapidly twisting and sliding it the rest of the way.

Tapping: A technique whereby very specific vibration is sent vertically into the body by tapping one stone directly down onto a placement stone.

Teetering: A technique that utilizes draping on a very specific part of the body.

This chapter describes specific techniques for handling and using your stones skillfully and effectively. While learning these techniques and incorporating them into your work, be careful that you don't abandon the principles that ground them. Instead, fuse these techniques to the underlying principles, and you'll produce a powerful modality for releasing your clients' most deeply held tensions.

The techniques included in this chapter apply to using the stones as tools, using the stones above the client's body, and using the stones beneath the client's body. Each group of techniques is discussed in its own section for easy reference.

TECHNIQUES FOR WORKING WITH TOOL STONES

The following techniques are meant for use with tool stones. Tool stones are stones with particular sizes and shapes useful for working very specifically on injuries, muscles spasms, trigger points, small areas of tension, and around bony protuberances. You can also use them to create and deliver specific types of **energetic vibration** (this will be discussed in the Energetic Stone Vibration section).

When you use a stone for a tool, the stone is the only thing that makes contact with your client's skin—there is no contact from your hand at all. Except for stone placement, this is the only case in which you should use a stone on its own. Otherwise, your hands should always accompany the contact of the stone to the skin.

Tool stones need to be warmer than other working stones for two reasons. As tool stones are used for working on very specific small areas of the body, only a very small portion of the stone makes contact with the skin. Although a stone may feel hot when applied to the body in its entirety, the effect is lessened when only a small portion of it is applied. As a result, the temperature of a tool stone needs to be slightly higher. Additionally, when a tool stone is used for deep work, its heat helps to alleviate the discomfort of the increased and specific pressure. To ensure that tool stones remain hot throughout their use, replace them with new hot ones more frequently than you do other working stones.

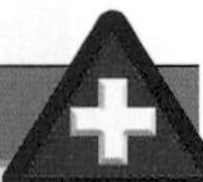

CAUTION

Remember, a cool stone is a hard stone. Unheated tool stones can also leave residual soreness and even bruising. The more specific and deep the work, the hotter the stone should be.

Because traditional massage tools made of wood or glass are not heated, they can be painful to clients. The beauty of using a stone for a tool is that it can be heated. Its heat not only reduces or eliminates the pain that usually accompanies deep work, but it also prevents residual soreness or bruising.

Using a Pointed Tool Stone

A **pointed tool stone** is useful for deeply working trigger points and very specific areas of tension. Tips of different shapes serve different purposes. The sharper the point on the tip, the deeper and more specific the penetration will be (Fig. 9-1). A slightly broader point on the tip will widen the area of penetration. When an area of tension or a trigger point is located deep within the client's muscle, it is optimal to use a stone with a sharper point. When an area of tension or a trigger point is not buried quite as deeply in a muscle, or when a client cannot tolerate as much pressure, a slightly broader tip is preferable.

TIP

In either case, adding the mother hand to the father tool stone will soften the entrance and allow for deeper penetration with less pain.

To use a pointed tool stone, first locate with your fingers or thumb the specific area that requires deep penetration. Once found, place the tip of the stone on the area and drop your weight slightly into the area, asking the client if you are on the right spot. If the client approves, sink your weight even more into the area while bringing the mother hand in to soften the sensation of the deep penetration. Once you have reached the appropriate and desired depth, move the stone around slightly to break open the trigger point or the contracted fibers of the muscle. After approximately 1 minute of held pressure, lighten up with the stone, allowing blood and oxygen to fill and cleanse the area. Repeat as many times as necessary to offer relief to the client.

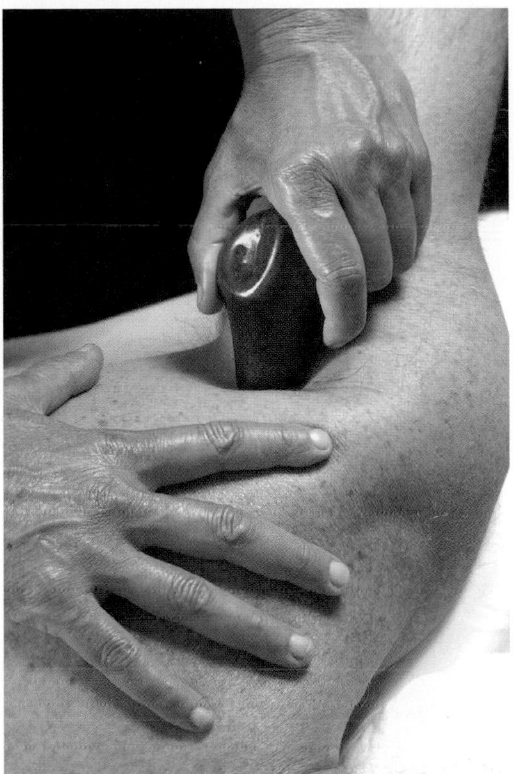

Figure 9-1 Using a Pointed Tool Stone. A sharp point on a stone allows deep and specific penetration. Use the mother-father technique to ease the penetration of the stone.

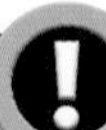

TIP

Sometimes the best course of action is to work a specific point for approximately 5 minutes and then leave the area. Return to work the point again later in the massage. This allows the muscle some recovery time and enables you to go to a deeper level. After working a specific area, use a warm working stone in a broad fashion to soothe and flush the area.

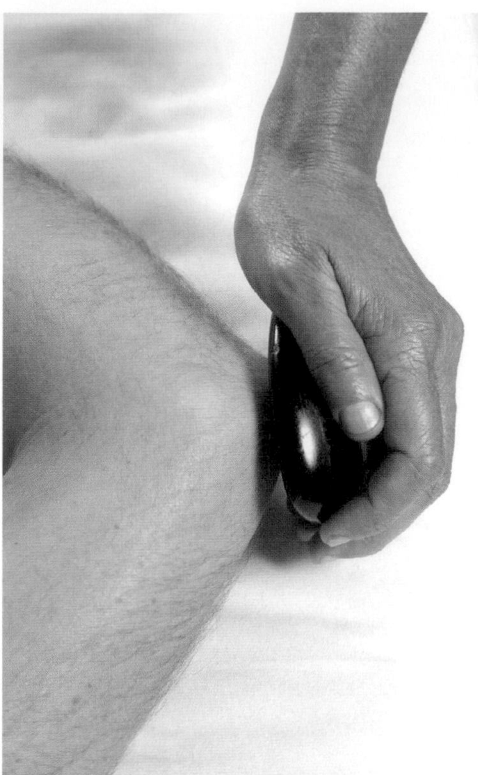

Figure 9-2 Using a Concave Tool Stone. The dip in this tool stone allows the therapist to hug the bony protuberance of the elbow.

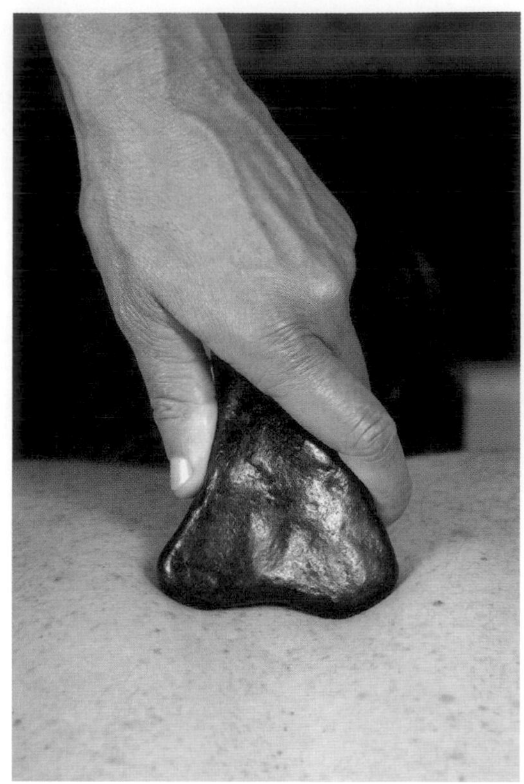

Figure 9-3 Using a Curved Tool Stone. With a curved tool stone, you can glide down the client's spine without making contact with the vertebral processes.

Using a Concave Tool Stone

When working over bony protuberances, such as an ankle, knee, elbow, or shoulder, use a **concave tool stone**; that is, a stone with a concave or indented surface that accommodates the contours of the bones (Fig. 9-2). Using the round or flat side of a stone on a bony protuberance is useless, as only a tiny part of the stone's surface will make contact. The concave surface of the stone should be very smooth, and you should be careful to enter with the stone gradually, beginning with the edge before gliding into the full indentation. As soon as it's in place, move the stone in slow, small circles around the ankle, knee, elbow, or shoulder.

Using a Curved Tool Stone

A **curved tool stone** allows you to match the contours of the client's body. For example, a stone with a slight curve in its end or edge can be useful for gliding along either side of the spine (Fig. 9-3). The curve does not need to be pronounced. Place the curved stone perpendicular to and flat against the spine. Its slight curve will keep the stone from hitting the spinous processes as you glide it down the client's back, making simultaneous contact with both sets of erector spinalis muscles.

A stone with a sharper curve can be used for sharper angles. You can use a sharply curved stone along the spine to massage the more proximal edges of the erector spinalis muscles or to massage the lateral edges of the multifidus muscle. A stone with a broad curve is useful for matching the shape of a curved area of the body like the shoulders, as shown in Figure 9-4.

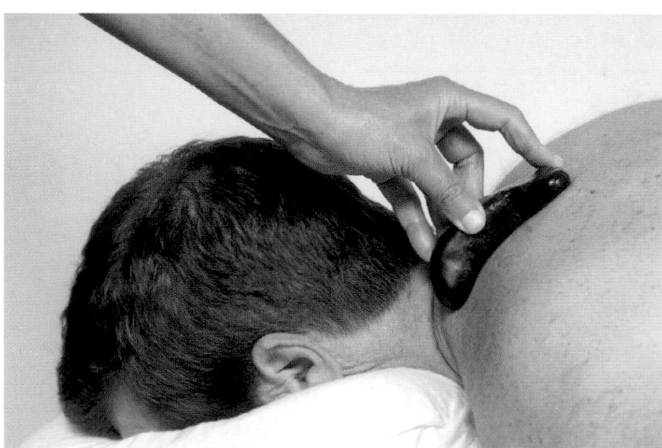

Figure 9-4 Matching a Curved Stone to the Body's Curves. A long curve on the side of a stone allows it to match the angle of the body.

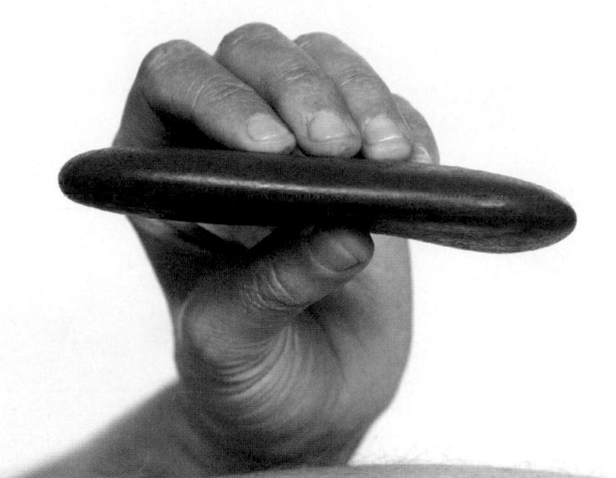

Figure 9-5 Using a Narrow Edged Tool. A stone with a very narrow edge is useful for edging.

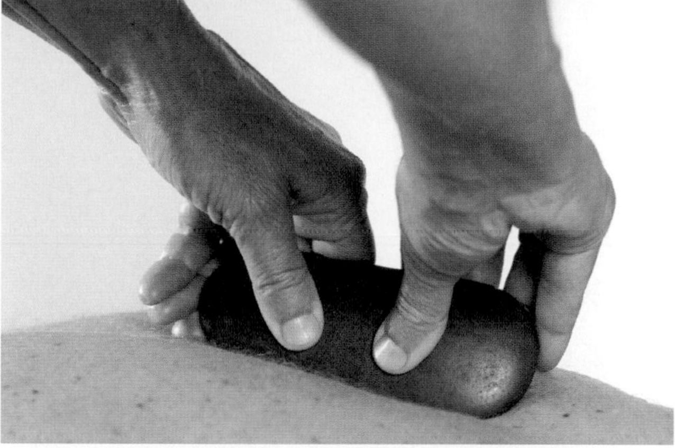

Figure 9-6 Edging. The therapist places the edge of the stone in the spinal groove and uses both hands to rock its edge back and forth as she moves slowly along the spine.

Sometimes, a pointed stone will also have a curve to its tip, making it useful as a pointed, concave, and curved tool stone.

Edging

Edging is a technique that opens a muscle by using the edge of a stone to push or "scrape" the muscle fibers into submission. A very narrow edge—between 0.125 and 0.25 inch—is required (Fig. 9-5). The 0.125 inch edge is useful for narrow areas and the 0.25 inch edge is best for larger surfaces of the body.

To edge along the spine, locate the laminar groove found just lateral to the transverse processes. Using both hands, place the edge of the stone in the groove, as shown in Figure 9-6. Once in place, drop the edge deeper into the groove and push the muscle away from the spine with a sweeping motion while maintaining the deep pressure. Repeat this motion in a rhythmic fashion up and down the spine.

TIP

If the groove is narrow, use the thinner edge. If the client is very sensitive to deep pressure, use the thicker edge.

To edge along large surface areas such as the sides of the back or the thighs, use the edge of the stone to make broad sweeping motions, dropping down and pushing out along or across the muscle fibers. Use a sweeping motion 2 to 4 inches in length before continuing down the muscle. Repeat this motion along the entire surface of the muscle or in particularly tight parts of it.

TIP

For edging on these larger surfaces, use a stone with a wider edge.

Compression

Compression is a simple technique that utilizes the weight of an additional stone or sand bag, which is laid on top of the placement stones, as shown in Figures 9-7 and 9-8. Compression can be increased

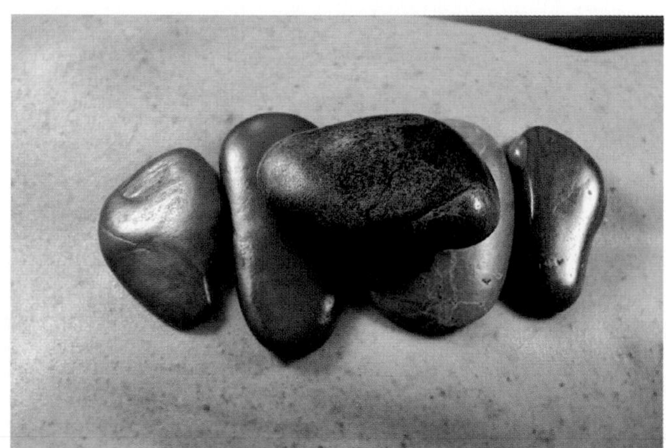

Figure 9-7 Compression with a Stone. Compression can be created by the weight of a stone laid on top of the placement stones.

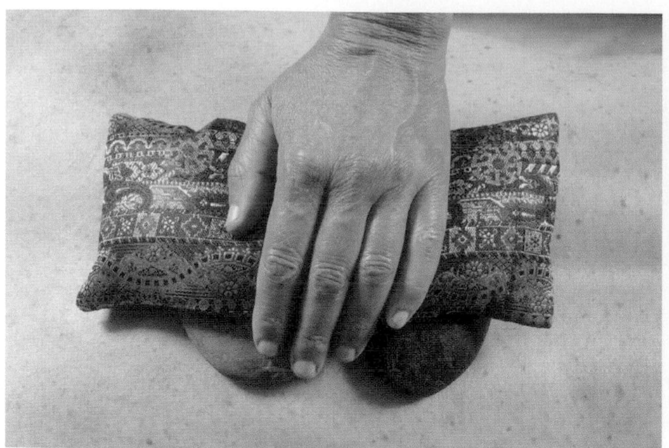

Figure 9-8 Compression with a Sand Bag and Hands. Compression can also be created by the weight of a sand bag. Press on the top of the sand bag to increase the compression.

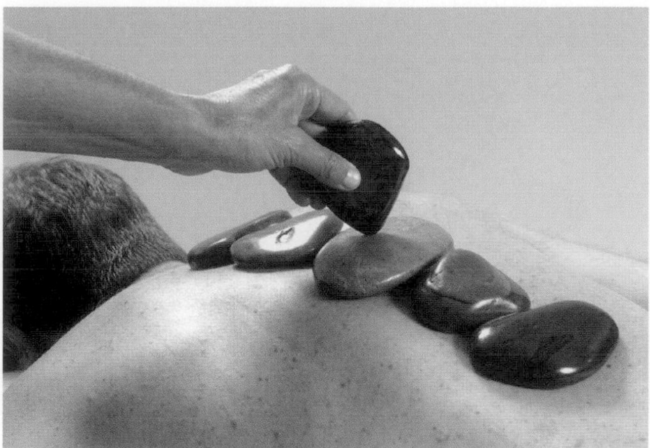

Figure 9-9 Tapping. Tapping a stone into other placement stones feels like a gentle jackhammer sending vibrations directly into the body.

by adding pressure from your hands. Compression feels safe and grounding to clients who have suffered trauma or have difficulty relaxing during a massage. It is very calming.

Compression can also be done using several stones to create patterns on an area. For instance, if you have four stones in a circle on the belly, you can press on adjacent stones one at a time to make a circle pattern or alternate stones to make a cross pattern. Experiment with other designs and sequences. As long as compression is performed slowly, it will create a peaceful, grounding experience for clients.

Energetic Stone Vibration

Use stones to transmit a subtle energetic vibration, not unlike sound waves, into the client's body. The sensation this produces invites the client's body to relax on a different level than muscular manipulation. Three techniques for producing energetic vibration are tapping, clanking, and rubbing.

Tapping

Tapping is a technique whereby very specific vibration is sent vertically into the body by tapping one stone directly down onto a placement stone with a motion similar to a gentle jackhammer (Fig. 9-9). The strength of the impact from the tap is determined by the height from which the stone begins its descent. It is done in a percussive manner, staying on one stone at a time for approximately 25 seconds before moving on to the next stone. You can also tap on just one stone as you move it slowly up and down the spine.

TIP

Tapping is helpful for releasing deeply held tension in a trigger point or a specific muscle spasm; however, it does make noise. Many clients like the musical sound, but it is not for everyone at every moment. For example, tapping is useful for helping the client "come back" at the end of a massage. In contrast, in the middle of a massage, if your client is in a deep state of relaxation, it may be too jarring. If you feel the vibration will be beneficial to the client but the sound will be too jarring, you can always place a small washcloth over the top of the stone before you tap.

Clanking

Clanking is a technique whereby the edges of placement stones are struck against one another. This can be done with just two stones at a time, for a very specific effect, or in a group or line of stones for a broader effect. For clanking to be effective, the height and shape of the stones need to match, and you should situate them so that there is no space between them. If the stones do not match in height or shape or if there is too much space between them, as shown in Figure 9-10, they will not make contact when you try to strike them against one another and the technique will fail.

To clank two stones together, simply take two adjacent same-sized stones and bring the sides of them apart and together, striking them against each another. This will create a vibration into the area directly beneath the two stones.

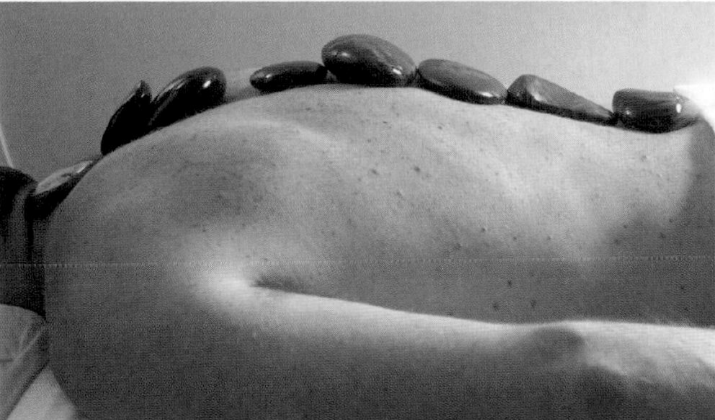

Figure 9-10 Improper Height of Stones for Clanking. Stones used for clanking must be about the same height or they will miss each other. This photo shows a line up with unmatched stones. You can see how the stones would miss each other or tumble over each other when being clanked.

For a broader effect, you can clank a group or a line of stones against one another at the same time. To do this, place your hands at either end of the line of stones. Pressing down, push the stones slightly towards one another (Fig. 9-11), then quickly pull your hands apart, stretching the stones away from one another, and then let the stones fall back together, clanking against each other. Repeat this action rhythmically, using an accordion motion. An alternative approach is to stand at the client's head and gently push on the shoulders rhythmically, letting their rocking motion produce the clanking of the line of stones. When the proper rhythm is found, the stones create a wavelike motion when they clank. This sends a tingling vibration along the client's spine that is simultaneously invigorating and relaxing. As with tapping, you'll need to judge whether the sound of clanking will be too jarring for the client and use the technique only when it feels appropriate.

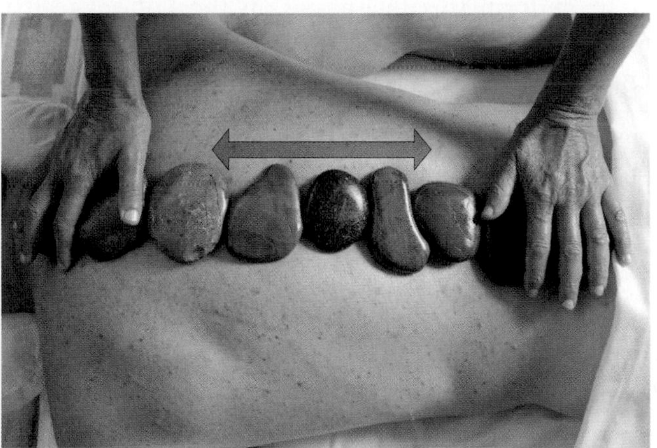

Figure 9-11 Clanking. To clank a line of stones, place your hands at either end of the stones and pull the stones apart. Then, release your hands and let the stones drop back against each other in a rhythmical fashion. Notice that the height of the stones is about equal for optimal contact.

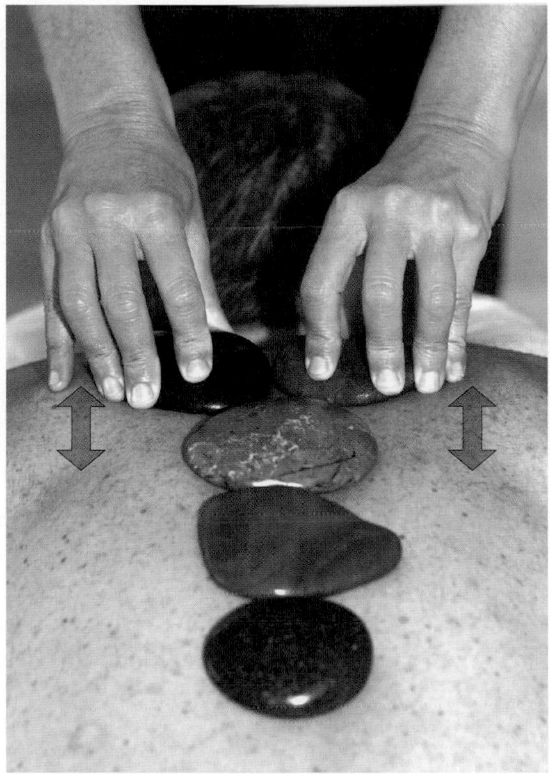

Figure 9-12 Rubbing. Vigorously rubbing two stones against each another sends vibration and heat directly into client's body.

Rubbing

In the **rubbing** technique, the sides of two stones are vigorously scrubbed against each other. As with clanking, the two stones need to be the same size and height for optimal surface contact. Place the stones flat on the body right next to each other and simply rub them back and forth together to create friction (Fig. 9-12). When the stones are rubbed at the appropriate speed and for the proper length of time, they will smell like burnt caps or phosphorous. The friction of rubbing creates vibration and heat, which are transmitted directly to the body tissues beneath the stones.

CAUTION

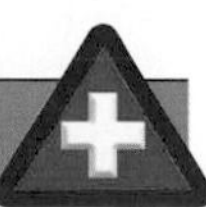

Be careful not to pinch the client's skin between the two rubbing stones.

Friction

Friction is similar to rubbing, but rather than scrubbing the stones against each other, you scrub them back and forth against the client's skin. Just like friction with your hands, friction from stones helps to increase circulation and break up dense, contracted tissue.

To perform friction, place the edges (stones are on their sides) of two stones against the client's body about 2 inches apart from each other. Be sure your thumbs are on the inside of the stones with your index fingers on the top edge and the rest of your fingers curled on the outside to frame and stabilize the stones, as shown in Figure 9-13. Once you are in this position, drop the stones vertically into the body and, alternating hands, create quick, up-and-down motions approximately 1 to 2 inches long. This motion creates the friction. Use the amount of depth and speed desired by your client. Stay in one place for 10 seconds and then move about 1 inch up or down the body and repeat. Remember to stop using the stones when they are no longer hot.

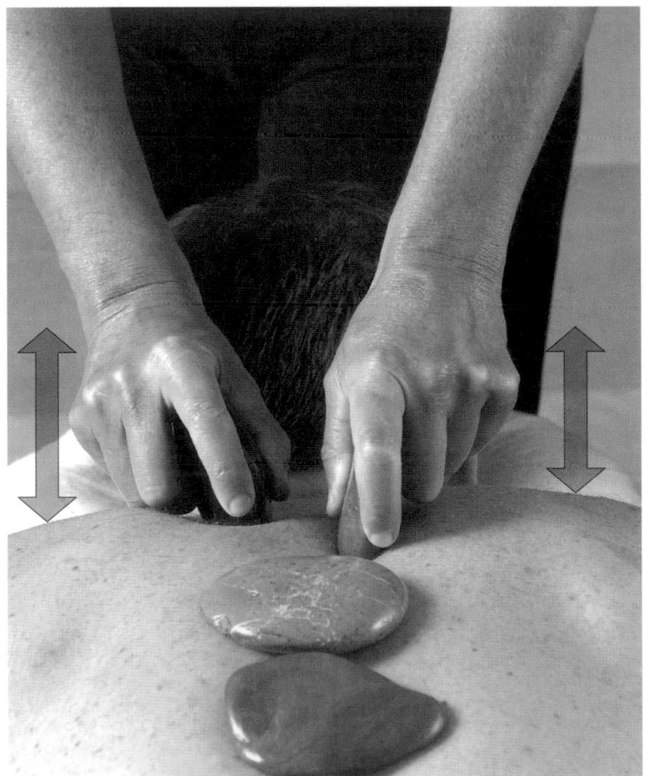

Figure 9-13 Friction. Making quick, firm back and forth motions with the stones against the skin creates friction that releases deep tension in the muscles.

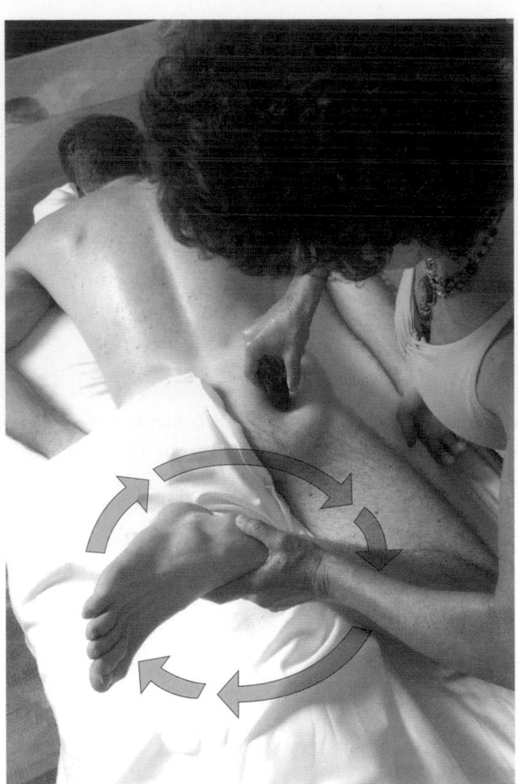

Figure 9-14 Pin and Stir. After the tip of the stone is pinned in place, lift the limb and begin the "stirring" motion.

Pin and Stir

Pin and stir is a technique that involves pinning the tip of a stone in place on the belly of a muscle and moving the limb around the pinned stone. This serves to open the muscle from the inside out. Some examples of this are pinning the buttocks and stirring with the leg, pinning the neck and stirring with the head, or pinning the biceps and stirring with the forearm.

To perform this technique on the buttocks, first find an area of tension in the belly of the gluteus maximus muscle with your hand. Using a pointed stone with a broad tip, place the tip on that spot. Gently press down with the stone tip to be sure you are in the right place. After the client affirms your location, press the stone in a bit deeper and hold in place while you raise the client's foot, as shown in Figure 9-14. Rotate (or "stir") the raised foot in slow circles around the pinned stone. You can circle the foot in both directions or go back and forth in place.

TIP

Improvise your stirring motion based on what is needed to release the tension in the area beneath the stone. After approximately 1 minute, or when the muscle feels as if it has released, move to another spot in the same proximity. Work as many areas as required, conferring with the client. After you have completed an area with the "pin and stir" technique, use broad strokes to soothe and flush out the area.

Snaking the Spine

In the technique I call **snaking the spine**, you use the point of a stone to carve an S-curve down the spine. The shape you make is similar to that made by a skier going down a slalom course. Begin by placing the tip of your pointed tool stone on either side of the client's spine. Now, slowly "snake" it in and out of each vertebra, back and forth along the spine, as shown in Figure 9-15. Do this motion up and down the spine. It is very liberating for the spaces between the vertebrae and to encourage circulation of the cerebrospinal fluid.

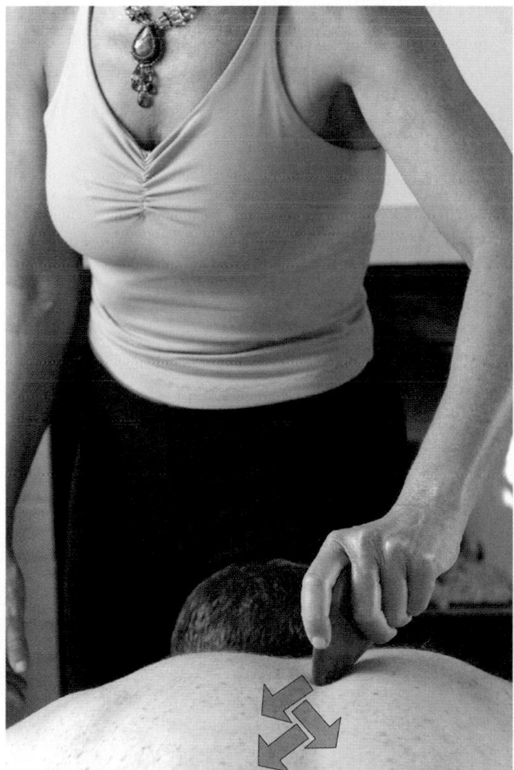

Figure 9-15 Snaking the Spine. Snake the stone down the spine in and out of each vertebra as you would ski down a slalom course on a ski slope.

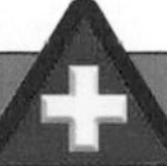

CAUTION

Be careful not to hit the spinous processes along the way, as this would be painful for the client. Also, make sure that the tip of the stone is sufficiently heated.

TECHNIQUES FOR USING STONES ABOVE THE BODY

Although three-dimensional hot stone massage emphasizes the use of hands on both sides of the body, certain techniques are done on the topside of the body only, in both the supine and prone positions. The following stone techniques are meant for performing above the body, rather than below.

Gliding

Gliding is simply sliding the hot oiled stone along the muscle in a long, sweeping motion. It is akin to an effleurage stroke but done with a stone. Gliding is the most common and basic stone technique. It is generally performed across an entire limb or body part, but you can also restrict it to smaller areas. Gliding is an excellent technique to use for your first and last stroke on each body part.

It is critical when gliding to make sure your fingers contact the client's skin along with the stone, as shown in Figure 9-16. Proper stone entrance is also imperative when gliding because it is a technique that is used so

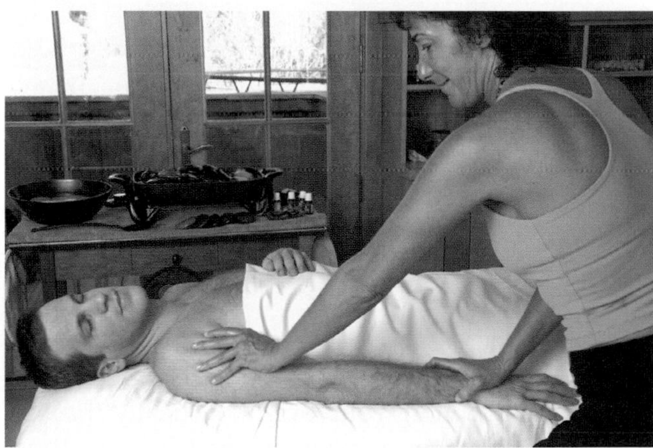

Figure 9-16 Gliding. Gliding is the most basic technique for sliding the stone in long broad strokes up and down the body. Be sure to make contact with the fingers and the stone as you glide along the skin.

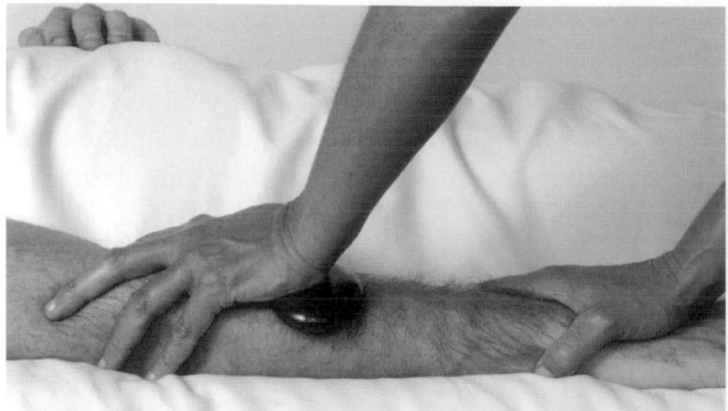

Figure 9-17 Heeling. Heeling is similar to gliding but done with more direct pressure from the heel of the hand.

frequently throughout the massage; thus, the quality of entrance will make the difference between a relaxing and a jarring massage. The amount of pressure you use in a glide should reflect the preference of your client.

Heeling

Heeling is a deeper, slower, more specific variation of gliding. Rather than simply gliding the stone along the limb or body part, you drop your weight vertically into the client with the heel of your hand, as shown in Figure 9-17, and then push the stone along.

Even though the focus of heeling is the stone just below the heel of your hand, it is still important to make contact with the rest of your hand as well. Use heeling in just a section of the limb or body part rather than throughout the entire limb. It is great for opening the tissue on a deeper level and is a nice technique to follow gliding.

CAUTION

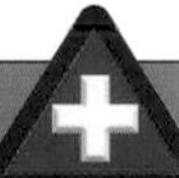

Because heeling involves deeper pressure than gliding does, it is important to pay careful attention to each area of the client's limb when using this technique, as various parts of the tissue may have a different tolerance for pressure. Adjust your pressure accordingly.

Circling

Circling is dropping your weight vertically through your hand and then making circles with the stone. Circle slowly, going up and out a few inches, moving across the top of the circle, and coming back down to where you started, as shown in Figure 9-18. Make a few circles in the same area and then slide up the body a few inches and make more circles. Try circling following heeling to help eliminate tension in a wider area.

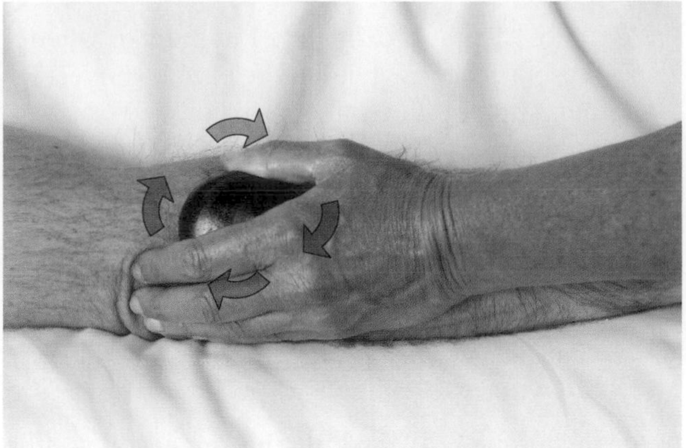

Figure 9-18 Circling. With weight dropped vertically, make slow circles with the stone.

Paws Digging

Paws digging is a technique for softening tissues. It resembles the action of a dog digging in the sand with its two front paws. Use the same motion, hand after hand, and dig away with the stones (Fig. 9-19). Make

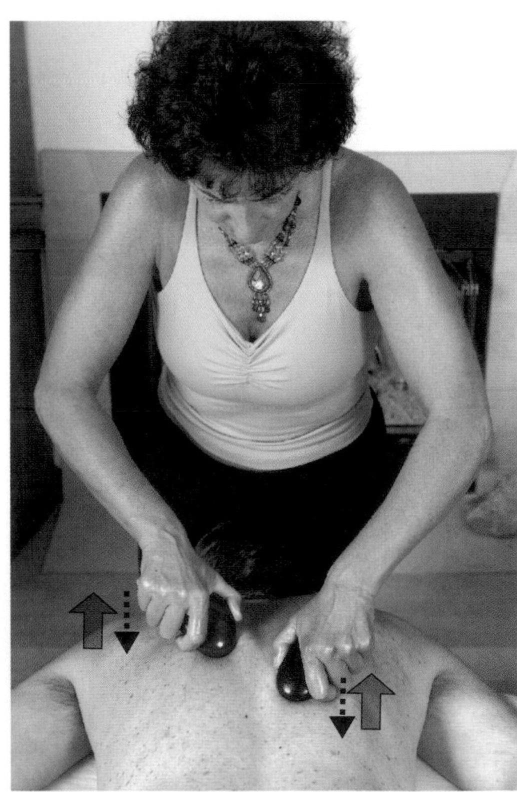

Figure 9-19 Paws Digging. With this technique, you move your hands up and down like a dog's paws digging in the sand.

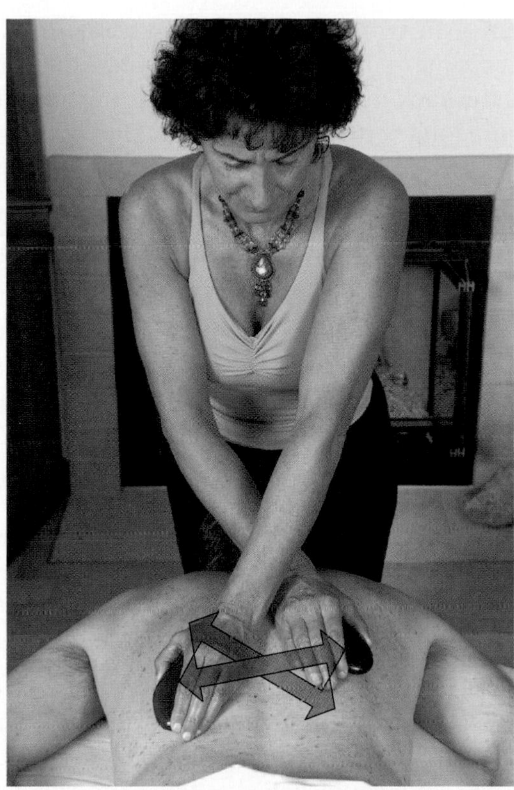

Figure 9-20 Crisscrossing. Begin with stone-filled hands that are crossed, then uncross, cross, and uncross them again up and down the back or legs.

only a minimal amount of finger contact with the body during this technique.

Paws digging is great for freeing up tense areas in the back, especially in the muscular areas of the upper thoracic region. You can also use it on the neck, lower back, buttocks, side of the torso, and either side of the thigh. It is difficult to do in more petite, less muscular areas of the body. Use paws digging wherever it feels good to your clients, using the depth and speed they desire.

Crisscrossing

Crisscrossing is similar to gliding, but is done in crossing patterns. Begin with stone-filled hands that are crossed, as shown in Figure 9-20, then uncross, cross, and uncross them again as you move up and down the client's back or legs. You can make different shapes with your hands, such as a figure-of-eight or an X shape, and vary your speed and depth.

Rolling

Rolling is as simple as it sounds. You just roll the stone back and forth or up and down the client's body. For

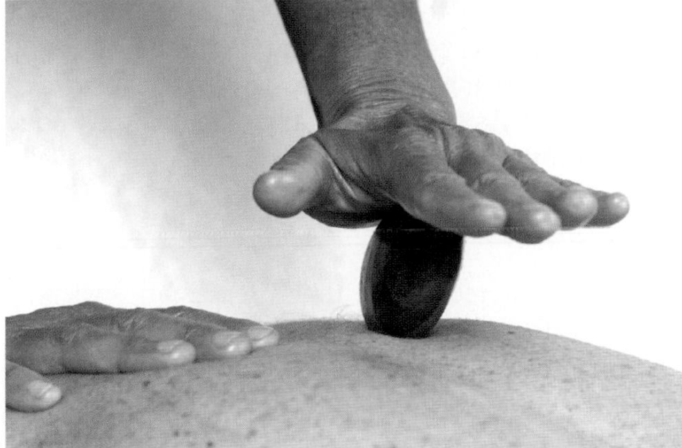

Figure 9-21 Rolling. Place a round stone in the center of your palm and slowly roll it back and forth in place or up and down the length of an area.

this technique to be successful, however, you need to use a very round stone. I have a few round stones that I reserve specifically for this purpose. Place the round stone in the center of your palm and slowly roll it back and forth in place or roll it up and down the length of an area of the body. Rolling can be done with one hand on top of the round stone, as shown in Figure 9-21, with two hands on top of the stone, or with one hand on either side of the stone. It is a useful technique for breaking up tension in a very calming way.

Elephant Walking

Elephant walking is like compression with movement. Using medium to large stones in each hand, alternately press the stones into either side of your client's back, as shown in Figure 9-22, or down the backside of both legs. As you press the stones, drop

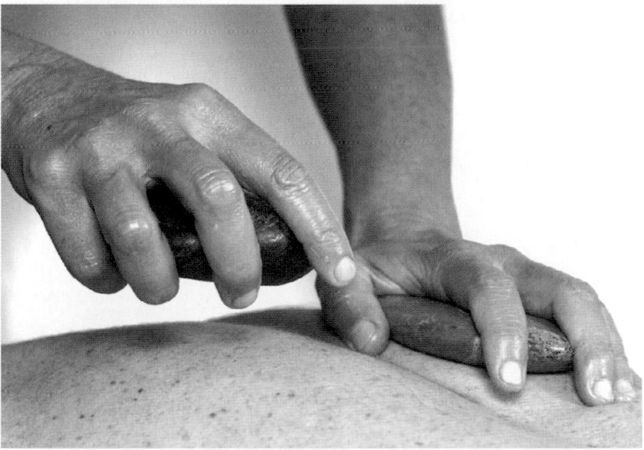

Figure 9-22 Elephant Walking. With medium to large stones in each hand, alternate pressing the stones up and down the length of the client's back or legs slowly, like an elephant walking.

your weight into the client's body, imagining your hands are the feet of an elephant. Walk the stones up and down the length of the body part slowly and rhythmically. As simple as it appears, this technique has a profoundly releasing effect.

Flushing

Flushing is a technique that uses light, sweeping strokes with a large flat stone to soothe and "clean out" an area that has just received deep specific work. Use it to increase circulation to a large area, bringing fresh blood and oxygen to flush out toxins that your deep work released. It feels great to the client and also serves as a wonderful way to close a massage.

To flush an area, use a very large placement stone to cover as much surface area as possible. If the stone you choose is too large for your hands to embrace, you can still make hand contact with the client's body along the edges of the stone. Incidentally, you can also do a more limited version of flushing on smaller areas with smaller stones.

To flush the back, first make long sweeping strokes with your large, flat stone up and down the spine (Fig. 9-23). After going up and down the spine a few times, you can then twirl the stone slowly along the back. After twirling, you can make long flushing strokes across the back to either side. End the flushing with a few more long vertical strokes along the spine.

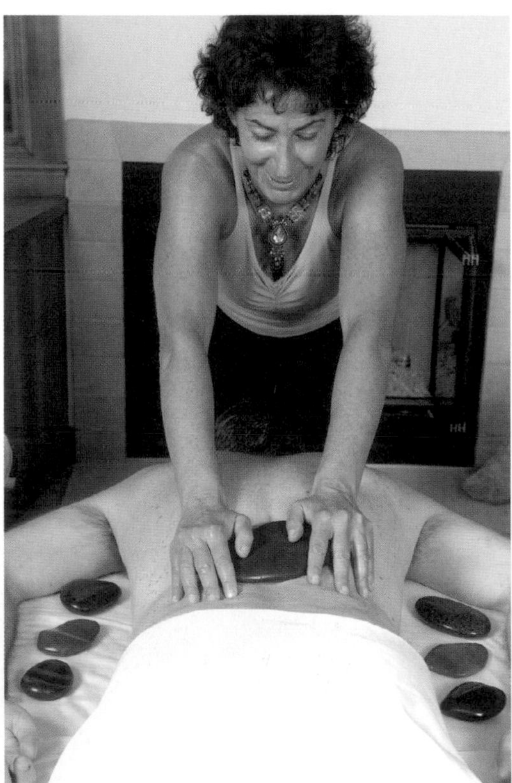

Figure 9-23 Flushing. Using a large, flat placement stone, make long sweeping strokes fairly quickly along the entire length of the back. Move the stone sideways as well.

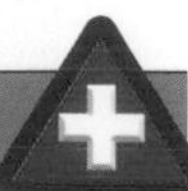

CAUTION

If your client's spinous processes stick out, it is advisable to avoid going over the spine and instead flush up and down either side of the spinal column, using a stone of a lesser circumference. Use your judgment and explore gently.

TECHNIQUES FOR USING STONES BENEATH THE BODY

The following stone techniques are performed from beneath the body or from both sides of the body at once. They thereby contribute to the three-dimensional nature of the massage and bring it to a deeper level than you could achieve using the "above the body" techniques alone.

Alternating

Alternating is a technique that involves alternating your stone-held hands beneath a body part. It can be done on any part of the body. Alternating creates, for the client, a continuous sensation of stones being dragged across the body part from beneath. This flowing warmth is deeply soothing.

The technique for alternating beneath the client's shoulders, back, arms, or legs is straightforward: Simply alternate the hands, holding a stone in each, to achieve a continuous flow of strokes.

When alternating on the neck, in addition to alternating your hands, you must hold the weight of the client's head. This makes the technique a bit trickier. As shown in Figure 9-24, as one hand drags the stone across the back of the client's neck, your other hand, in addition to holding a stone, holds the client's head. At the end of each stroke, slide your working hand up to the top of the neck and switch places with the holding hand. Continue alternating your hands across the neck from below in a slow, rhythmical fashion. If it is difficult for you to hold the head up with your hand, you can rest the top of the client's head against your abdomen to support it while you alternate hands back and forth across either side of the neck. When you cross the

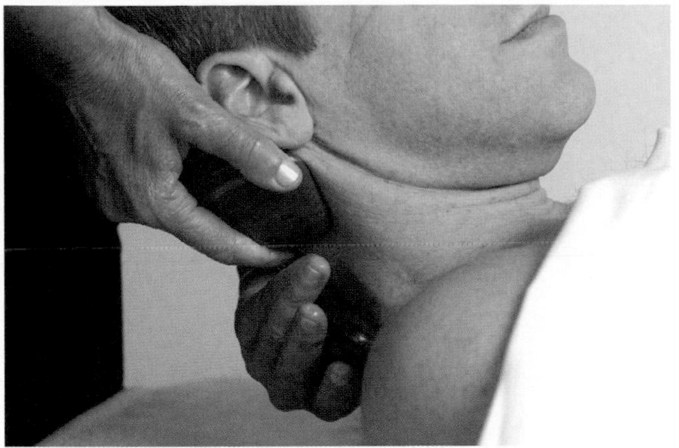

Figure 9-24 Alternating. With a medium-sized stone in each hand, alternate hand over hand making sweeping strokes up and across the neck.

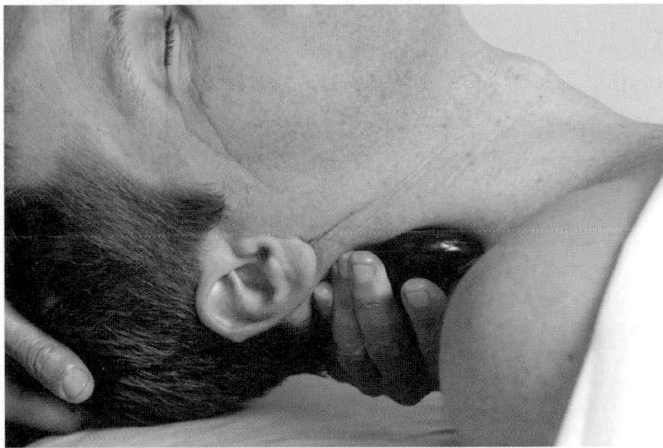

Figure 9-25 Draping. Allow the client's neck, limb, shoulder, or other body part to fall over your stone-filled hand.

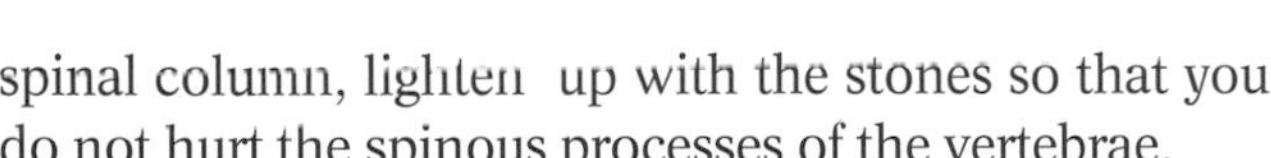

spinal column, lighten up with the stones so that you do not hurt the spinous processes of the vertebrae.

Draping

Draping (not to be confused with draping the sheet) is a technique for allowing the client's body weight to drape over the stone. It is both more effective and more soothing to the client than attaining the same deep pressure by means of pushing the stone into the body. To drape, simply lift the part of the body you wish to penetrate with the stone and place the stone beneath it. Then, slowly allow the weight of the body part to fall over the stone. For instance, when draping the neck, lift the client's head with one hand, place the stone on the outside of the neck with the other, and then allow the head to fall toward and over the stone as you gently lift your stone-filled hand up and glide it across the gravitational pull of the neck (Fig. 9-25). To drape the low back, bring client's knees up and then roll them away from you, exposing the client's low back. Place a stone-filled hand beneath the low back, and then slowly lower the body back over the stone-held hand. Use the weight of the torso to gain the depth needed for the stone's penetration. This method allows the stone's heat to penetrate deeply without causing pain or discomfort to the client. It is also easier on your arms and hands. Explore draping with every part of the body.

Teetering

Teetering is a technique that adds movement to the stone that is being draped. To do it, first place a stone beneath a body part in a way that maintains some space around it and will allow you to create movement with the stone. Once in place, flip the stone back and forth in a slow rhythmical fashion.

For example, when performing teetering on the rhomboids, locate the area just inside the medial border of the scapula and place the stone with its long edge against this area. It is best to use an oblong stone with 0.25 inch edge for the most comfortable and effective teetering. Position the stone at the base of your fingers and grasp it between your thumb and finger pads (Fig. 9-26). After the stone is in its proper position, keep it planted against the body and wiggle it back and forth in place, as if the body part is teetering on top of the stone. This motion is very effective in opening the muscles and releasing deep tension from the area.

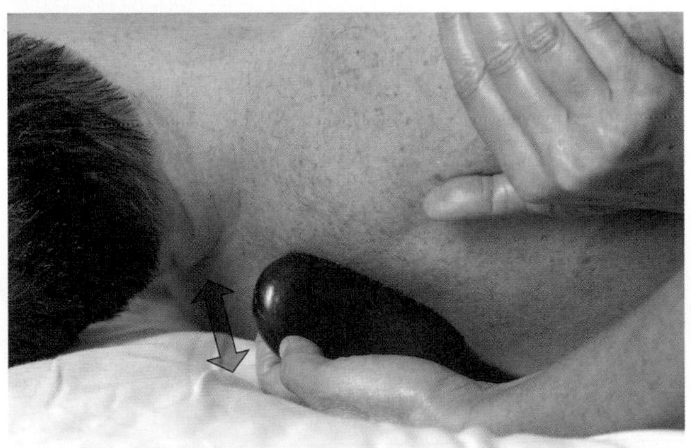

Figure 9-26 Teetering. When teetering the stone beneath the shoulder, make sure the stone is completely on its side, or the technique will be painful for both you and your client.

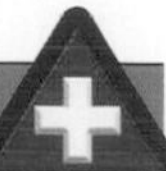

CAUTION

It is critical that you hold the stone completely upright in the side position, as shown in Figure 9-26, to achieve the teetering effect. If you're not holding the stone completely upright, you will not create an effective teetering motion and you might hurt your hand attempting to produce it. When the stone is held completely upright, the teetering motion is easy to do and feels great to both you and your client.

Squeeze, Twist, and Slide

Squeeze, twist, and slide involves squeezing a stone up from beneath a body part and then rapidly twisting and sliding it the rest of the way. The technique feels particularly good on the upper trapezius muscles, but you can perform it in other areas of the body as well. On the trapezius, slide a stone beneath the upper trapezius and then squeeze it between your thumb and the client's body. As you squeeze the stone against the body, pull it toward you, allowing it to twist and then flip to its other side, as shown in Figure 9-27. After the stone has twisted and flipped to its other side, slide the stone up the length of the neck. Repeat this technique on the upper trapezius and neck several times. The twisting and flipping of the stone puts momentary deep pressure into the trapezius, just before it slides off. The combination of deep pressure followed immediately by the fluid slide serves to relieve long-held tension in a luxurious way.

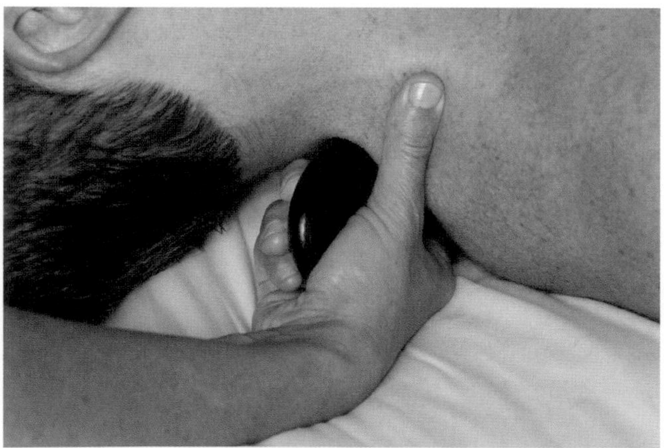

Figure 9-27 **Squeeze, Twist and Slide.** As you squeeze the stone up against the traps, pull it towards you and allow it to twist and then flip to the other side. End by sliding the stone up the length of the neck, then repeat.

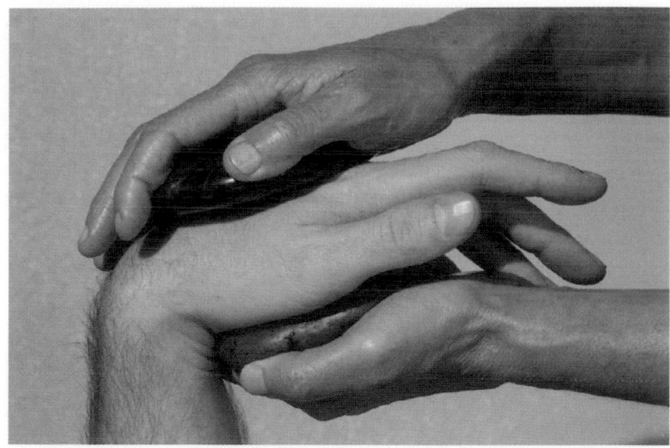

Figure 9-28 **Sandwiching.** Using stones on both sides of the body at the same time allows the body to feel completely met. This technique can be done on practically every part of the body except the head.

Sandwiching

Sandwiching is an easy technique that uses stones on both sides of the body at once to envelop the body in warmth, as shown in Figure 9-28. You can use it on most any part of the body except the face. Rather than stopping to place two stones on the body before beginning to massage, work with one stone at first and then seamlessly add the second stone while continuing to massage. You can use the stones in a similar fashion and direction or move them in opposite directions from each other. As long as you move the two stones with awareness of their relationship, the precise direction in which you work them does not matter. Sandwiching the stones like this doubles their effect and helps to dissolve tension twice as fast.

Lift and Drag

Lift and drag is a technique that involves lifting a stone against the underside of the body so that it drags rather than glides along the muscle. This simple technique can be done anywhere you are able to reach beneath the body with a stone. As you move the stone along the underside of the body, lift the stone to create tension so that it slowly drags against the client's muscle (Fig. 9-29). This deepens the tissue-softening effect of the stone beyond what you can achieve with gliding.

Sneaking Under

If you stop the massage to pick up a stone, it breaks the flow and lets the client know that another stone

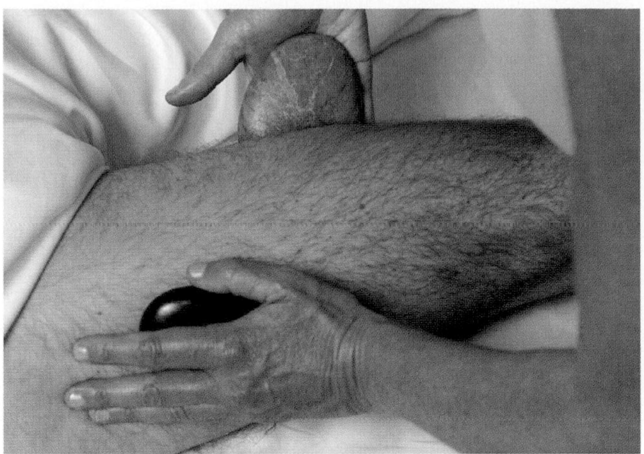

Figure 9-29 Lift and Drag. Lift the stone up into the posterior thigh and then drag it slowly across the hamstrings. You can also use this technique on many other parts of the body.

is coming. Instead, use the **sneaking under** technique to pick up a second stone while you are massaging with another stone on top of the client's body. Slide this second stone beneath the body midstroke. With sneaking under, entry of the stone is so smooth and subtle that the client is not aware of where it came from. It seems to appear out of nowhere.

When entering from beneath the body, it is important to enter with the stone where there is a natural space such as the joint areas, like the lumbar region, the back of the neck, or the knees. You can also rotate or push on a body part, such as the shoulder, in a way that creates a slight opening beneath the body, as shown in Figure 9-30. Another trick for easy stone entrance from below is to strategically place your stones on the massage table so that they are there waiting for you when you need them. So, for instance, you would leave a stone on the table near the top of the client's shoulder so that when you reach under the armpit and beneath the shoulder, you can grab the stone with your hand from below and simply slide it beneath the shoulder on your down stroke.

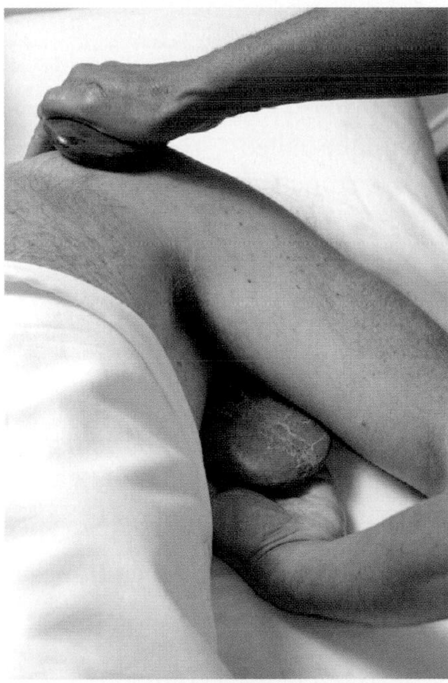

Figure 9-30 Sneaking Under. Pushing back and down lightly on the shoulder creates a slight opening for easy entrance under the shoulder. This allows you to sneak the stone in with no effort.

Sneak in with a stone whenever you can. This technique adds to the seamless, flowing quality characteristic of three-dimensional hot stone massage.

SUMMARY

There are techniques for working with tool stones, using stones above the body, and using stones beneath the body. Each has its own purpose and effect.

The three types of tool stones are: pointed, concave, and curved. Techniques for working with tool stones include edging, compression, friction, pin and stir, and snaking the spine. Energetic vibrations can be produced by using these techniques: tapping, clanking, and rubbing. Because only a part of the tool stone is felt against the client's body, its temperature must be higher than it would be if the whole stone were being used. A tool stone that is not hot enough will cause discomfort to the client.

Techniques for using stones above the body include gliding, heeling, circling, paws digging, crisscrossing, rolling, elephant walking, and flushing. If these techniques were the only ones used, the massage would feel flat; adding the techniques for using stones beneath the body produces a three-dimensional massage.

Techniques for using stones beneath the body include alternating; draping; teetering; squeeze, twist, and slide; sandwiching; lift and drag; and sneaking under. These techniques allow you to use the client's weight for depth, which not only feels wonderful to the client but also requires less strength than working from above. These techniques promote the feeling of a three-dimensional massage.

When incorporating the techniques for using stones into your massage practice, remember to ground them in the principles discussed in Chapter 8. The combination of principles and techniques will prepare you for effectively performing the three-dimensional strokes that you will learn in the next and final chapter.

REVIEW QUESTIONS

TRUE/FALSE

1. When you are using a tool stone, your hands do not contact the client's body, but just hold the upper part of the stone.

   Circle: True False

2. A concaved stone is used to work the concaved areas of the body.

   Circle: True False

3. Edging is a technique that requires a stone with a narrow edge ranging from 0.25 to 1 inch thick.

   Circle: True False

4. Tapping, clanking, and rubbing are ways to create energetic vibrations with the stones.

   Circle: True False

5. Friction differs from rubbing in that with friction, the stones are rubbed against one another, and with rubbing, the stones are rubbed against the client's body.

   Circle: True False

MULTIPLE CHOICE

6. When an area of tension is deep, it is best to use a pointed tool stone with a:
   a. Broad, wide tip
   b. Sharp, narrow tip
   c. Flat tip
   d. Narrow edge
   e. Curved tip
7. The following technique is performed above the body:
   a. Snaking the spine
   b. Alternating
   c. Crisscrossing
   d. Draping
   e. Both a and c
8. The following technique is performed from below the body:
   a. Gliding
   b. Tapping
   c. Elephant walking
   d. Lift and drag
   e. Flushing
9. Sneaking in involves:
   a. Entering the massage room without the client knowing it
   b. Entering with slow speed
   c. Leaving a working stone on top of the body as a placement stone
   d. Using your pile system well
   e. Entering with a stone beneath the body invisibly
10. Techniques need to be grounded in:
    a. A particular order
    b. The geology of the stones
    c. The underlying principles
    d. The proper use of oil
    e. None of the above

SHORT ANSWER

11. A technique of continually changing the stone-held hands that are beneath the client's body is called ______________.
12. The technique called ______________ adds stone movement to the more fundamental technique of draping.
13. Introducing the stones that will be used below the body in a seamless way so that they seem to appear out of nowhere, is called ______________ ______________.
14. Adding the ______________ hand to the pointed tool stone softens the entrance.
15. The technique called ________________ requires you to use stones of the same height and shape.

MATCHING

a. Paws digging c. Heeling e. Flushing
b. Pin and stir d. Gliding

16. A technique done with a tool stone.
17. Pushing with the heel of the hand.
18. A technique similar to something a dog does.
19. Cleans out toxins after doing deep specific work.
20. One of the most common techniques used in hot stone massage.

Answers to Review Questions can be found in Appendix D.

CHAPTER 10

Strokes Used in Three-Dimensional Hot Stone Massage

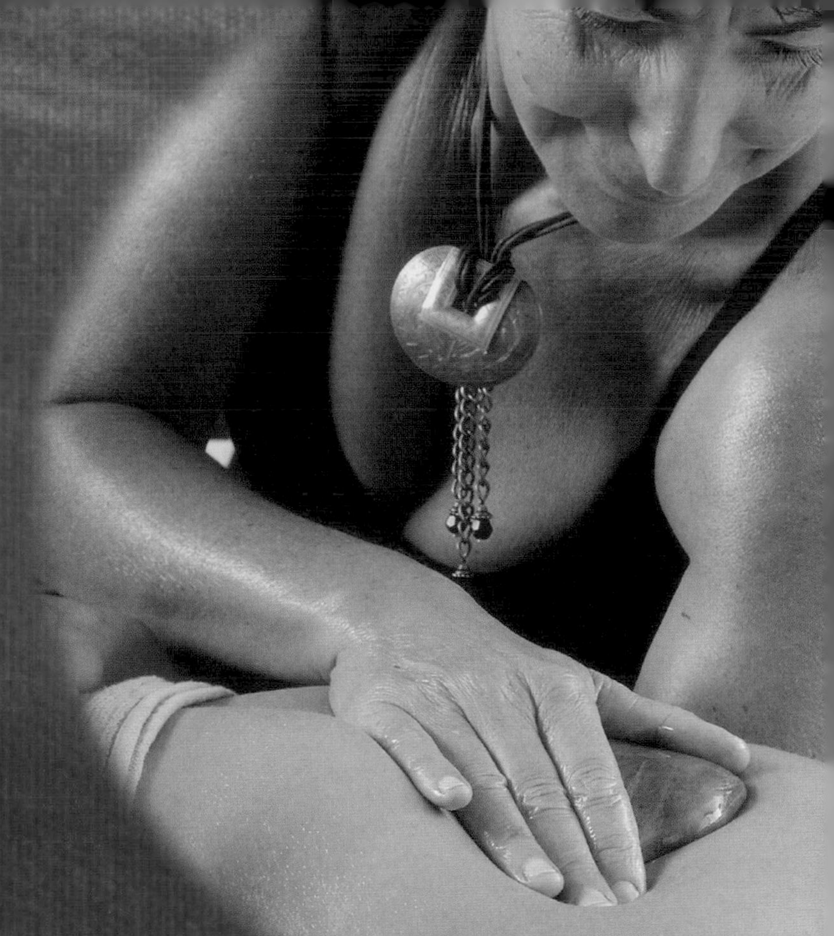

Outline

Three-Dimensionality and Draping

Opening Strokes

- Heart and Belly Stone Breath
- Head Stone Cradle

The Face

- Face Flush
- Infiniteye
- Jaw Melt

The Neck

- Waterfall
- Neck Drool
- Neck Over
- Rock n' Roll

The Arms and Shoulders

- Three-Dimensional Arm Effleurage
- Altar-nater
- Hand Scrunch
- Lat Pump

The Torso

- Rag Doll
- Lumbar Torque
- Undertow
- Belly Waves

The Legs—Supine

- Three-Dimensional Leg Effleurage
- Foot Scrunch
- Leg Over Sequence
- The Frog
- Hip Flip

Turning the Client Over

The Back

- The Fullback
- Forearm Frenzy
- Chicken Wing
- Teres Tango
- Reverse Belly Wave
- Hip Hop

The Legs—Prone

- Three-Dimensional Leg Effleurage
- Shortened Ham Pump
- Calf Mush
- Reverse Frog

Closing Strokes

- Calf Up-Arm Down
- Bubbling Spring/Palace of Weariness

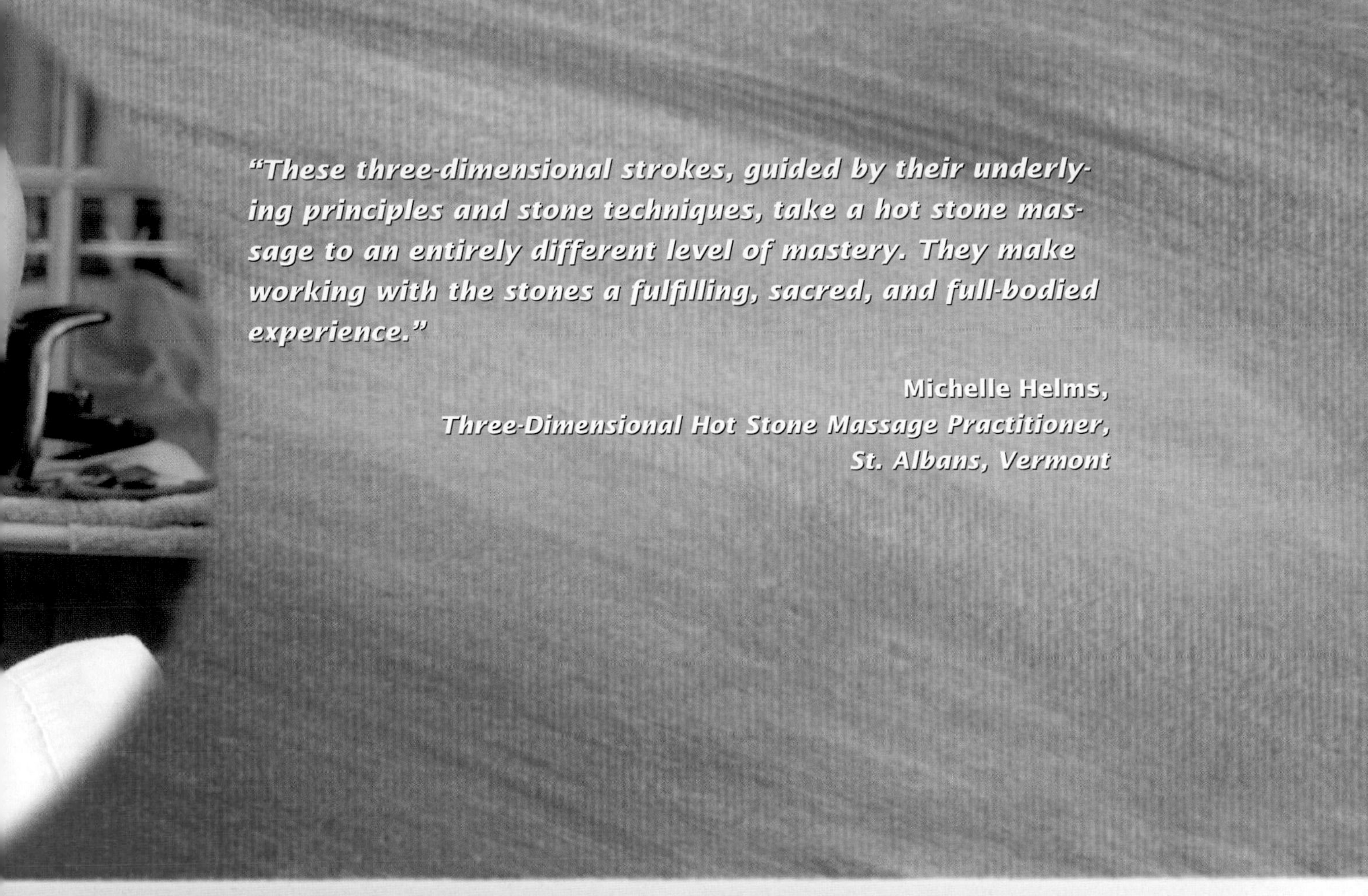

"These three-dimensional strokes, guided by their underlying principles and stone techniques, take a hot stone massage to an entirely different level of mastery. They make working with the stones a fulfilling, sacred, and full-bodied experience."

Michelle Helms,
Three-Dimensional Hot Stone Massage Practitioner,
St. Albans, Vermont

Objectives

After reading this chapter, you should be able to:

- Explain why draping is particularly important when providing three-dimensional hot stone massage.
- Become familiar with each of the three-dimensional massage strokes described in this chapter.
- Incorporate hot stones with each stroke described in this chapter.

Key Terms

Bubbling spring: The acupuncture point kidney 1, located at the ball of each foot. Holding this spot at the end of a massage is very calming and grounding.

Deltoid: A thick triangular muscle covering the shoulder joint used to raise the arm from the side. It originates on the lateral third of the clavicle, acromion process, and spine of the scapula and inserts in the middle of the lateral surface of the humerus.

Erector spinae: The largest muscle mass of the back. It lies near the vertebral column and runs along the length of the spine. It is divided into three longitudinal columns—the iliocostalis, longissimus, and spinalis muscles—and assists in extension, lateral flexion, and rotation of the spine.

Foot-hand or arm: The therapist's hand or arm that is closest to the client's foot when facing the side of the table.

Gastrocnemius: The largest and most prominent muscle of the calf, which acts to extend the foot and bend the knee. It originates by two heads on the lateral and medial condyles of the femur and it inserts into the calcaneus at the same place as the soleus muscle, joining tendons to make up the *Achilles* tendon.

(Continued)

Key Terms *(Continued)*

Gluteus: A broad and thick fleshy mass made up of three gluteal muscles (gluteus maximus, minimus and medius) and otherwise known as the buttocks.

Hamstrings: The three tendons that insert behind the knee and connect to the muscles located in the back of the thigh, referred to as the *semitendinosus*, *semimembranosus*, and the *biceps femoris*.

Head-hand or head-arm: The therapist's hand or arm that is closest to the client's head when facing the side of the table.

Hogu: A large-intestine acupuncture point located in the middle of the meaty part of the webbing of the thumb. This spot is known to relieve headaches when worked. It is often very painful to work.

Humerus: The long bone of the upper arm that runs from the scapula to the radius and ulna.

Iliac crest: The long curved upper border of the wing of the ilium or the upper part of the bony pelvis. It is thinner at the center than at the extremities.

Iliotibial band: A thick, wide fascial layer that runs from the iliac crest of the pelvis to the knee joint. It is often referred to as the *IT band*.

Infraspinatus: A thick triangular muscle that originates from the infraspinous fossa of the scapula and inserts laterally to the greater tubercle of the humerus. It is a lateral rotator of the glenohumeral joint and an adductor of the arm.

Inside hand or arm: The therapist's hand or arm that is closest to the client when facing the client's head or feet.

Laminar groove: The groove that runs along either side of the entire spinal column. Made of paraspinal tissue, it is the crevice that exists between the transverse process and the erector spinae mass.

Latissimus dorsi: A pair of fan-shaped muscles extending across the middle and low back that attach to the arms and the spine and work to adduct, extend, and medially rotate the arm. They are often referred to as the *lats*.

Masseter: A thick, somewhat quadrilateral muscle, consisting of two portions, superficial and deep, both originating from aspects of the zygomatic arch and inserting into aspects of the mandible. It aids in chewing (masticating).

Occipital ridge: The region at the back of the head where the base of the skull meets the cervical spine.

Outside hand or arm: The therapist's hand or arm that is furthest from the client when facing the client's head or feet.

Palace of Weariness: The acupuncture point pericardium 8, located in the center of the palm of both hands. Holding this spot at the end of a massage is very calming and grounding.

Pectoralis: Two muscles, one major and one minor, located on the lateral edges of the upper chest just medial of the shoulders. They originate from the sternum, clavicle, and ribs and insert on the greater tubercle of the humerus and the coracoid process of the scapula. They serve to flex, adduct, and medially rotate the arm, as well as elevate ribs and aid in inspiration.

Quadratus lumborum: A muscle that is irregularly quadrilateral in shape, broader below than above. It originates from the iliolumbar ligament at the iliac crest and inserts into the lower border of the last rib for about half its length and into the transverse processes of the upper four lumbar vertebrae.

Quadriceps: The large four-part extensor muscle at the front of the thigh often referred to as the *quads*. The four parts of this large muscle mass are: rectus femoris, vastus lateralis, vastus medialis, and vastus intermedius.

Rhomboid(s): Two muscles that originate on the spines of the seventh cervical and upper thoracic vertebrae and supraspinous ligaments and insert into lower half of the posteromedial border of scapula. Their purpose is to retract the scapula, rotate it inferiorly, and stabilize it.

Rotator cuff: A set of muscles and tendons that secures the arm to the shoulder joint and permits rotation of the arm. It is composed of four muscles: supraspinatus, infraspinatus, teres minor, and subscapularis.

Soleus: A broad flat muscle in the calf of the leg that lies deep to the gastrocnemius muscle and plantar flexes the foot. It originates on the superior posterior tibia and fibula and inserts in the calcaneus at the same place as the gastrocnemius muscle.

Temporal: A muscle that originates in the temporal fossa and fascia and inserts in the coronoid process of the mandible. Its location is normally referred to as the *temples*, and its purpose is to close the jaw.

Temporomandibular joint (TMJ): The joint between the head of the mandible (lower jaw bone) and the tubercle of the temporal bone.

Teres minor: A narrow, elongated muscle of the rotator cuff that originates from the axillary border of the scapula and inserts into the greater tubercle of the humerus. It stabilizes the shoulder joint and medially rotates and adducts the arm.

Trapezius: A muscle, commonly known as the *trap(s)*, extending from the occipital bone and nuchal plane to the clavicle and inferiorly to the spines of the thoracic vertebrae. Its purpose is to draw the scapula backward and rotate it to raise shoulder.

Key Terms (Continued)

Vastus lateralis: A muscle that originates from the posterior ridge of the femur as far as the greater trochanter and inserts into the tibia to extend the leg.

Zygomatic arch: A paired bone of the human skull that articulates with the maxilla, temporal bone, sphenoid bone, and frontal bone. It forms a part of the orbit and is commonly referred to as the *cheekbone.*

This chapter will introduce you to a sample of three-dimensional massage strokes you can use during a hot stone massage. Part of my Phenomenal Touch Massage (PTM) modality, these strokes add a new dimension to the experience of giving and receiving massage, with or without stones. Many of the strokes involved in Phenomenal Touch Massage are too complex to convey in words and photos; thus, the strokes included in this chapter are just a sampling of the multitude of three-dimensional strokes that you would learn in a PTM workshop.

Even the strokes included in this chapter can be difficult to learn from a printed page. It is advisable, therefore, to practice them without stones in your hands first. Once you feel comfortable performing the strokes with just your hands alone, you can add the stones. When you do add stones, take it slowly. Because hot stone massage is a complex art that involves stone entrance, proper temperature, timing, stone flow management, and finesse, it can be challenging to combine stones with these three-dimensional strokes. Wait to use the stones with the most complex of these strokes until you've really become comfortable handling them. You can also use the principles and techniques you learned in earlier chapters of this book to invent your own strokes.

As you work, keep in mind the guideline of always making your initial contact with each body part with stone-free hands. This allows you to get a feel for what is happening in the muscle before bringing in the stones. After you have made your initial contact with your hands on a body part, it is then optional to use stones with all of the strokes you do on that particular body part.

Also, don't forget the body mechanics principles discussed in Chapter 8. The more dynamic the three-dimensional stroke is, the more important it is for you to use intelligent body mechanics. Specific instructions on body mechanics will be provided only for those strokes that require a unique approach. Otherwise, make a general practice of enforcing the proper body mechanics taught in Chapter 8 while learning each stroke. This will not only enable you to protect your body, but it will also enhance the client's experience of the strokes.

As you read on, you'll notice that some of the strokes have seamless transitions into the next stroke described; however, because of the limited number of strokes included, gaps do exist between other strokes. Be sure to fill in the gaps with strokes from your normal repertoire, as well as new ones that you develop based on the principles of three-dimensionality.

And finally, before we begin, you'll need to understand the terms used in this chapter to designate which hand/arm you should use. When you are standing on the side of the table, facing the table, your hand or arm that is closest to the client's head will be referred to as your **head-hand** or **head-arm**, and your hand or arm that is closest to the client's feet will be referred to as your **foot-hand** or **foot-arm**. However, when you are standing on the side of the table and facing the client's head or feet, your hand or arm that is closest to the massage table will be referred to as your **inside hand** or **inside arm**, and your hand or arm that is furthest from the massage table will be referred to as your **outside hand** or **outside arm**.

THREE-DIMENSIONALITY AND DRAPING

Proper draping with the sheet is important for all types of massage; however, it is especially important when using three-dimensional strokes, which often require you to move the client's body in space. Without careful attention to draping, this can result in inadvertent exposure, which in turn can leave your client unable to relax and fully absorb your work.

Be especially careful with strokes that involve sideways movements of the torso and legs, as these are more likely to dislodge the sheet from the breast and groin regions.

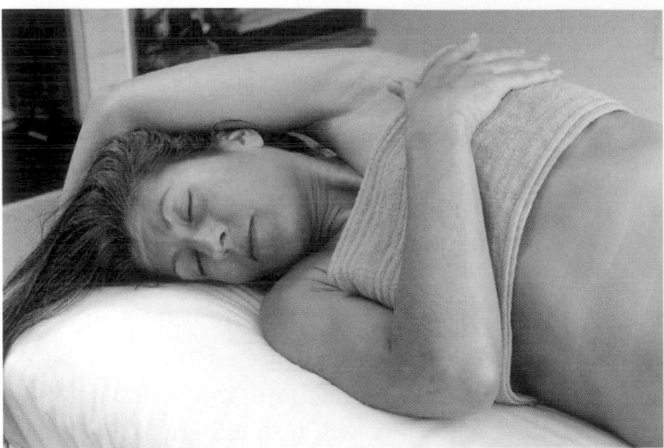

Figure 10-1 Involve Client with Draping. Placing the client's hand over the sheet/towel gives the client a sense of control over the draping and is especially reassuring during sideways movements.

TIP

In particular, during sideways movements with a female client, it is appropriate to place one of the client's hands over the sheet/towel (Fig. 10-1) or hand a piece of the sheet to the client to hold for a short while. This can give the clients a sense of control over their body's level of exposure.

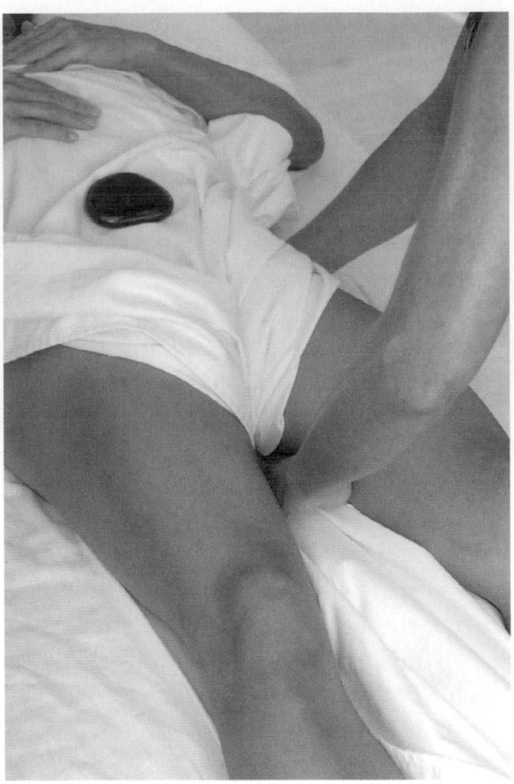

Figure 10-3 Prepare for Your Stroke. Tuck the sheet in between the client's legs and into the groin area before lifting the knees up.

With strokes that involve close proximity of the client's body against yours, it is even more important to drape proficiently to keep clear boundaries with the client (Fig. 10-2). A small pillow or towel can be placed between you and the client if body-to-body contact is an issue for either of you. The level of closeness that can result from cradling a client on both sides of the body at once can sometimes be misunderstood by the client as a sexual invitation. Paying attention to the draping can create clarity for clients and help them to relax into the massage.

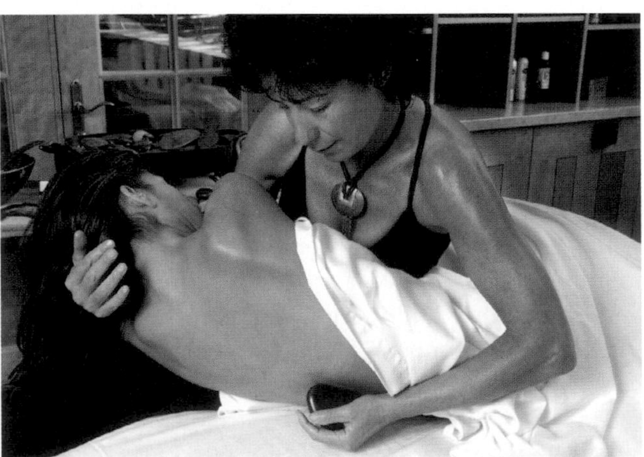

Figure 10-2 Create Safety with Draping. Make sure the sheet is covering the client when doing an intimate stroke that requires body-to-body contact.

Think ahead and take the necessary precautions with the sheet before an exposure occurs. For instance, if you know you are going to do a stroke that involves lifting the client's knees up or moving them laterally, prepare for this stroke by tucking your sheet in between the client's legs and into the groin area before lifting the knees up, as shown in Figure 10-3. While you are in the midst of a stroke, check your draping to be sure that the sheet has remained in place over the groin, buttocks, or breast area (Fig. 10-4). Sometimes, you may have to hold your sheet in place to avoid an inadvertent exposure, as shown in Figure 10-5. Rather than stopping a stroke to hold the sheet in place, try to make the draping be a part of the move, as demonstrated in Figure 10-6. Always drape in as flowing a fashion as possible.

Because of the three-dimensional nature of these strokes, it is important that you make sure your

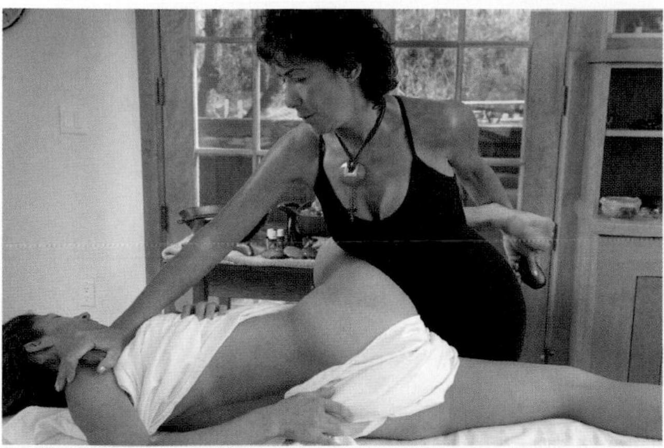

Figure 10-4 Check Draping. Make sure the sheet stays in place over the client's groin and breasts when the client's leg is around your body and the torso is twisted.

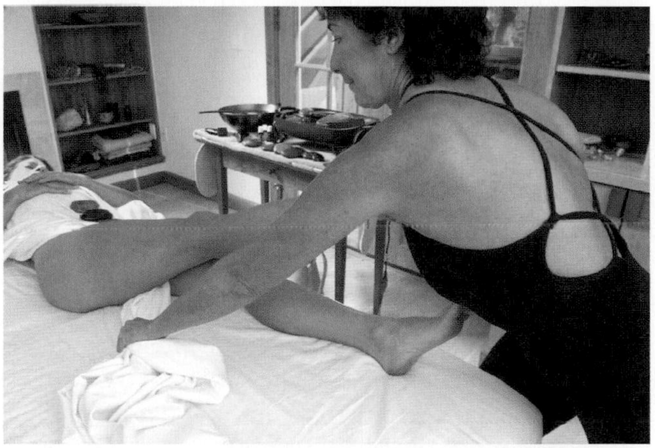

Figure 10-6 Make Draping a Part of the Stroke. Pull the sheet down and across the groin area as you move the client's body in space.

bottom sheet is pulled snugly on the table. Otherwise, you will not be able to get your hand or arm underneath the client without it getting caught in the loose sheet. Tighten the bottom sheet prior to the client lying on the table. Place a sheepskin, fleece, or rubber yoga mat between the massage tabletop and the sheet to help keep the sheet in place without being tied. To further secure the sheet, try one of the following options. You can open the piece of wood on the outside of each table leg (used for adjusting the table height) and slide the sheet between it and the leg, then snug the wood up against the leg to hold the sheet in place. You can tie each corner of the sheet individually in a knot to itself or around each table leg. You can take both of the corners at each end of the table, tie them together in one knot, and then pull the end snugly over the table. You can use an adjustable strap or an elastic rope and wrap it snugly around all the sides and ends of the sheet as it falls off the table. The goal is for your sheet to fit snugly on the table so that you can reach your hand or arm beneath the client without getting caught in its folds. It is worth taking the time to do this before the session begins, or otherwise you will spend much of the massage fighting with the sheet!

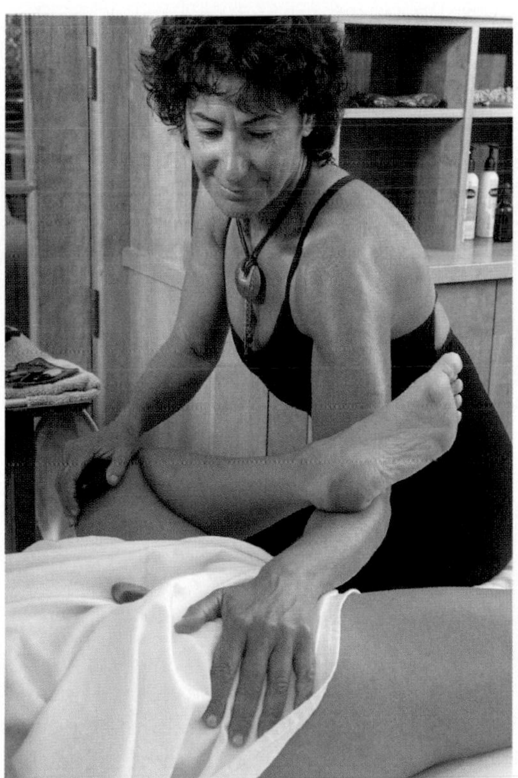

Figure 10-5 Hold Draping in Place. Make sure the groin area remains covered by the sheet when the client's leg is folded open laterally.

As important as draping is, it is also as important to avoid fixating on it. If too much of your focus is on making certain that there are no inadvertent exposures, some clients might feel you are focusing more on the sheet than them. Use your judgment and try to find the right balance between sufficient draping and adequate connection with the client. If an inadvertent slip of the sheet happens, simply fix it right away in a calm manner.

In the following description of the strokes, directions on draping will be included only when there is a specific need for extra care. Otherwise, use common sense and employ appropriate draping for each stroke you perform, giving extra care with sideways positions and movements that involve undulation or lifting.

OPENING STROKES

This chapter begins with descriptions of strokes with the client in the supine position. I often begin my massages with clients lying on stone placements beneath their back. This gives the back muscles a chance to soften and relax before I begin working on them. The supine position also enables me to work more three-dimensionally earlier than I could if the client were in the prone position. However, if you prefer to begin massaging your client face down, start with the strokes listed for the back and then return to the beginning of this section when the client is supine.

The following two opening strokes are particularly effective for promoting relaxation and centering within both the client and the therapist.

TIP 

Experiment with the stones and see what you can create to start your massages. But keep in mind that, for a gentle beginning, slow and simple is best.

Heart and Belly Stone Breath

Heart and belly stone breath is a stroke that offers both you and your client a chance to become fully present with each other and yourself as you prepare for the onset of the massage. After you have done a stone placement on top of the body, stand to the side of the client and place one hand on the heart stone and one hand on the belly stone, as shown in Figure 10-7. Put a slight amount of pressure on each stone and simply breathe in silence with your client, lifting your hands slightly on the in breath, and compressing slightly on the out breath.

After a few minutes of silent matched breathing and slight stone compression, lift your hands slowly off the stones and slide them onto the client's skin to begin massaging with your warmed hands, before you introduce the stones into the actual massage.

Head Stone Cradle

The head stone cradle is another very simple way to begin a massage. It is very helpful for shifting gears from the outside world to the inside world. It is extremely calming for the client's nervous system, and it encourages both you and the client to take nice full breaths. First, lay your stones on top of your client's body. Then, place small warm stones on the face, including the forehead, eyes, and cheeks. Take a medium-sized stone in your hand and hold it beneath the client's head at the **occipital ridge**.

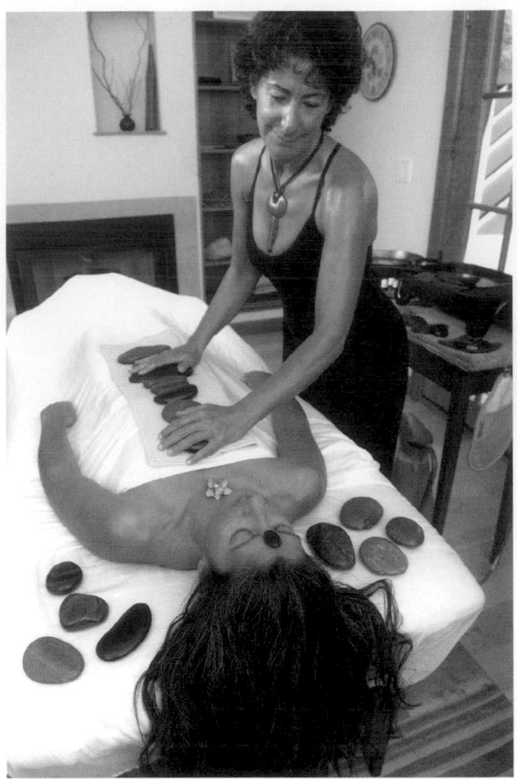

Figure 10-7 Heart and Belly Stone Breath. Open the massage by gently holding your hands on heart and belly stones while matching your breathing with that of your client.

Place your other hand over the stone on the forehead and cradle the head with both hands. Breathe with your client as you hold gentle pressure on both sides of the head (Fig. 10-8).

After cradling the two stones on either side of the head for a few minutes, slide the occipital ridge stone to the bottom of the neck where it meets the back and leave it there. Begin massaging the head with stone-free hands before you integrate your stones into the actual massage.

THE FACE

After you have made contact with the face with stone-free hands, you can perform the following massage strokes with stones. Feel free to go back and forth between stone-filled and stone-free hands while working on the face. Small to medium-sized working stones are best to use for massaging the face. The face strokes are most commonly done from a sitting, rather than standing, position, but choose whatever is most comfortable for you.

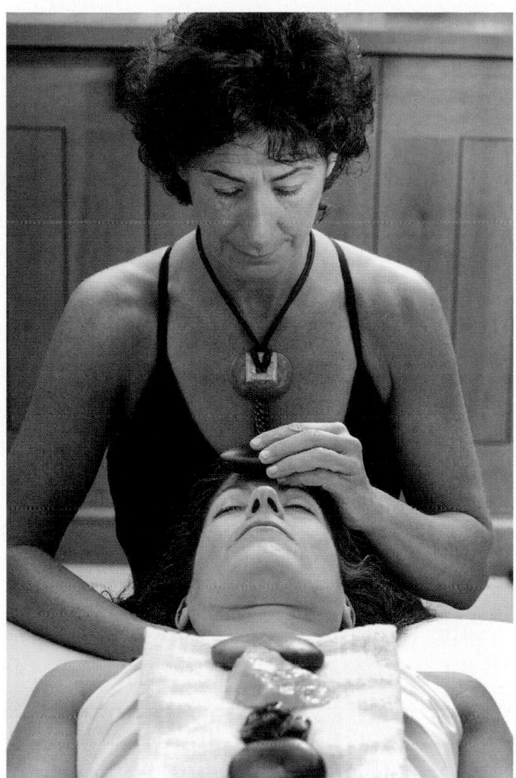

Figure 10-8 Head Stone Cradle. Cradle a stone at the client's occipital ridge and forehead. Sit and breathe with your client in silence.

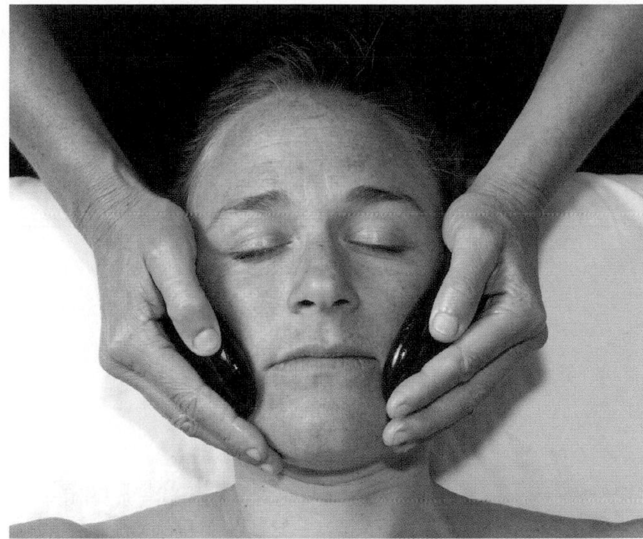

Figure 10-9 Face Flush. With slight pressure, move stones around the entire circumference of the client's face.

TIP

Be sure that your client's head is all the way to the edge of the massage table so that you do not have to bend your back to work the face. This may seem insignificant at first, but over time, it will cause your back to ache.

Face Flush

Face flush is a simple stroke that works the face in a broad fashion. It is great for making initial contact with the stones to the face. Feel free to begin this stroke at any place on the face (Fig. 10-9).

With two medium-size warm stones, use proper entrance of fingertips, edge of stone, then entire stone, to make contact with the face. After you've made full stone contact, press the stones slightly into the face and make slow broad sweeping strokes around its entire surface.

When you reach the ears, hold the stones over them for a moment rather than just sweeping by. If the client is not wearing contact lenses, gently go over the eyes with the stones.

When you reach the forehead, allow your hands and the stones to cross over one another, glide down the sides of the face, and then uncross at the chin.

Repeat this soothing flushing motion over the entire face approximately four times before beginning to work the face with more specific detail. Return to this stroke after you have done more detailed techniques on the face. This utilizes a principle known as "broad to specific to broad."

Infiniteye

Infiniteye (pronounced in-FIN-i-tai) is a stroke in which you make opposing circles around the edges of the client's eyes. The motion of alternating circles creates the shape of a sideways "figure-of-eight" or an infinity symbol, thus the name. Very small, flat, round rocks are best, and they can be either cold or warm: Cold produces a reduction in inflammation and a refreshing feeling, and warm creates a relaxing, soothing experience. Alternating cold with warm is also a delightful option.

CAUTION

Avoid this stroke if the client is wearing contact lenses.

Begin by placing two small stones gently over the eyes.

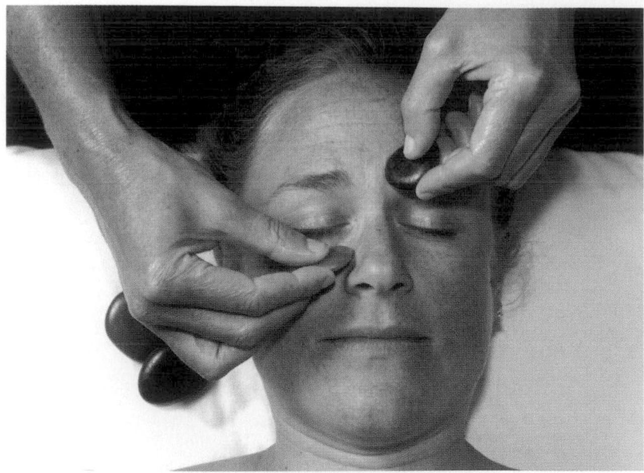

Figure 10-10 Infiniteye. Create simultaneous alternating circles around the eyes.

Move one of the stones off the eye by slowly sliding it down the inside of the eye next to the bridge of the nose. Continue moving that stone slowly to the outside of the eye, while bringing the second stone over the other eye to the inside of the bridge of the nose.

Keeping the stones flat and using some pressure, create alternating circles simultaneously around the eyes, being sure you go over the **zygomatic arch** on the lower sweep of the circle and just above the eyebrows on the upper sweep of the circle. You can do this stroke with the edge rather than the flat side of the stone for more precision (Fig. 10-10). This is desirable for the clients who prefer deeper and more-specific vertical pressure around the eyes. If you do use the edges of the stones, it is important to end with a broad sweep with the flat side of the stone for a soothing effect.

TIP

To be sure your circles continue to alternate, keep the stones at opposite ends of the eyes at all times as you circle. Create a rhythmic motion with gentle pressure, as you simultaneously circle around each eye.

Even though this is a small movement, it is important to still "be the wave." Allow the movement of your hands to stem from the movement of your body. As you move your hands left and right, your body should be making a slight back-and-forth movement as well. As you circle around the zygomatic arch, your body should make a semi-circular motion.

CAUTION

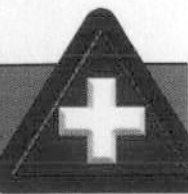

Dragging the stones directly over the eyebrows is uncomfortable for the client so be careful to stay just above them.

Jaw Melt

Jaw melt is a stroke used for releasing tension held in the client's jaw area. Begin by holding small hot stones flat against the client's **masseter** muscles. Make slow, broad circles with the stones around the entire area of the jaw.

After the **temporomandibular joint** has been warmed up and softened, turn the stones so that the most pointed parts of their edges are against the belly of the masseter muscles. Use the stones to do trigger point work in this area, holding vertical pressure, making tiny circles, and creating cross fiber in the masseter muscles.

CAUTION

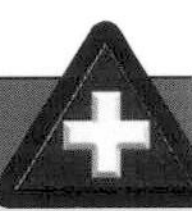

Be careful to avoid applying pressure over the client's teeth. This is painful to the client and could cause injury.

After you have worked the jaw muscles, either one at a time or simultaneously, in a deep and specific fashion, use the flat side of small, cool stones to work the masseter muscles in a broad fashion, helping to reduce any inflammation and discomfort prompted by the deep work. You can ask the client to open and close his or her mouth, as shown in Figure 10-11, and move the jaw left and right to help release tension from its joint.

TIP

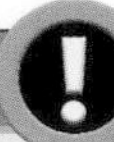

It is often helpful to work the temples after doing jaw release, as tension released from the temporomandibular joint will often move to the **temporal** muscle.

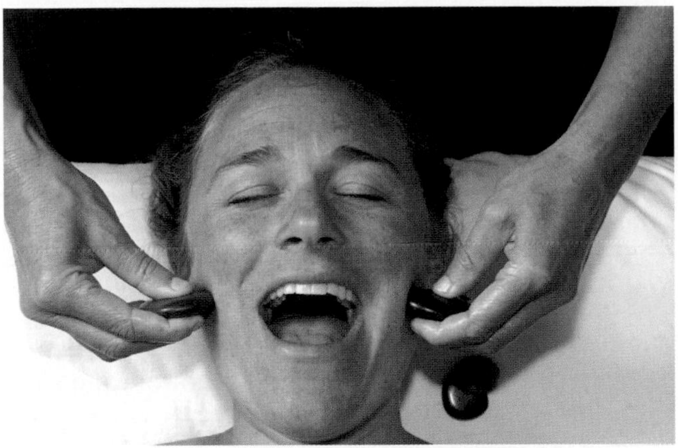

Figure 10-11 Jaw Melt. Use the edges of small stones to work the muscles of the jaw more specifically.

Figure 10-12 Waterfall. Allow the client's head to fall back over the edge of the stone. Just before the head falls all the way back, lift it again and let it fall over the stone once more.

THE NECK

With stone-free hands, use long, scooping and squeezing motions to warm up the neck. After you have used your hands to detect any areas of tension in the neck, you can introduce stones. Small- and medium-sized working stones are best. First, work the neck with stones in a broad fashion, using such techniques as gliding; alternating; and squeeze, twist, and slide (see Chapter 9). After the neck is thoroughly warmed up, you can introduce any of the following strokes.

Waterfall

Although tricky to master, when done correctly, waterfall is a delightful stroke for freeing up the client's cervical vertebrae. Begin by lifting the client's head up onto your abdomen. Hold a flat, oblong stone perpendicular to the base of the client's neck with a hand on either side, as shown in Figure 10-12.

Allow the client's head to begin slowly falling back over the stone, like water falling over the edge of a cliff.

Almost immediately, slide the stone smoothly up the neck and lift the head back up against your abdomen.

TIP

Timing is critical in this stroke. Experiment to find the perfect equation for a smooth drop and lift.

Repeat this stroke two or three times if the client seems to enjoy it. The smoother the fall and lift, the more enjoyable and effective the stroke will be.

CAUTION

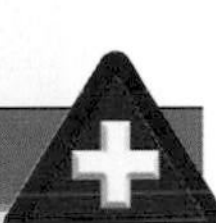

If not done correctly, waterfall can be experienced as abrupt and can even cause injury. Do not attempt this stroke on clients who have experienced trauma to the neck or who are suffering from a migraine or inflammation. Also, do not attempt it with any client until you have reached a satisfactory level of proficiency in practice sessions.

Neck Drool

Neck drool is similar to waterfall but performed on the side of the neck, adding an oppositional force to the drop and lift. Like waterfall, it can be challenging to learn, but it's well worth the effort. After you've mastered the timing and opposition, you'll find it easy to perform and your clients will find it delightful to receive.

Begin neck drool by lifting the head with a stone-free hand.

Move sideways across the back of the client's neck with your other (stone-filled) hand until it is just past the edge of the neck.

Allow the client's head to slowly fall back and then toward the side of the neck where the stone is (Fig. 10-13). As you do so, simultaneously lift the stone-filled hand up against the neck so that it pulls upward.

The "drool" happens from the oppositional contrast of the head falling back toward the table at the same time the neck is lifted up. This move needs to be

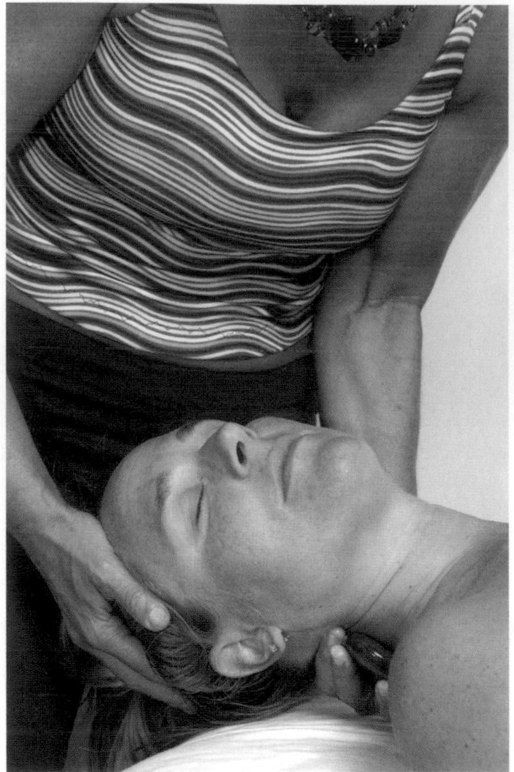

Figure 10-13 Neck Drool. Allow the client's head to slowly fall back and to the side as you simultaneously lift the neck with the stone, creating a "drooling" sensation.

done very slowly, like molasses dripping over your hand. Allow the full weight of the head to fall back while you lift the neck. Do this stroke with a rhythmic, rather than staccato, movement of your hand.

TIP

It is important to keep the thumb of your stone-filled hand nested against the rest of your hand rather than protruding out. If you keep your thumb out, you limit how far the stone-filled hand can reach under the neck. You want to be able to reach all the way across the neck before the drool begins in order to get optimal range from this movement.

CAUTION

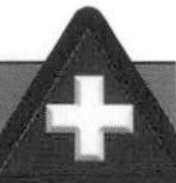

The most common mistake beginners make with this stroke is to lift the client's neck from the upper part of the neck (base of occipital ridge). This does not allow the head to fall back against the neck lift because the hand blocks the head-neck hinge. You also want to be sure you find the right balance between the drop and the lift so that the client's head does not hit the massage table, although it does come rather close when the stroke is performed correctly.

After you have done one neck drool on one side, drop the stone into your other hand as your hands meet at the neck.

Continue on up the head with your stone-free hand while the other hand (with the stone) becomes the new neck lifter.

Practice slowly until you can perform this switching of stones smoothly.

Neck drool is a perfect stroke for clients who find it difficult to release control of their head. Because the gravitational pull of the head is enhanced by the oppositional pull on the neck, it becomes almost impossible for the client to hold up his or her head. The slower you go, the more the client will be able to fully release. This stroke offers some clients their first experience of letting go of the weight of their head and can be extraordinarily rewarding.

Neck Over

Neck over is a stroke that provides deep, specific point work on the muscle groups along and around the cervical spine. Because it is done slowly, with the muscle in its shortened position, and utilizes gravity and the weight of the client's body rather than your strength, it is not only easier on your hands than normal point work, but it is also much easier for the client to receive.

Begin by lifting the head and turning it away from the hand with the stone.

While the neck is in the open and extended position, locate a point on the neck that you would like to work with the tip of a pointed tool stone, but do not apply pressure to that spot yet (Fig. 10-14).

Making sure that your forearm is resting on the table, create an altar with your hand and stone to support the weight of the head as it falls over the stone.

Allow the head to slowly fall toward the stone in a controlled fashion, as shown in Figure 10-15.

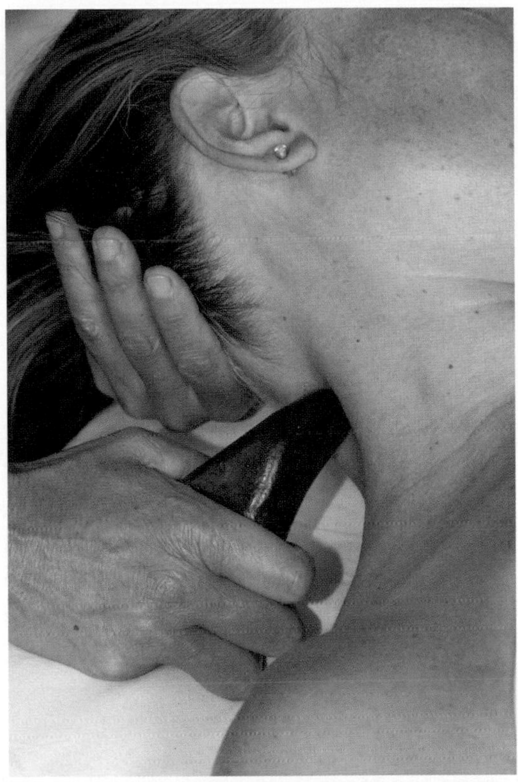

Figure 10-14 Neck Over (Step 1). With the client's neck in a lengthened position, locate a spot on the neck with the anchored stone, but do not enter the muscle.

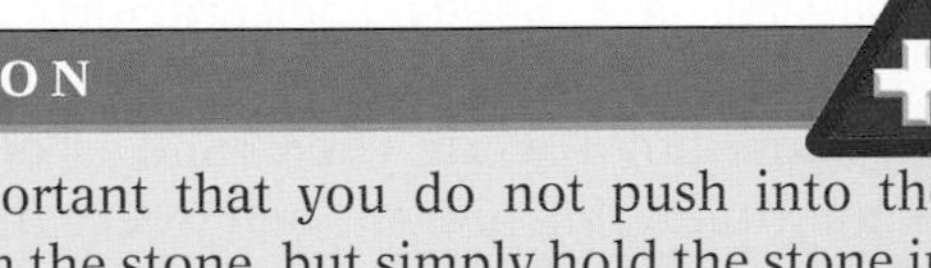

CAUTION

It is important that you do not push into the neck with the stone, but simply hold the stone in place as the head rotates toward it and drops over it. Be sure you do not let the stone slip. If it begins to slide and point down toward the **trapezius** muscle, the client will not feel enough pressure or depth from the stone. Keep the stone pointing straight toward the spine as the head falls over it and the neck moves into the short position.

After you have held the stone in place with the weight of the client's head over it for approximately 5 to 10 seconds, allow the head to rotate laterally away from you, opening the neck again, so that you can move to a new location. Choose a new spot on the same side of the neck and then allow the head to close again over the stone for a deep penetration.

Once the head has fallen over the same side of the neck approximately four times, switch hands

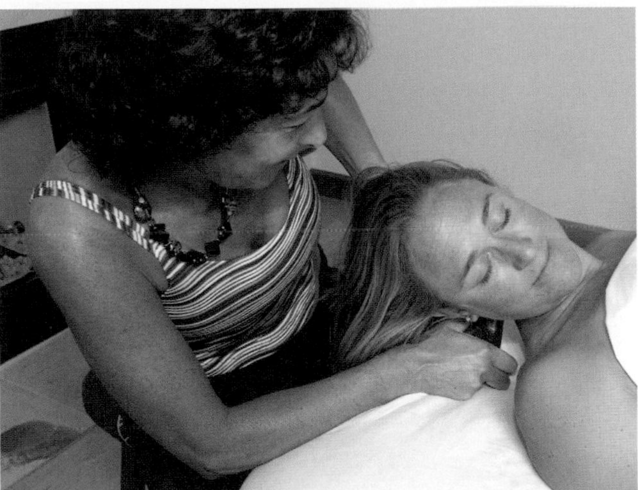

Figure 10-15 Neck Over (Step 2). Once the stone is in position, allow the head to slowly fall over the stone and penetrate the muscle.

and repeat the same action on the other side of the neck.

Some variation in the placement of the stone is certainly possible; however, it's usually most effective to place the stone in the **laminar groove,** right next to the spine, as that is the most receptive part of the muscle.

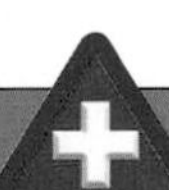

CAUTION

If you are too lateral, the muscle will tend to "kick you out" and your client will experience pain, even in the shortened position. And if you are too close to the vertebrae, you could injure the client.

The ideal placement can vary anatomically, so check with your client to be sure you have found the best spot. After you have found the right location for your first placement of the tip, move the stone up and down the neck along this line with each stroke.

Rock n' Roll

Rock n' roll is a stroke that adds a rocking movement to the normal static neck stretches and turns them into a gravitational dance, which enables the client to more easily receive the stretches. Grounded in the principles of fulcrums, being the wave, and using the client's weight (see Chapter 8), rock n' roll is as enjoyable to perform as it is to receive.

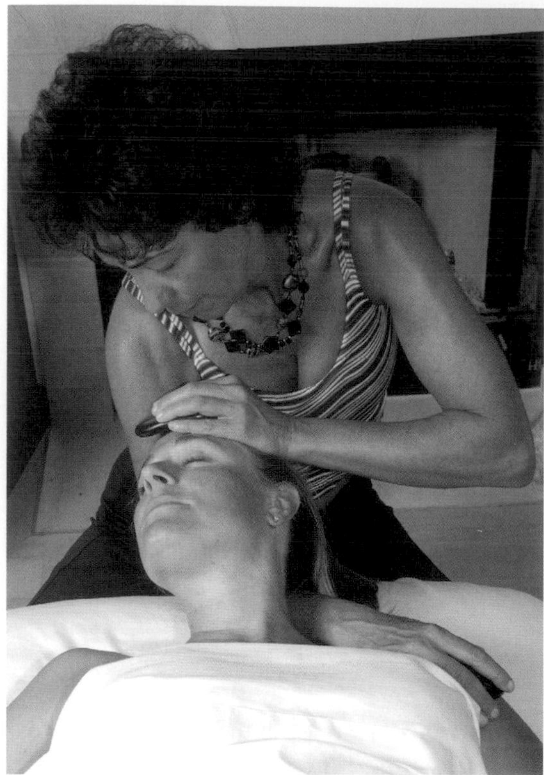

Figure 10-16 Rock n' Roll. Fulcrum your hand off the client's shoulder and use your elbow as a lever to raise and lower the head, allowing it to slowly roll over your arm. Switch sides seamlessly to create slow wavelike motions with the head and neck.

Begin by lifting the client's head with one hand and placing the occipital ridge in the crook of your other elbow.

Place your hand (from the same arm) on the client's shoulder.

Using the client's shoulder for leverage, push off the shoulder with your hand while you straighten out your elbow, allowing the client's head to lift up high on your upper arm, as shown in Figure 10-16.

Open and close your elbow, as you simultaneously slide your hand down and then up the client's upper arm, allowing the head to move up and down.

Slide your hand further down the client's upper arm to increase the range of motion. Also, try moving your body to the left and right, letting your arm slide up the back of the client's head and then sideways across the lowest part of the neck to allow for every possible motion of the client's head. Be sure the client's chin moves up, down, left, and right so that all possible directions of movement are included.

Use your other hand to lightly guide the head as it rolls over your arm.

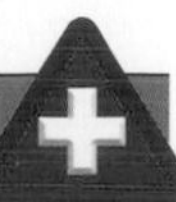

CAUTION

It is important that the client's head rest either in the crook of your elbow or on your upper arm. Although the head must roll over the top of your forearm from time to time, do not allow the head to remain there for an extended period of time, as it is not very comfortable. Never turn your forearm up so that your bone is against the client's head. This is very painful.

TIP

Be sure that the hand that is guiding the head does not exert excessive pressure. Allow the head to make its own movement and use the guide hand as a safety precaution to keep the head from hitting the table or to gently assist the natural motion the client's head.

Integrate the stones into rock n' roll as follows: After you have spent some time opening and closing your elbow and letting your hand slide up and down the client's shoulder, let that same hand slide down to the massage table. Slide it back and forth on the table for a variation in effect.

At some point while your hand is on the table, pick up stones from pile one and weave them into the stroke. Continue to do rock n' roll with a stone in each hand, as shown in Figure 10-16.

After approximately 1 to 2 minutes, switch arms to continue the stroke from the other direction. Switching arms needs to be as much a part of the stroke as the rock n' roll motion. To do so, lift the client's head as high as possible to allow space for your other arm to enter. Allow the head to gently ooze over your new arm. Avoid abruptly stopping the flow of movement.

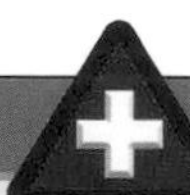

CAUTION

Be careful not to catch or pull the client's hair as your first arm comes out. To avoid this, try lifting the arm you are removing toward the sky, rather than pulling it back toward you.

Continue the rock n' roll motion until it is time to switch back to the original arm. Practice switching arms until it becomes as smooth as the rest of the stroke.

Do this stroke for approximately 5 minutes, unless the client is resisting you.

TIP

Be sure you go very slowly with this stroke and vary the movements; otherwise, the client could become dizzy or nauseated. Pay attention to the organic unfolding of the client's own head movement rather than imposing your own design or speed. Pause from time to time, allowing the client a chance to breathe and keep up with the motion. Let the shape of the movement be unique each time you open and close your arm.

If you heed all of the precautions identified here, your clients will receive this stroke with gratitude and profound release. It has proven to be one of my clients' favorite strokes.

THE ARMS AND SHOULDERS

Medium-sized flat stones are excellent for working the arms and shoulders. These parts of the body can easily be worked with two stones at a time (one on either side), or by one stone if you are seeking a more specific effect.

Three-Dimensional Arm Effleurage

Three-dimensional arm effleurage differs from a regular arm effleurage in that it works both sides of the arm at once, relies on your weight for pressure, incorporates opposition, goes beyond the shoulder and neck, and lifts the head and shoulder up in space. Adhering to the principle of seamless transition, this arm effleurage flows uninterruptedly from the last neck stroke right into the arm.

Here is how to make a seamless transition from rock n' roll into a three-dimensional arm effleurage on the client's right arm. With your right arm beneath the client's neck, bring your left arm parallel to your right arm and slowly slide your right arm out, allowing the head to gently fall onto your left arm.

Now, bring your body to the left side of the table where the client's right arm is.

Slowly pull your left arm across the neck and under the client's right shoulder as your right arm grasps the top of the client's right arm.

Sandwiching the arm between your two hands, pull down on the arm with all of your weight.

Once you reach the client's hand, leave your foot-hand at the client's wrist (to avoid jamming the shoulder) while the head-hand continues back up the arm and beneath the shoulder to the neck.

When you reach the neck, push up on the base of the head while you pull down on the hand, creating a pleasant opposition of the neck, shoulder girdle, and arm.

After the oppositional pull, release your hand from the base of the head, and let it slide under and past the neck to the massage table, where you can pick up a stone.

Drag the stone along the far shoulder and back across the neck.

While you are doing this, bring your stone-filled foot-arm underneath the client's near shoulder via the armpit.

Slide your entire forearm beneath the client's shoulder and lift it from both sides.

Massage the shoulder from both sides with a stone in each hand.

Finally, pull down the client's arm with a stone on either side, as shown in Figure 10-17. Use your body weight to lean back as you come out of the arm effleurage.

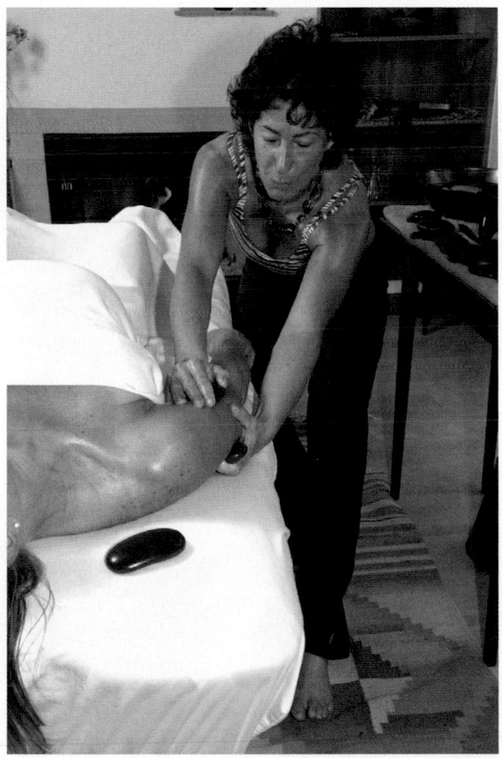

Figure 10-17 Three-Dimensional Arm Effleurage. Sandwich the arm with stones on either side when going up and down the arm.

Repeat this stroke a few times before moving into the altar-nater.

Altar-nater

You can move right into the altar-nater from the arm effleurage. The altar-nater is a stroke that involves alternating the hand and stone "altars" beneath the shoulder, while pushing from above with the other hand.

From the last arm effleurage, allow the stone-filled hand of your outside arm to continue up past the shoulder, beneath the neck and across to the opposite shoulder, as demonstrated in Figure 10-18.

At the same time, slide your other stone-filled hand beneath the armpit and underneath the client's shoulder nearest you.

Use the armpit (inside) hand to lift the client's shoulder high so that you can slide your outside arm back beneath this shoulder and make a sideways (parallel to spine) altar with the stone in the belly of the **rhomboid** and **erector spinae** muscles, as shown in Figure 10-19.

Once the altar is firmly in place, allow the hand that was under the armpit to slide back out and come to the top of the shoulder or **pectoralis** muscle.

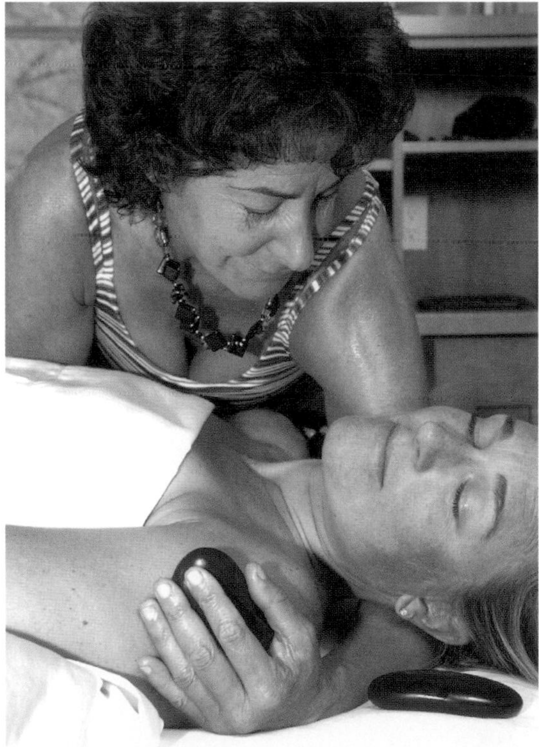

Figure 10-18 Transition from Arm to Shoulder. Let your hand and arm go all the way under and across the client's neck and lift the shoulder closest to you from beneath to transition seamlessly into the altar-nater.

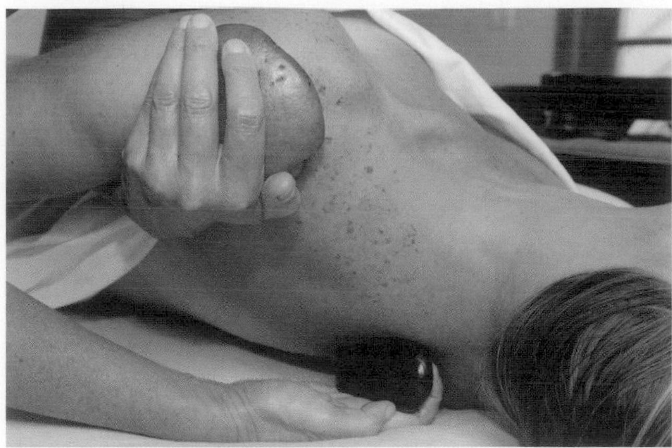

Figure 10-19 Altar-nater (Altar 1). Lift the client's shoulder with one hand. With your other hand, create a stone altar beneath the client's shoulder and parallel to the spine.

Push down on the pectoralis muscle while rocking back and forth in a sideways motion (teetering) with the altared stone from beneath. Sometimes it is more comfortable to kneel down on one knee for this movement.

Do this motion for approximately 10 seconds before alternating your stone altars. To make the switch, slide the hand that was below the shoulder up the neck.

Using momentum, slide that same hand (with its stone) back down beneath the outside of the shoulder, and lift it high enough to create space for the arm that was on top to now go back under the armpit and beneath the shoulder.

Using the stone from this hand, create an altar that is perpendicular to the spine in the meaty area of the trapezius and rhomboid muscles, as shown in Figure 10-20.

Place your other hand on top of the lateral edge of the shoulder's surface (top of **humerus**), being careful not to push too hard into the bone.

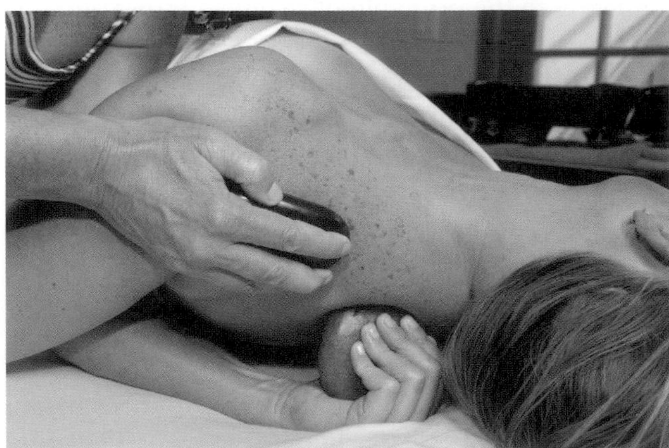

Figure 10-20 Altar-nater (Altar 2). Switch stone altars and make a new perpendicular altar with the stone in the other hand.

Rock the altared stone slightly up and down while you pull out on the shoulder top. Depending on the client, you may also be able to gently pull out on the clavicle bone while rocking.

This stroke is wonderful for releasing deeply held tension and trigger points in these muscles. Alternate your altars approximately four times before continuing. To come out of this stroke, you can do a three-dimensional effleurage stroke.

Hand Scrunch

Hand scrunch is a catchall name for the ways in which you can use the stones to massage the client's hands. One possibility is to sandwich the hand between two stones, squeezing the stones toward one another as you slowly slide them down the hand, toward the fingers. You can use more pressure by heeling both stones into the hand, as shown in Figure 10-21.

Use the tip or edge of a stone to do specific point work in the palm of the hand. Bending the hand toward the stone will create a subtle shortening of the muscles and add a "mother" effect, softening the pointed penetration.

You can also use the point of a stone to precisely work the tender ***Hogu*** spot in the thumb webbing.

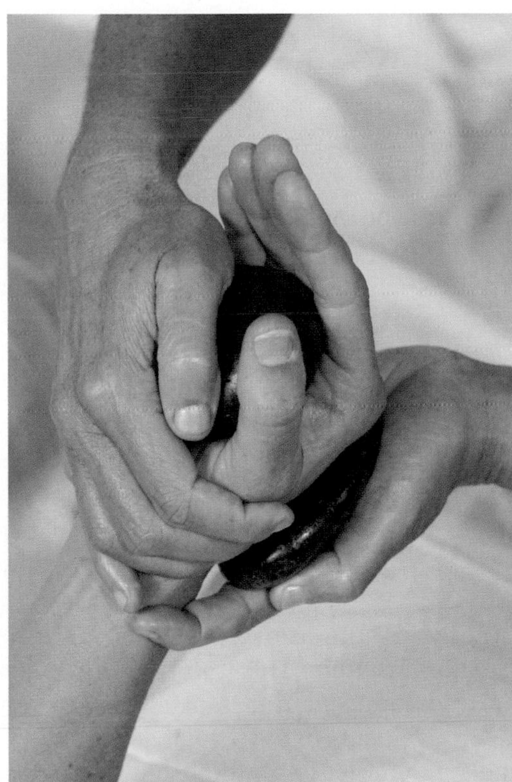

Figure 10-21 **Hand Scrunch.** Use the heels of your hands to create pressure with the stones.

TIP 

Be creative and find all the ways you can use the stones on the hands.

Lat Pump

Lat pump is a simple stroke for releasing tension in the **latissimus dorsi** muscle by working it in the shortened position with a pointed tool stone.

Kneeling next to the table, use your head-hand to lift the client's arm up above the head, or as high as you can go without straining the client's arm.

Using your foot-hand, place the pointed edge of a stone in the belly of the lat muscle without creating any pressure. Slowly, lower the client's arm, shortening the lat muscle, as you begin to penetrate with the stone, as shown in Figure 10-22.

Continue down the arm, as far as you can go, for full penetration in the short position.

Bring the arm back up, letting up on the stone penetration, and repeat the stroke several times, creating a pumping motion with the arm.

When you are done with the stroke, you can leave the stone beneath the armpit, and continue on to the next arm, or remove the stone and proceed directly into the strokes for the torso. Either way is fine.

THE TORSO

Find a seamless way to transition from the arm into the torso. You can massage the arm and torso on one side of the client's body and then go to the other side, or you can do both arms before moving to the torso. Either

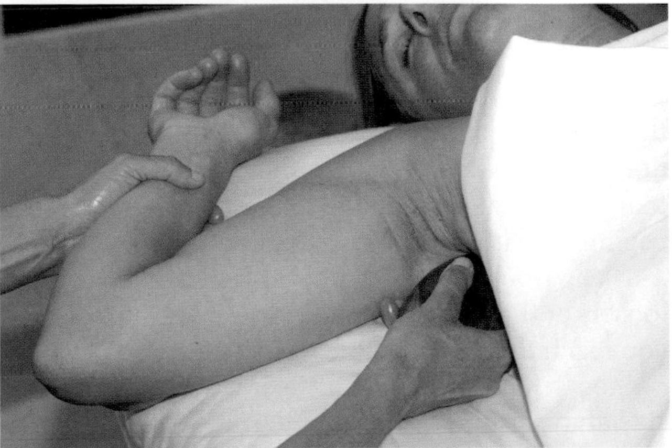

Figure 10-22 **Lat Pump.** With the client's arm in raised position, place the edge of the stone against the latissimus dorsi. Slowly lower client's arm as you penetrate the lat in its shortened position.

way works well, as long as you make your transitions smooth. Begin the torso without stones and then add them when ready. Medium- to medium-large–sized working stones are best to use for massaging the torso.

The following series of strokes works well together as a sequence. Once you learn them individually, I would then recommend using them in order, seamlessly transitioning from one into the other during the massage.

Rag Doll

Rag doll is a stroke used for stretching the torso in a fluid, undulating fashion that opens the spine on a deep level. As one of the most dramatic strokes in three-dimensional hot stone massage, it requires extensive practice with the help of an experienced PTM practitioner, or in a three-dimensional hot stone massage training course (see Appendix C). Words and photos are of limited value in capturing this technique; however, a description is included here to convey a general sense of what it involves and to serve as a reference following training.

The preliminary steps of rag doll are very similar to the ones you use to remove stones from beneath the client's body (see Chapter 6), and thus you should already be familiar with these steps. Rag doll then continues into a magnificent undulating dance that, when done properly, allows the client to feel as fluid and loose as a rag doll.

Begin rag doll by standing on the side of the massage table. If you are planning to use this stroke as a means to remove the stones from beneath the client, then begin on the opposite side from where the skillet sits. If not, you can stand on either side of the table to perform this stroke. Ideally, you want to do it from both sides in order to stretch the spine in both directions, but it does not have to be done consecutively.

There are four preliminary steps to get the body in the sideways position before you begin the undulations. For the sake of clarity, these directions assume that you are starting on the left side of the client and beginning with his or her right arm.

Using your outside hand, take the client's hand loosely at the wrist and walk toward the head. When you reach the client's head, the following steps begin:

Step 1: Grasp the client's elbow from the bottom side at the crook with the hand from your inside arm, as shown in Figure 10-23.

Step 2: Lift the client's elbow upward first and then toward you as you reach behind the upper thoracic area of the client's back with your foot-hand, as shown in Figure 10-24.

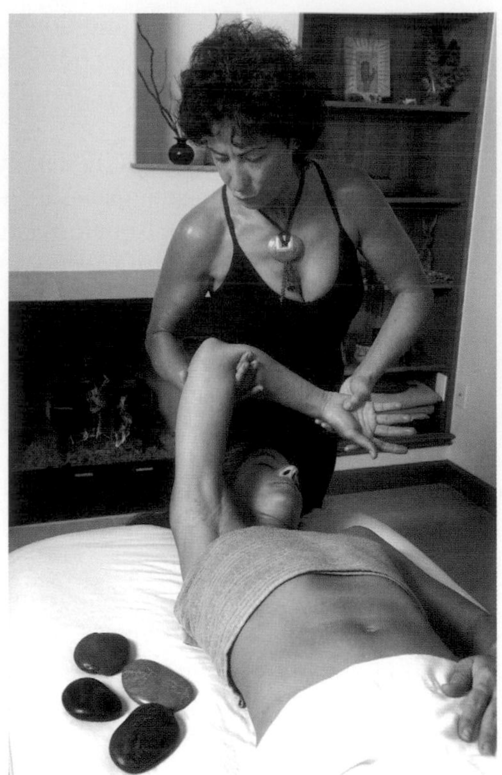

Figure 10-23 Rag Doll (Step 1). Grasp the client's elbow at the crook with the hand from your inside arm.

Step 3: Replace the foot-hand on the upper back with your head-hand and lift the torso even higher toward you, as shown in Figure 10-25.

Step 4: Bring your foot-hand to the lumbar region of the client's back as you raise the client's body even higher toward you, as shown in Figure 10-26. You are now in position to either remove the stones from beneath the client or to begin the undulation part of rag doll.

Once in this position, take a stone in each hand and begin the undulations in the following manner:

Allow the client's hip to drop away from you while keeping the client's shoulder toward you. Just before the hip reaches the table, gracefully catch it with your stone-filled foot-hand and pull it up toward you as you gently push the shoulder away from you, as shown in Figure 10-27.

Repeat these motions over and over, following the client's natural rhythm. This is not a stagnant stretch. It is an undulating motion that alternates hip and shoulder movements in a rhythmic fashion.

Make sure you let go of the client's hip for a second so it can fall back away from your hand before

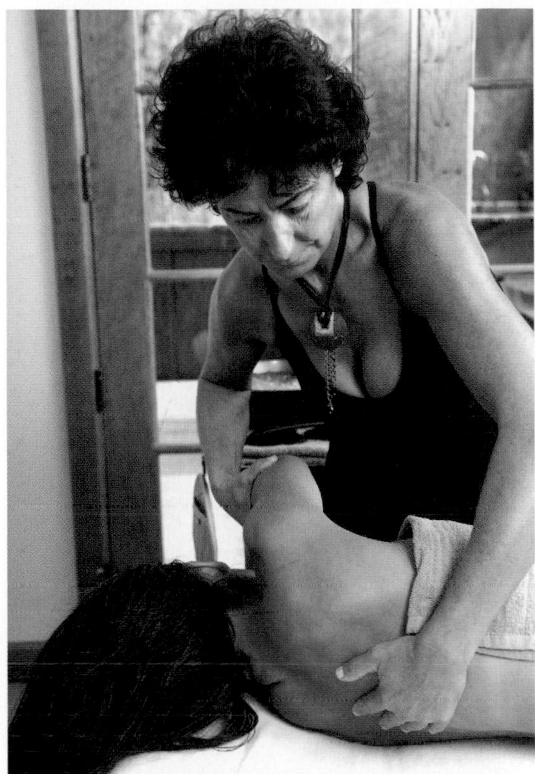

Figure 10-24 Rag Doll (Step 2). Lift the client's elbow up and then toward you as you reach behind the upper thoracic area of the client's back with your foot-hand.

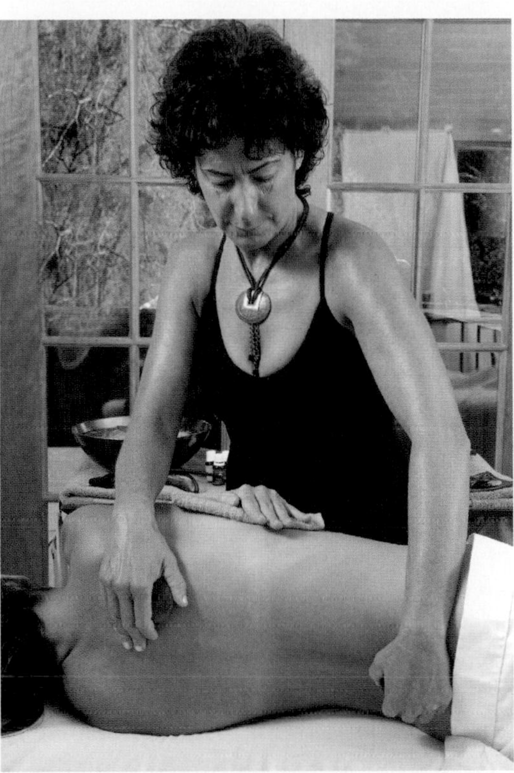

Figure 10-26 Rag Doll (Step 4). Bring your foot-hand to the lumbar region of the client's back as you raise the client's body even higher toward you. You are now in position to either remove stones from beneath the client if they are there, or to begin the undulation part of rag doll.

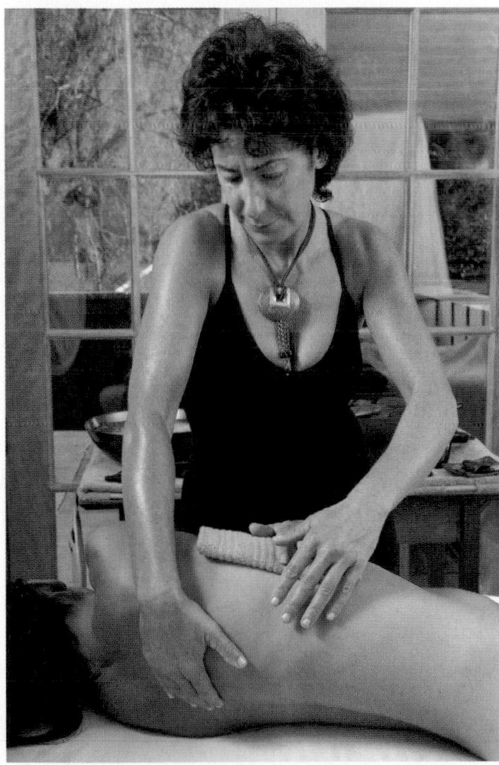

Figure 10-25 Rag Doll (Step 3). Replace the foot-hand on the upper back with your head-hand and lift the client's torso higher toward you.

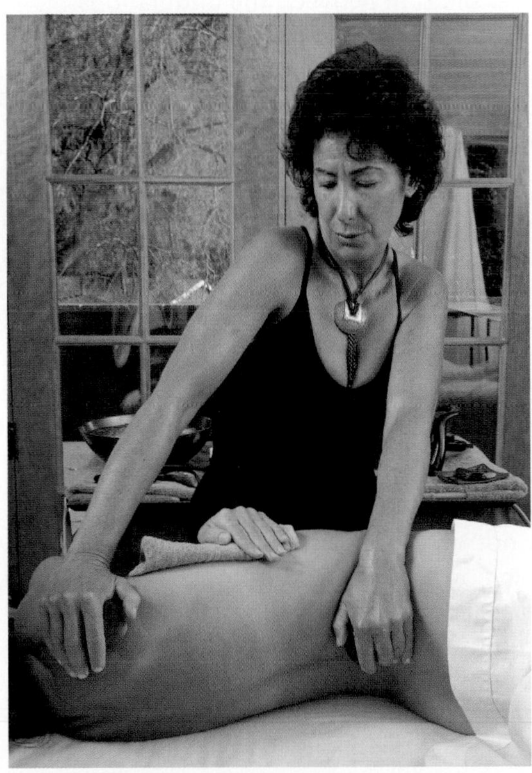

Figure 10-27 Rag Doll Undulation. Undulate the torso back and forth with stone-filled hands for the actual rag doll stroke.

you catch it to bring it back up. In this way, you get the client's full weight. It is important to mimic the movements of the client's body with your own body, allowing your own hips to move in a similar fashion. Brace one of your legs against the massage table to help you catch the weight of the client. Bring your other leg away from the table and point your toes of this leg. This gives you a better pivot point to move your own hips forward and back. Deciding which leg to put forward and which to put back to gain optimal movement of your hip is an individual choice.

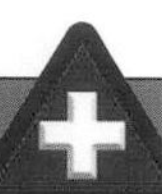

CAUTION

Do not do this undulating motion too fast or the client will get nervous about falling off the table. Listen carefully to the client's body for the exact speed and rhythm required. Make sure you use the entire range of motion available in order to slow the movement down. Do not repeat the undulation motion more than approximately 10 times to prevent the client from getting dizzy.

To keep clients from gripping the table, you can place your upper hip slightly against their body, to assure them that they won't fall off. You can also pause at times in between the undulations.

TIP

If the client tries to help you get his or her body into the sideways position by scooting the hips over for you, you will not be able to do the undulation part of this stroke very well as it relies upon using the client's weight for the hips to fall back. If this happens, you can reach underneath the hips and slide them back toward you, or you can restart the stroke and kindly ask the client not to help you, explaining that you need the weight of the body to perform it effectively.

To not tire out the client's low back, slightly vary the location of your hand from time to time. You can also use your fingers or the stone to dig into the spinal muscles and pull them toward you as you pull the hip toward you. This relieves deep held tension along the spine.

When you have completed rag doll, keep the client in the sideways position to seamlessly transition into lumbar torque.

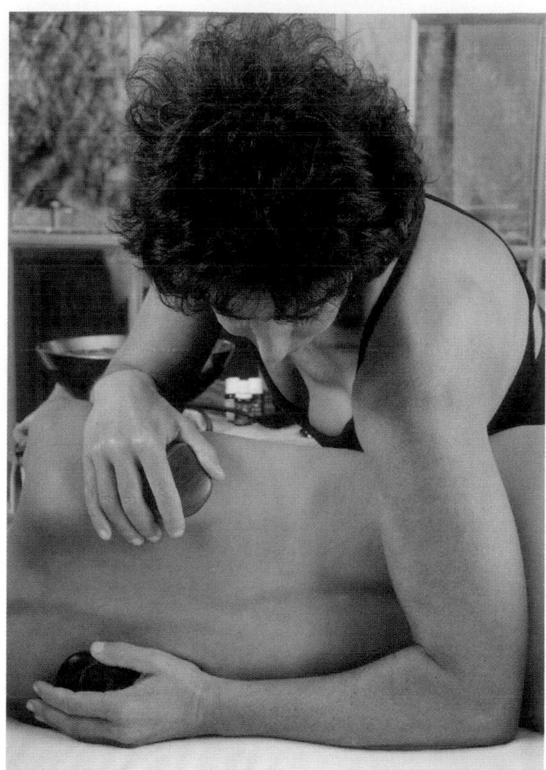

Figure 10-28 Setup for Lumbar Torque. From rag doll, plant your forearm parallel on the table, while your upper arm stays straight up like a bar and pushes against the client's lower back, holding it in a sideways position.

Lumbar Torque

An effective stroke for stretching and releasing tension in the lower back, the lumbar torque is also a wonderful completion to rag doll. From the sideways position, bring the client's torso all the way up so that it is perpendicular to the massage table.

Create a vertical bar against the client's lumbar region with the upper part of your foot-arm, as shown in Figure 10-28. Make sure there is a stone in your hand and that your forearm rests on the table.

Continue to hold your bar arm vertical while you slowly lower the client's upper torso down and over your forearm. Gently guide the client's arm and shoulder all the way over your stone-filled hand without applying any pressure to the arm.

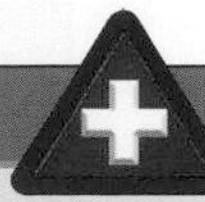

CAUTION

Applying pressure to the arm in this position can cause a shoulder to dislocate, so take care to avoid applying pressure.

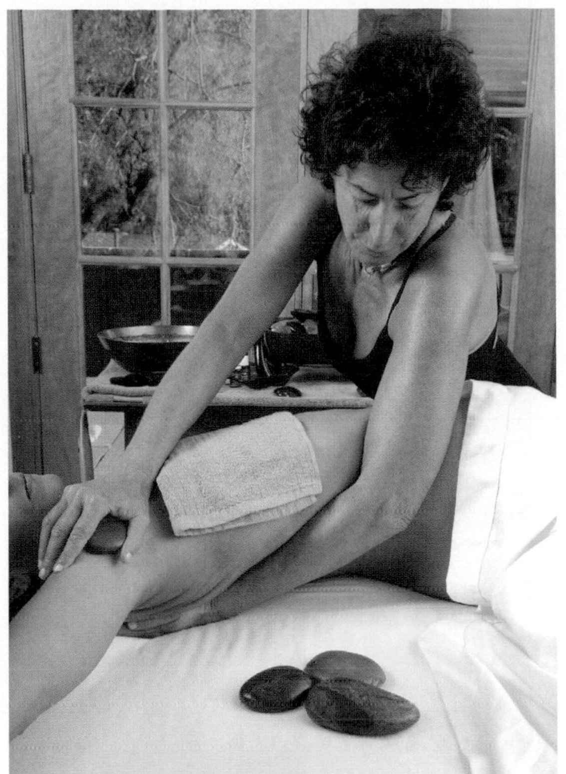

Figure 10-29 Lumbar Torque. From the set up position, push the client's shoulder (at the armpit) to the table while simultaneously (and with equal force) pulling the client's lower back up and toward you with your forearm and hand.

Once you have the upper torso fully resting on your upright forearm and stone-filled hand, place your other hand, with a stone, on the client's armpit and begin the oppositional push and pull of your two hands.

Continue to hold pressure against the client's armpit as you simultaneously lift and drag your forearm against the client's midback in a long, slow sweeping motion, as shown in Figure 10-29, until it reaches the client's **iliac crest**. From here you will begin undertow.

Undertow

Undertow is a useful stroke for straightening out the body after lumbar torque, as it creates the reverse stretch, helping to balance the client's body. In addition, your hands are already in place for the seamless transition into this stroke.

From lumbar torque, with your foot-hand already resting on top of the client's iliac crest, bring your head-hand (that was previously pressing on the client's armpit) toward the side of the client's body most proximal to yours, and begin sliding it underneath the lumbar back.

To gain momentum and have your weight behind you, bring the same leg that corresponds to your head-hand back in a staggered stance so that your legs mimic the formation of your arms.

Straighten your head-arm, lower your body (by bending your knees, not leaning over) with a slight pull against the iliac crest for a counter resistance, and slide your stone-filled hand all the way across the curve of the lower back with momentum. Go all the way until the crook of your elbow is below the middle of the client's lower back.

Now, push down on the client's iliac crest (be careful to move the stone away from the bony protuberance) while you straighten your elbow from below. This causes an upward motion of the client's lumbar region.

Continue to straighten your elbow, increasing the lumbar lift, as you simultaneously pull your arm slowly toward your torso and straighten the client's body, as shown in Figure 10-30.

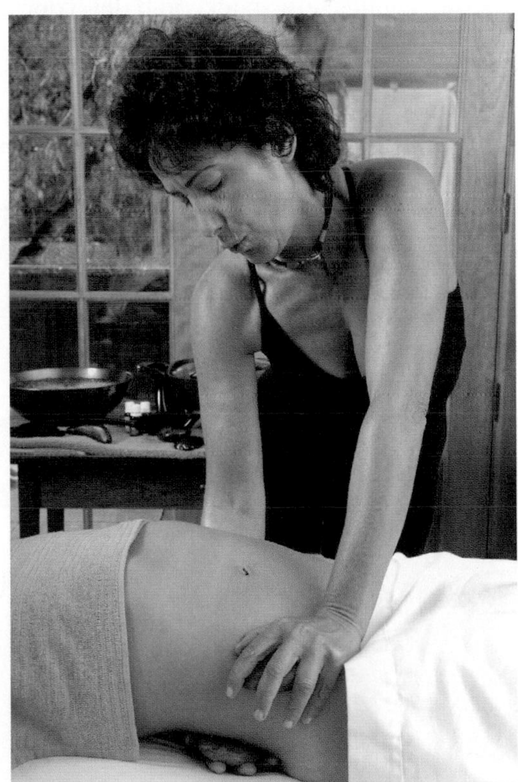

Figure 10-30 Undertow. Slide your head-hand under and all the way across the client's lower back with momentum. Now, push down on top of the client's hip with your foot-hand while pulling your head-hand across and lifting up at the elbow, creating a stretch in the client's low back.

TIP 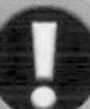

Undertow can be used any time in the massage when the body needs to be straightened out or balanced from a counter stretch.

Belly Waves

Belly waves are two strokes that encompass the belly and the low back at the same time. There is a small belly wave and large belly wave; both consist of wavelike motions formed from the hands below and above the belly; however, the small belly wave makes small vertical waves, and the large belly wave makes large horizontal circular motions.

Because of the dynamic of the two hands relating to one another, many clients who normally have a difficult time receiving belly work can receive belly waves with no problem. This stroke can offer relief from constipation, menstrual cramps, and low back pain.

Small belly wave can be done with either the head-hand or the foot-hand beneath the client's body. Slowly slide the stone-filled hand of your choice beneath the client's low back, and let your other stone-filled hand slide over the top of the belly, as shown in Figure 10-31.

Once both hands are in the center of the belly and low back region, begin to make slow vertical wave-like motions.

You can vary the "wave" with circular and side-to-side motions as well as by squeezing and dragging the stones in various directions in relationship to one another. Be careful not to push up directly on the spine. Working one side of the belly and back at a time—or both sides of the spine and belly at the same time—with a curved stone feels wonderful.

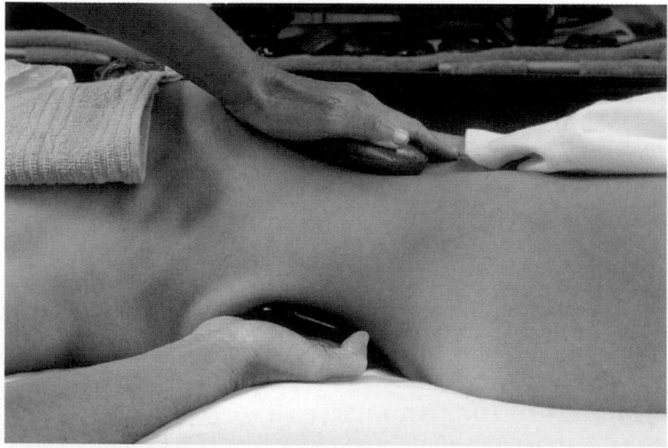

Figure 10-31 Small Belly Wave. With one hand above and one hand below the client's belly, make small circles and wave-like motions.

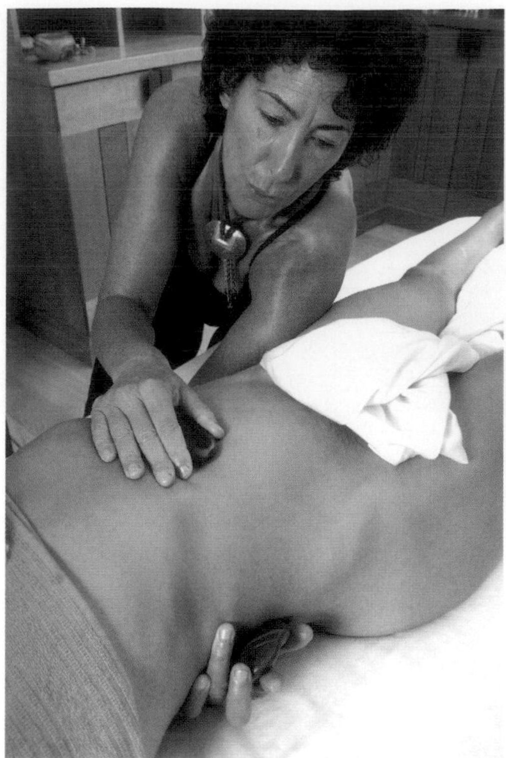

Figure 10-32 Large Belly Wave. Torque your upper arm against the client's hip and pull your body back and toward the client's feet as you make large circles on the belly and low back at the same time.

Large belly waves should only be done with your stone-filled foot-hand beneath the client's low back and your stone-filled head-hand on top of the belly. Start with your foot-arm all the way under and past the low back (so that your hand peeks out the other side of the body) and the upper part of that same arm nested against the client's hip, as shown in Figure 10-32.

Now, make large clockwise circles (following the natural direction of the intestinal flow) on the belly with the head-hand while the foot- hand makes long slanting strokes beneath the low back. The key to this stroke is to lean your body back with momentum and torque off the client's hip with your arm as you make each circle.

Body mechanics are important in this stroke. At the start of the stroke, when you are sliding your hand beneath the lower back, the same leg as the arm needs to be staggered straight back behind you as you face directly into the side of the table. Use a straight arm, a lowered body, and momentum to slide your arm underneath the low back. When you begin the circular motion on the belly, you need to bring that same leg forward toward the table and then up in the air to gain momentum for the downward pull of the upper circle and lower slant. When you do your downward pull, lean in against the client's hip and let the weight of your body fall back, as you step that leg toward the client's feet, pull down, and torque against the client's body. The leg motion is similar to that of a pitcher winding up for a pitch.

You can do large belly waves from either side of the table as long as your circular motion follows the clockwise intestinal flow, and you use your leg closest to the client's foot to make the leg motions. Experiment with the motions to discover what allows you to create the smoothest circles.

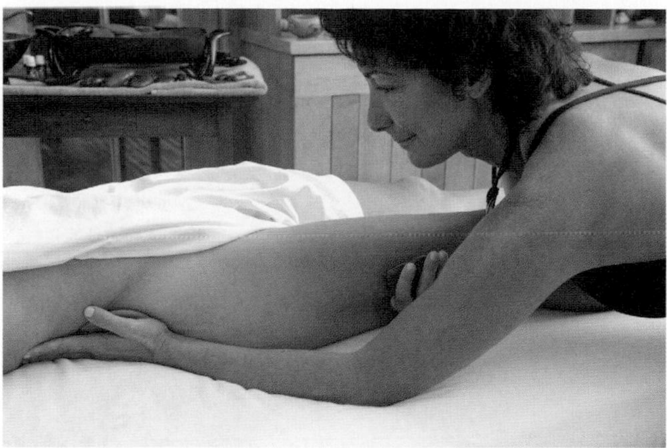

Figure 10-33 Three-Dimensional Leg Effleurage. Let your inner arm slip beneath the client's thigh to work on both sides of the leg. Continue gliding your outside arm up and beneath the client's back to the shoulder.

THE LEGS—SUPINE

The legs offer opportunities for using two stones at one time in long, sweeping strokes, some of which can continue up under the torso and back down the arms. Medium to medium-large working stones are best to use for massaging the legs.

Three-Dimensional Leg Effleurage

Three-dimensional leg effleurage differs from a regular leg effleurage in that it works both sides of the leg, uses levers and fulcrums, moves the leg in space, includes opposition, and continues all the way up the back and down the arm.

From large belly wave, continue backward down the leg, allowing your hands to sandwich either side. Once you reach the client's foot, glide back up the leg with one hand on either side of the calf.

When you reach the client's thigh, let your inner arm slide beneath the inside of the leg to the backside, and fulcrum off the table to lift the thigh.

Use both hands to sculpt the thigh from either side.

Now, you can pick up two stones and slide back down the leg.

Once you reach the foot, use the same two stones to glide back up the leg, sandwiching the calf.

Once at the thigh, allow the stone-filled inner arm to loop beneath the thigh from the inner side, and reach across the bottom to the outside of the thigh, while the stone-filled outer arm continues up beneath the back, as shown in Figure 10-33.

Once you reach the shoulder, you can leave a flowing placement beneath it with the stone you just used. With your hand still beneath the client's shoulder, pick up another stone from the massage table (that has been strategically placed at the top of the shoulder ahead of time) and slide over the shoulder and then down the arm (Fig. 10-34) while, with your other hand, you begin the slide down the leg.

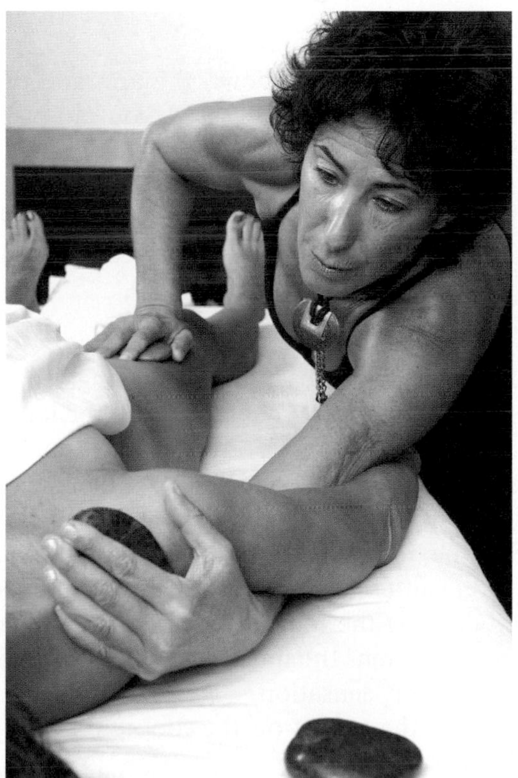

Figure 10-34 Include Arm in Leg Effleurage. When your hand emerges at the shoulder, pick up a stone on the table and slide it over the top of the client's shoulder and down the arm with one hand while you begin the slide down the client's leg with your other hand.

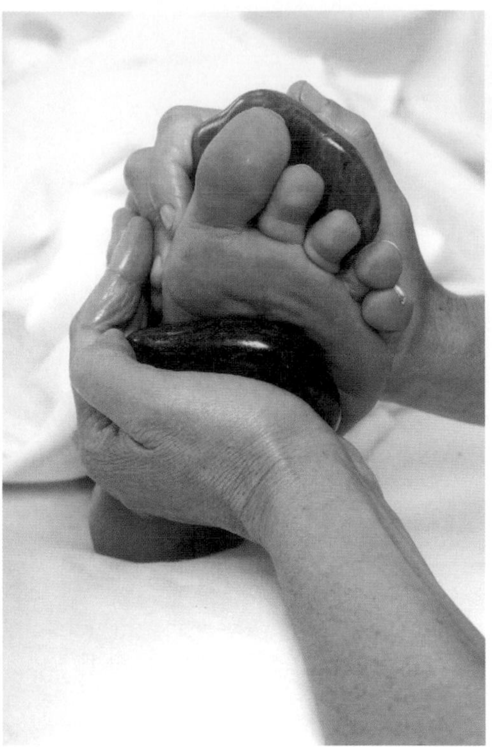

Figure 10-35 Foot Scrunch. When you reach the client's foot, massage the top and bottom at the same time, squeezing the stones toward one another.

Continue all the way down the arm and the leg. When you reach the client's hand, you can place the stone you've been using to massage the arm into the client's hand and pick up a new stone from the massage table to continue massaging down the leg.

Continue down the leg until you reach the foot.

Foot Scrunch

The foot scrunch is useful for relieving tension in both sides of the foot. When you reach the foot, massage both the top and bottom at the same time, squeezing the stones toward one another, as shown in Figure 10-35.

After the foot has been warmed up from both sides, you can use the pointed edge to work specific points. Pushing the foot down and toward the bottom stone shortens the muscle a bit, creating a slight "mother–father" sensation.

Play with the stones on the foot and create your own strokes as well.

Leg Over Sequence

Leg Over is a dynamic stroke that includes many stretches while massaging many different parts of the whole body. It requires extra attention to draping both during the entrance and exit of the stroke.

Begin by standing at the client's feet. Use your left hand to lift the client's right foot (which is on your left because the client is supine). Let the heel of the client's foot rest in the heel of your hand.

Hold the client's other leg with your right hand to keep it from sliding off the table.

Cross the raised leg over the down leg and begin to move forward, keeping it high to prevent the knee from buckling.

Continue moving forward, keeping the client's raised leg in a straight position.

TIP 

Do not allow your body to get in front of the client's leg or you will not be able to do the stroke. If you always stay behind the leg, it will naturally wrap around your body as it is supposed to.

When you can no longer easily walk forward, you will need to change hands. Bring your right hand up to the client's heel and switch hands, using your left hand now to prevent the client's lower leg from sliding off the table. Keep walking forward into the area between the two legs.

Check to make sure that the client is still draped.

Now, let go of your upper hand and allow the client's leg to wrap around your hip. Make sure that the crook of the client's knee is butted right up against your hip so that there is no space between the two body parts.

You are now in a position to begin some stretches:

First stretch: The first stretch requires that you face the side of the massage table. Push the top side (as it faces you) of the client's down leg away from you (careful not to push on the knee), while you pull the client's hip toward you. This creates a nice opposition and keeps the bottom leg on the table.

TIP 

As you do this stretch, make sure that you lower your body so that you position your body weight behind you, as you push forward with your lower hand. Getting low also allows your hand to push against the front of the client's thigh rather than on the inner thigh. This gives a much more solid placement for pushing. You can also put your elbow in the crook of your hip and use your hip movement to help push the client's leg forward.

Second stretch: Now, turn to face the client's feet for the second stretch. Slide your two hands down the inside of the client's leg, while you push your buttocks and lower back backward against the client's raised leg. Simultaneously lean your upper body forward.

TIP

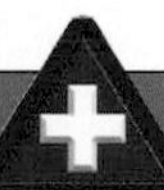

This strokes feels great on your own body as well, stretching out your lower back.

Third stretch: Turn to face the client's head for the third stretch. Put your foot-arm straight behind the client's ankle (of the leg that is wrapped around you), and place your head-hand on the client's shoulder. Create a stretch of the client's torso by pulling the client's knee away from the table with a lateral rotation of your hip (that is closest to the client's head), while stabilizing the client's shoulder with your hand.

CAUTION

Do not try and grip the client's foot with your hand to do this stretch. It can injure your shoulder and the client's knee. It is best to simply rest your upper forearm against the front of client's ankle to anchor the foot in place. It is also very important to create the stretch by the rotation of your hip rather than by pulling on the client's ankle or foot and bending it forward. This can cause discomfort to the client's ankle and knee.

TIP

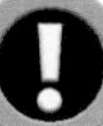

If you are not able to reach the client's shoulder to stabilize the upper body, then hold just below the breast on the rib cage, or the sternum, if the client is a woman, or hold right over the breast if the client is a man.

Once you have completed all three stretches, your hands are free to pick up stones from the massage table. Use these stones to massage the client's buttocks and the lateral side of the thigh, as shown in Figure 10-36. You can also massage the shoulders and upper back. Additionally, you can let the client's upper leg rotate toward you to give you access to the lower back, which you can now massage with the stones, as well as leave placement stones beneath it.

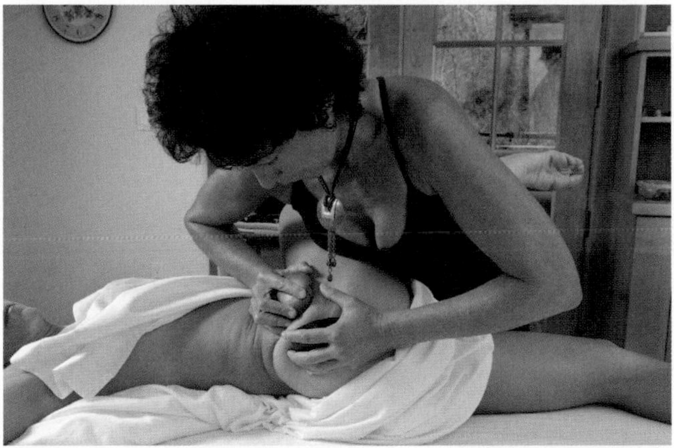

Figure 10-36 Leg Over. You can perform many different stretches and movements during leg over. Take advantage of the multitude of creative ways you can work both sides of the body from this position.

End leg over by massaging the buttocks area once again with the stones. As you back out of the stroke, make sure you pull the sheet with you in such a fashion that the client's groin does not become exposed.

The Frog

The frog is a single-legged stretch that can be done instead of or along with the hip flip (discussed next). It can be done from one side of the body only, as it involves movement in both directions. It is fine to do the frog on both sides of the body, but it is not critical.

CAUTION

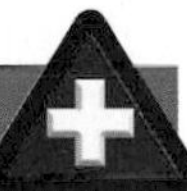

Make sure the client has not had a recent hip injury or surgery before attempting to do the frog or hip flip. If your client has had a hip injury, you may still be able to do these strokes depending on how recent the surgery or the extent of the injury. However, check with the client or his or her physician first, and if it is possible to do the stroke, go very slowly and limit the range you use.

To do the lateral part of frog, lift one leg from beneath the knee with your head-hand and from the

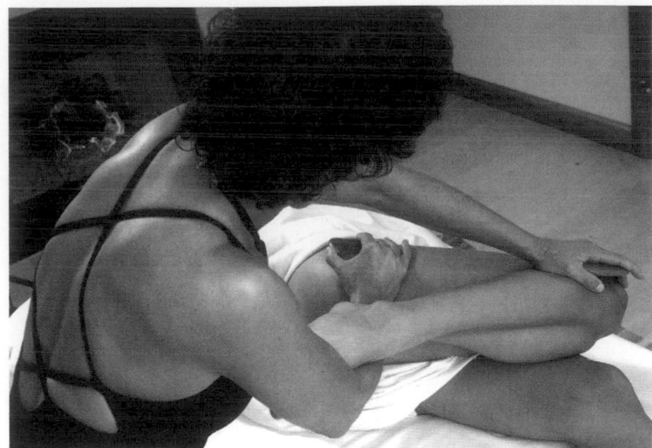

Figure 10-37 Frog. Frog utilizes fulcrums, levers, and your own body weight.

base of the foot with your foot-hand. Lift the knee toward the client's chest.

Now, place your head-hand on the front of the knee and hold the leg up as you place your foot-hand on the lateral side of the client's other thigh to stabilize it.

Gently lower the client's knee laterally and let the ankle rest on top of your foot-arm.

After the leg has rested in the lateral frog position for a moment, you can stretch it further by gently pushing down on the client's knee. Only do this if the client is able to receive a further stretch.

When you are done with this lateral aspect of frog, bring the client's knee back to center to prepare for the medial part of frog.

From the center position, wrap your foot-arm around the inside of the client's ankle and bring it toward the outside of the client's buttock.

Lean toward the client and push the knee away from yourself with your head-arm, as you lift the feet with the crook of your elbow, making a fulcrum with your hand on the buttock, as indicated in Figure 10-37.

If you want to increase the stretch, lift the client's foot up higher or bring your knee up on the massage table and lean further into the move.

Do this motion back and forth slowly a few times with one leg. It's up to you if and when you want to do it to the other leg.

Hip Flip

A double-legged version of the frog, hip flip stretches the client's hips and lower back even further. Like the frog, hip flip can be done from either one or both sides of the body.

Begin hip flip by placing the sheet between both of the client's legs and tucking it up under the groin.

Bring your stone-filled head-hand beneath the client's knees until the crook of your elbow rests below the center of the two knees.

Place your foot-hand at the base of the client's feet to help with the knee lift.

Bring the client's knees up toward the client's chest by lowering your body and allowing the knees to swing out to the side on their way up to center. This is much easier on your body than simply raising them directly up.

Once the knees are both up and in the center, remove your head-arm from below the client's knees and place your hand on the top of the knees.

Hold them in place as you move your foot-arm behind the client's ankles and place your hand on the outside of the client's buttock that is furthest from you.

Slowly lower the client's knees toward you as you lift up on the client's feet with the crook of your elbow and push off your hand that is acting as a fulcrum on the buttock (Fig. 10-38).

Straighten your elbow out even more and allow the knees to fall more forward to increase the stretch in the client's hips.

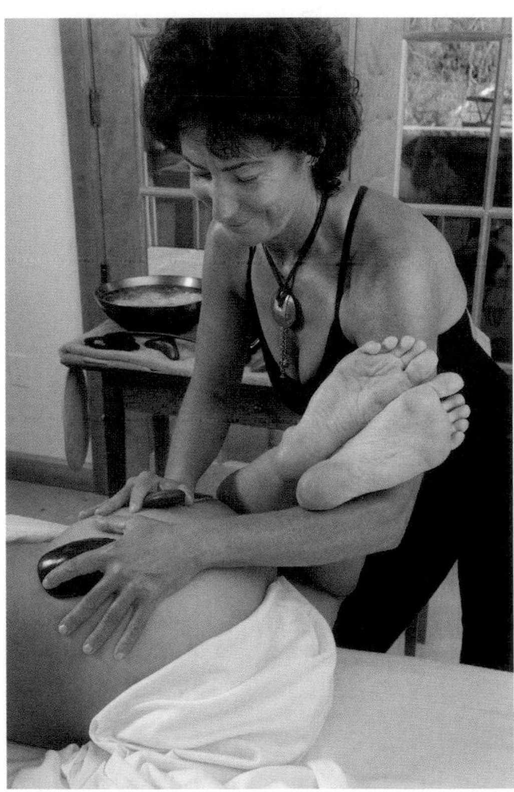

Figure 10-38 Hip Flip. Hip flip utilizes the same principles and creates the same motions as frog, but with two legs at once.

Bring the knees back to center, stabilizing them once again, with your head-hand. Rest for a moment. When ready, wrap your foot-arm around the inside of the client's ankles and bring your arm all the way to the buttocks closest to you. Make sure your hand is far enough up on the buttocks that the crook of your elbow, rather than your forearm, is beneath the ankles, as this could be painful to both the client and you. It is also important that your arm is low enough down on the ankles to get a proper stretch.

Once in position, use your head-arm to push the knees away from you.

Raise the client's feet higher and bring your knee up on the table to increase the stretch.

Before you come out of this stretch, you can place a stone beneath the client's lower back and then lift the client's knees in a circular fashion toward the head back up to center.

CAUTION

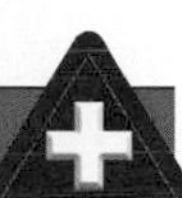

Be careful not to lose control of the client's knees and have them roll off the table too far. You may not necessarily lose your client to the floor, but you may have difficulty regaining your posture and returning the knees to the table without injuring yourself. Go slowly and stay within your safety zone. It is also critical to go slowly enough so that you can keep checking in with the client as you create the stretch. You can always go a little further if client requests, but if you go too far too fast, you cannot undo the strain you have caused the client.

Repeat hip flip approximately two times on each side before placing your head-arm beneath the client's knees and slowly lowering them down to the table. When done properly, this stretch is very effective for releasing tension in the client's hips and low back.

TURNING THE CLIENT OVER

To massage the back, you must turn the client over or request that the client turn over. Clients report that having the massage therapist turn their body over is an extraordinary experience for them. When done slowly, and in stages, they have no idea what is happening. They simply experience lots of sideways stretching, and then suddenly they are on their other side. This ethereal technique also allows the massage to continue uninterrupted with little effort on the client's part.

However, turning the client over is only recommended when you can do it without straining or injuring yourself. Before attempting it with clients, practice with a friend who is very light weight. You may find you only want to do this with clients who are light weight, or you may only want to turn your client over part way. In time, you will find your own comfort zone with this move.

Before attempting to turn your client over, double check to make sure there are no placement stones left beneath or on top of the client. It is also important to have the face cradle ready before beginning the turn over. Start by getting the client into the hip flip position with the knees facing away from you. Pause.

Raise the client's arm (the one opposite from where you stand) above the head, making it into a stretch. Pause.

Reach through the small of the client's lower back until you reach the client's opposite hip.

With a flowing but strong motion, pull the client's hip all the way across the table toward you so the hips are almost off the side of the table. Stretch the client in this position. Pause.

Bring the arm closest to you across the client's chest. Now, lift the client's head with the forearm of your head-hand, while you use the foot-hand to simultaneously pull the shoulder (not the elbow) of the raised arm underneath the lifted head and toward your side of the table, as shown in Figure 10-39. Stretch the client's neck. Pause.

Raise the client's arm that is closest to you, up and over to the other side of the table. This will cause the whole upper body to turn over. Pause.

Now, gently push on the client's raised hip while pulling back on the newly turned shoulder. This turns the rest of the body over. Stretch. Pause.

The client might be slightly disoriented, so allow time for reorientation. Then, ask the client to slide up into the already upturned face cradle.

Feel free to create any variation that suits you, as long as it feels good to the client and is easy on your body.

THE BACK

Now that you have turned your client over, or have asked your client to turn, you can continue the massage by working the back and then the legs. Medium

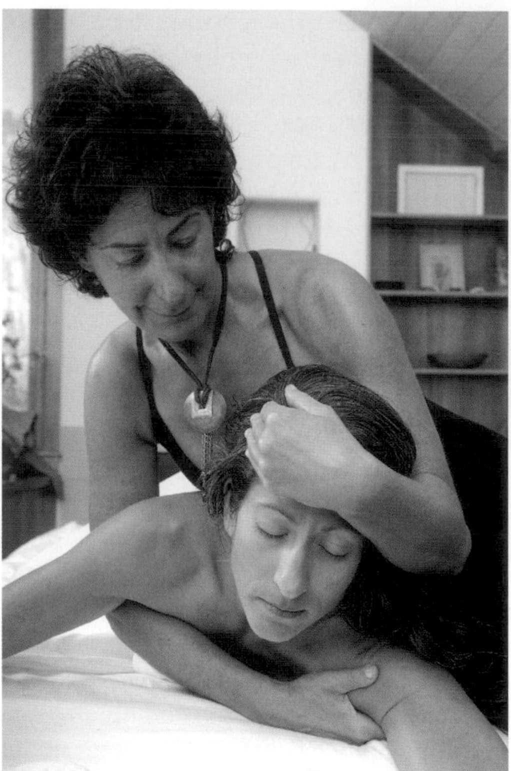

Figure 10-39 Turning the Client Over. Turning the client over as a part of the massage maintains the flow of the massage and involves the client as little as possible.

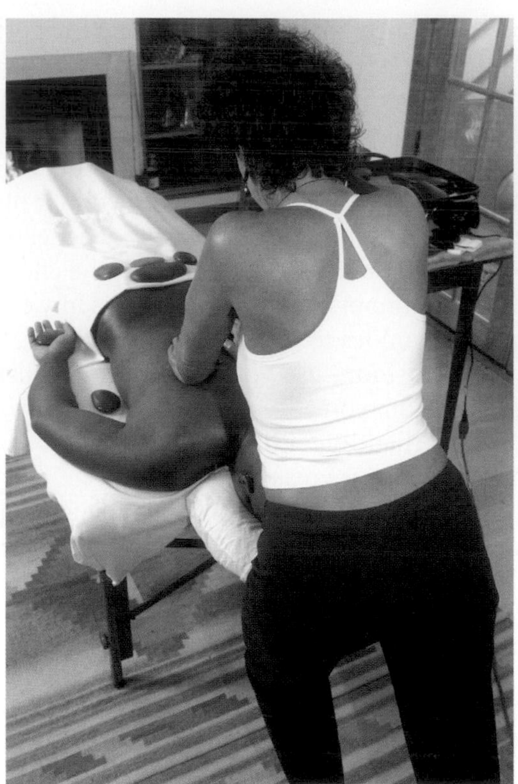

Figure 10-40 Fullback. Drop your entire weight vertically into the client's back and maintain this vertical drop as you begin your slide down.

to medium-large working stones are best for massaging the back. Large placement stones can also be used at the end for flushing the entire surface of the back.

The Fullback

The fullback is an enriched three-dimensional effleurage. It differs from most back effleurages in that it begins at the uppermost portion of the trapezius muscles, pressing forward into the perpendicular angle of the upper shoulders, before going up and over the horizontal angle of the back. It is not uncommon for most back effleurages to leave out the upper shoulders and begin contact a third of the way down the upper back, leaving an unsatisfying gap between the therapist's chosen starting point and the back's natural origin.

With fullback, your work extends into the buttocks on the way down and beyond the upper back into the neck on the way back up. You also work three-dimensionally because, rather than remaining on the surface of the back, you slide your hands on the sides of and beneath the client's belly and front of the shoulders.

In fullback, you drop your weight vertically into the upper thoracic region rather than sliding by that area before deepening the pressure, as indicated in Figure 10-40. As you perform this stroke, pay attention to your body mechanics. In particular, make full use of your weight to effortlessly gain depth into the client's back.

Begin fullback with a staggered stance so that you can lower your body by bending your forward knee. You need to lower your body for the entrance into fullback to get right behind the upper trapezius muscles, which lay perpendicular to the back. The more you can lower your body, the more you will be able to use your weight for depth.

Enter with your finger pads at the traps and then hook the traps with the heels of your hands and thrust your pelvis forward to help apply pressure. Pause here for a moment.

Now, bring your forward leg back to join your other leg. With both legs parallel and approximately 3 to 4 feet back from the client's head, straighten your arms out as you drop all your weight vertically.

Slide slowly down the back, making sure to penetrate with your whole hand (including your finger pads) and drop your weight straight down into the convex aspect of the thoracic region. As you continue down the back, bring your leg forward again into the staggered stance. Use the heels of your hands to drop deeper into the **quadratus lumborum** muscles.

TIP 

You will know if you are dropping all of your weight into your client if you would fall flat on your face if the client were suddenly to vanish.

Do not stop at the base of the back; instead, continue on to the upper gluteus muscles. Slide the stones laterally off either side of the buttocks and beneath the client's belly in a sweeping motion.

Lift up against the belly slightly as you drag the stones out and to the sides of the back.

Rake the stones up the client's sides, using your weight to lean back, until you reach the midpoint of the torso, and then drag in toward the center of the back and up the erector spinae muscles.

Move your hands laterally across the scapulas and over the shoulders, then scoop down beneath the front of the shoulders and lift the shoulders up.

Slide your hands out from underneath the shoulders and rake up either side of the neck.

Slide back down the neck and, with a staggered stance, drop your weight forward and push your heels into the flat part of the traps.

Continue on down the back, repeating the same motions as before but penetrating a bit deeper with each run. After a few stoneless runs, reach down with both hands and pick up stones from pile two on the client's lower buttocks. Weave the stones into the stroke, making sure to wrap the fingers around the stones so that you enter fingers first. Do a few more runs down the back with stones before transitioning into forearm frenzy.

Forearm Frenzy

Forearm frenzy is a stroke that works just the upper thoracic region with your forearms, using a fair amount of broad depth. It should be done rhythmically at a speed of about 1 second per arm. If it is done much faster or slower than this, it will not feel as good to the client.

You can slide seamlessly into forearm frenzy from the fullback's exit off the neck. Begin with one arm at the top of the trapezius muscle, entering with a stone-filled hand at a medial angle.

Drop your weight as you slide your forearm medially at an angle across the meaty part of the rhomboids and other muscles between the edge of the scapula and the spine.

TIP 

Stones are used only for the entrance of each arm and not in the actual forearm movement; however, it is useful to have the stones in your hands, as you can return into a fullback at the end without having to stop and pick up stones.

Once you pass the medial angle of the scapula, rotate your forearm medially so that it is perpendicular to the spine and begin a downward lateral sweep, tracing the edge of the scapula.

As soon as your first hand begins to leave the back, enter in the same manner with your other arm, as indicated in Figure 10-41.

Trace the scapula with your second arm. As soon as it begins to leave the back, enter once again with your first hand. Create a rhythmical sweeping motion

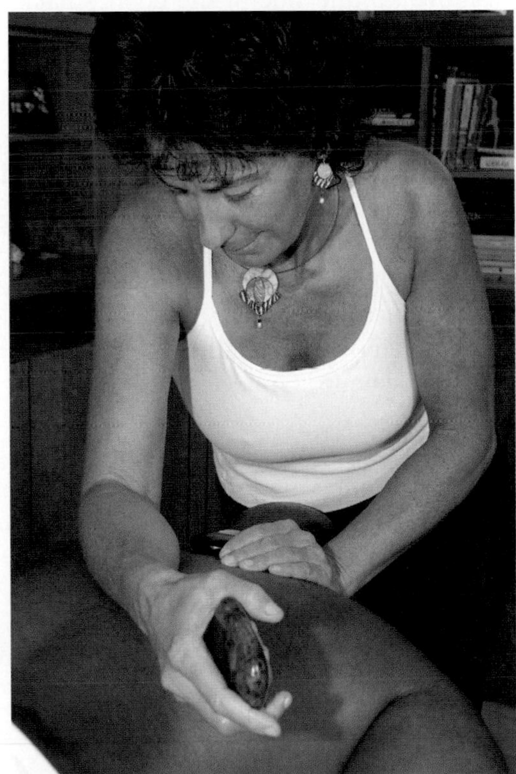

Figure 10-41 Forearm Frenzy. Alternate your forearms while rhythmically tracing the edges of the scapula.

with both arms alternating and slightly overlapping, one after the other.

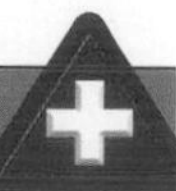

CAUTION

Avoid hitting the client's bone with your elbow as you trace around the scapula. This is very uncomfortable for the client. Be sure that your forearm turns appropriately to keep it in the meaty part of the muscle between the scapula and the spine.

Once you have done forearm frenzy several times, end with a nice slow fullback, integrating the upper and lower portions of the back. For more detailed work on the back, utilize the stone techniques described in Chapter 9.

Chicken Wing

Chicken wing is a two-part stroke used to stretch the muscles of the chest, particularly the pectoralis and the anterior aspect of the **deltoid,** in a three-dimensional fashion. If you slide right into it from a long sweeping forearm move up one side of the client's back, your momentum will aid in the initial lift; however, it can be done from a static stance as well.

Start by bringing the forearm or your head-arm to the top of the client's shoulder and sweeping it beneath the shoulder to begin the lift. Once the shoulder is lifted enough to create space, slip a stone-filled foot-arm underneath the armpit and front of the shoulder.

Continue moving your foot-arm forward until your hand reaches the far side of the client's occipital ridge and your elbow is beneath the front of the head of the humerus bone. Grab a stone with your free head-hand.

Gently push down on the client's occipital ridge as you straighten your elbow to lift the client's shoulder up high. Stabilize the shoulder by placing your stone-filled head-hand on top it.

TIP

Be sure to keep your forearm under the front of the head of the humerus bone. If you don't, the client's shoulder will tend to fall forward rather than stay up in the stretched position.

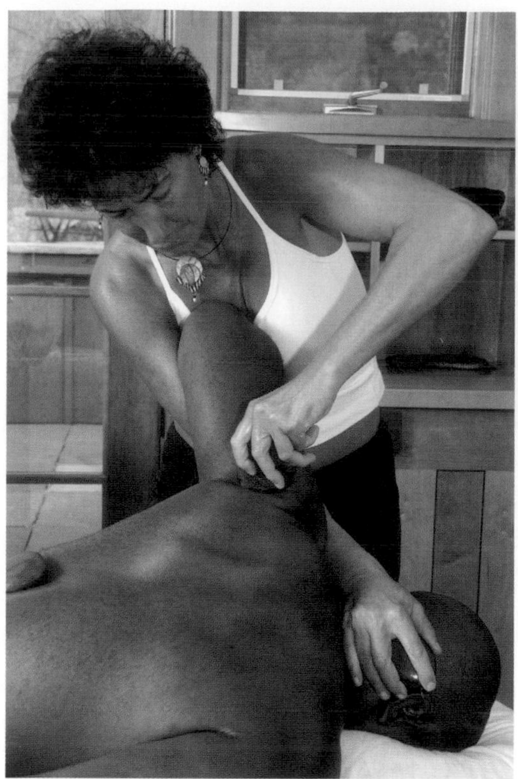

Figure 10-42 Chicken Wing (Part 1). Pivoting off of the client's occipital ridge, lift the client's shoulder up and back for a nice stretch.

While in the stretch, work the **teres minor** and **infraspinatus** muscles (which are now in the shortened position) with the stone, as shown in Figure 10-42. Use both the edge and the flat side of the stone, according to the amount of depth and specificity you would like to create in this area.

Transition into the second part of chicken wing by sliding your foot-arm off the client's head and bringing it beneath the crook of the client's elbow. Seamlessly switch arms by bringing your head-arm into the crook of the client's elbow, as your foot-arm simultaneously slides out.

Stretch your head-arm across the client's back until it rests with a stone on the client's quadratus lumborum.

Anchor the client's hand with your foot-hand as you push off from the client's back, creating a lever to lift and stretch the client's shoulder in a slightly different direction (Fig. 10-43).

Teres Tango

Teres tango is a stroke that works the teres and other muscles of the shoulder girdle in their shortened position and in a three-dimensional fashion by embracing

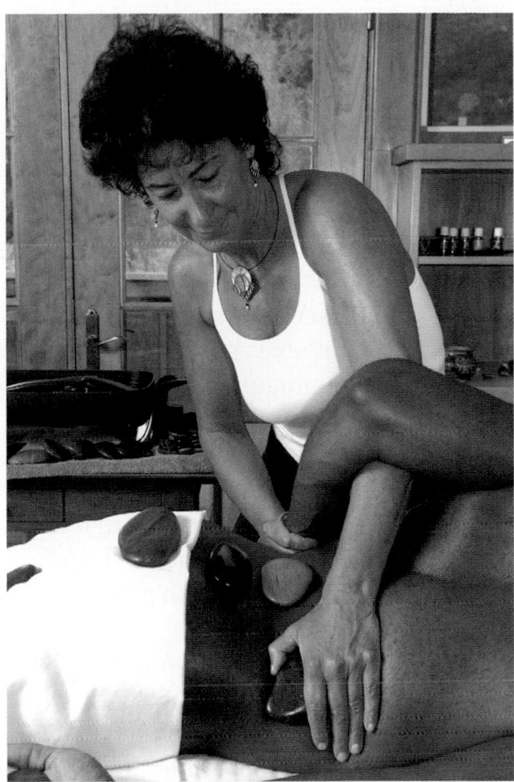

Figure 10-43 Chicken Wing (Part 2). Switch your arms and pivot off the client's back to lift and stretch the shoulder and arm in different directions.

the shoulder on both sides at once and adding movement to the normally static penetration of points.

Seamlessly glide into teres tango from chicken wing by lifting the client's arm up, out, and over your thigh with your head-hand, as you sit down on the table facing the client's head.

TIP

Leave a space between the client's shoulder and your thigh so that you can have easy access to the front of the client's shoulder and have room to shorten the muscles.

First, reach the hand from your outside arm beneath the client's shoulder and then place a stone in it with your other hand.

Cradle the front of the shoulder with your stone-filled hand while you place the stone-filled hand from your inside arm on top of the lateral edge of the client's scapula, creating a sandwich effect between the two hands.

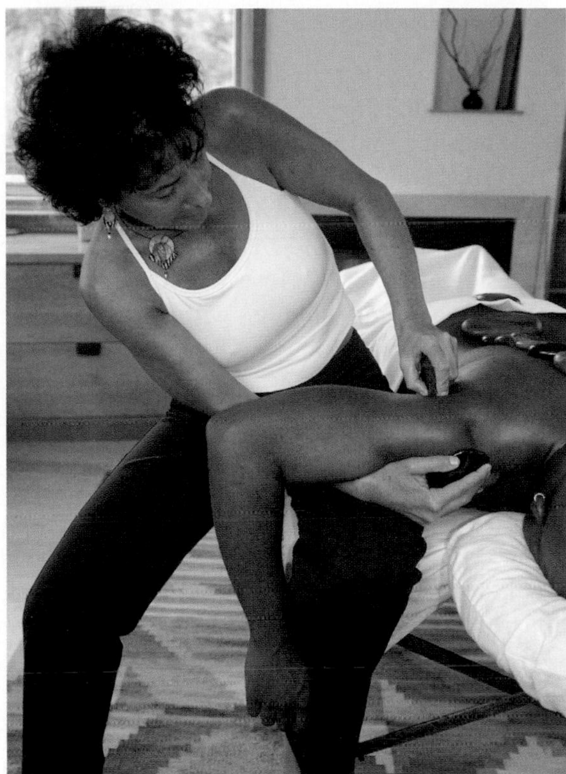

Figure 10-44 Teres Tango. Create a sandwich effect between your two hands: Work the teres minor and infraspinatus muscles with a stone in one hand, while lifting the front of the client's shoulder and making circular motions with a stone in the other hand.

Work the teres minor and infraspinatus muscles of the **rotator cuff** with the stone from above while lifting the shoulder from below to shorten the muscles with each penetration, as shown in Figure 10-44. Create a dance between the two hands.

TIP

The teres minor and infraspinatus muscles are best accessed by a perpendicular direction after you have entered in a vertical direction. Lean your body out to change your angle so that you can penetrate the muscles from the outside, pushing down first and then inward toward the spine.

Work specifically with the edge of the stones and then turn the stones flat to soothe the muscles with a broad stroke.

Once you complete teres tango, stand up and slide your hands down the back until you reach the middle of the torso where you can begin reverse belly wave.

Reverse Belly Wave

Reverse belly wave is a flowing stroke that frees both sides of the lumbar region at the same time. Position yourself standing on the same side of the table as you were for teres tango. Begin with a stoneless foot-hand.

Lower your body and, with a straight arm, slide your well oiled foot-hand beneath the client's belly from the side of the body closest to you. If you lift the client's opposite hip slightly with your head-arm, you'll make it easier for your foot-hand to slide in and across the belly.

Keep sliding your arm in until your hand is exposed on the other side.

Once your hand comes out the other side, place a stone into it with your head-hand, as shown in Figure 10-45, and then pick up another stone from the side of the table with your head-hand to use on the back.

Drag both your upper and lower hands with stones across the belly and lower back until you reach the center of the torso.

Create vertical waves with the two hands on either side of the belly. Straighten the arm that is below the belly to lift the hip up off the table. Improvise with different movements between the two hands and forearms.

To complete reverse belly wave, slide your lower arm out and bring it across the top of the client's low back to the opposite hip to begin hip hop.

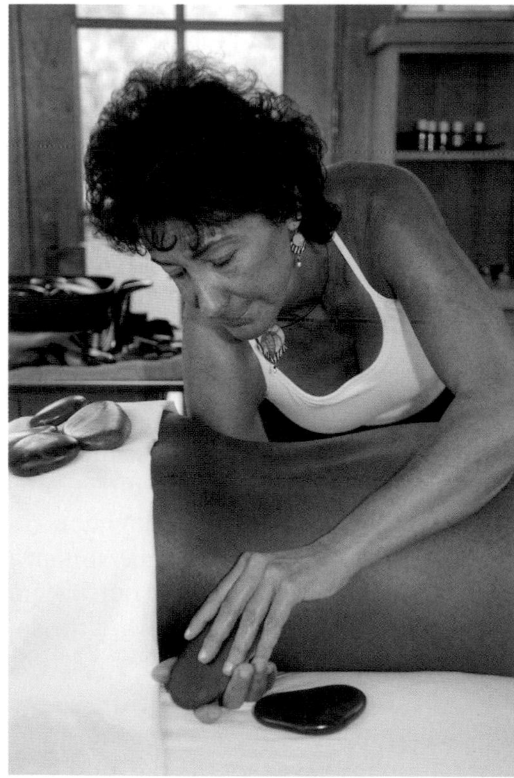

Figure 10-45 Reverse Belly Wave. Reach under the client's belly with a stoneless lower hand. As your hand emerges from beneath the client's belly, place a stone in it and one in the upper hand as well. Create small vertical waves with your two hands on either side of the belly and back.

Hip Hop

Hip hop is a stroke useful for stretching the low back with movement. It involves small rocking incremental lifts of the hip, culminating in a large oppositional torque (hop) of the hip and low back.

The rocking serves two purposes: It allows you to get your hand far under the iliac crest without pinching the client's skin or being abrupt, and it also offers momentum to lead into the torque or "hop."

From the side of the table, reach across the client's low back to the opposite hip.

Begin your first rock with your foot-hand flat against the side of your client's hip. Pull your hand toward you, gently lifting the hip.

As you slide this hand out, slide the other one in, letting the hip rock forward onto it.

Alternate your hands approximately five times, going further under the iliac crest with each rock.

On the final hand switch, your foot-hand should be squarely on the iliac crest. Without hesitation, lift the hip up high by pulling on the iliac crest, while you simultaneously push down (vertical) and up (horizontal) toward the head on the SAME side of the client's lower back with your head-hand, as illustrated in Figure 10-46. This creates the torque, or "hop," that makes the stroke.

Repeat the hop two or three times on each side.

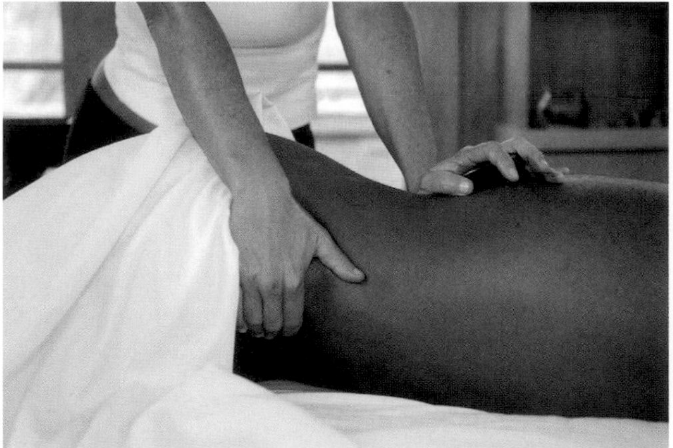

Figure 10-46 Hip Hop. Make sure you lift the hip at the same time as you push up on the low back toward the head. This simultaneous motion is what creates the "hop."

TIP

It is best to do hip hop on both sides right in a row, rather than waiting, for the sake of balance.

THE LEGS—PRONE

The legs, in their prone position, offer the largest surface area of the body for massage. In particular, the three-dimensional leg effleurage goes all the way from the foot, up the back and down the arm, thereby providing the longest easily uninterrupted stroke you can do with stones. For this reason, both clients and therapists love to use hot stones on the back of the legs.

Three-Dimensional Leg Effleurage

Like the supine version of three-dimensional leg effleurage, the prone version differs from a regular leg effleurage in that it embraces both sides of the leg, incorporates fulcrums and levers, extends beyond the leg, and lifts the leg in space. Because it involves and connects most parts of the body, it is a wonderful way to end a hot stone massage. Medium to medium-large working stones are best to use for massaging the back of the legs.

From hip hop, face toward the feet and seamlessly slide past the buttocks and down the leg to the foot.

Once you reach the foot, turn to face the client's head, drop your weight vertically, and glide up the leg with hands on either side of the calf.

When you reach the knee, create opposition by continuing up the thigh with your outside arm, as you pull down on the calf with your inside arm.

Repeat this accordion oppositional pull a few times before sliding both hands down either side of the client's calf and back to the foot.

Pick up two stones and glide back up the calf with stones on either side.

When you reach the thigh, work the **hamstrings** and **quadriceps** muscles at the same time with a stone in each hand.

After you have worked the thigh for the desired amount of time, massage the buttocks and then continue past the leg up the back with both stone-filled hands.

After reaching the top of the client's back, slide back down the back with one hand while you slide down the arm with the other, leaving a stone in the client's hand as you pass by.

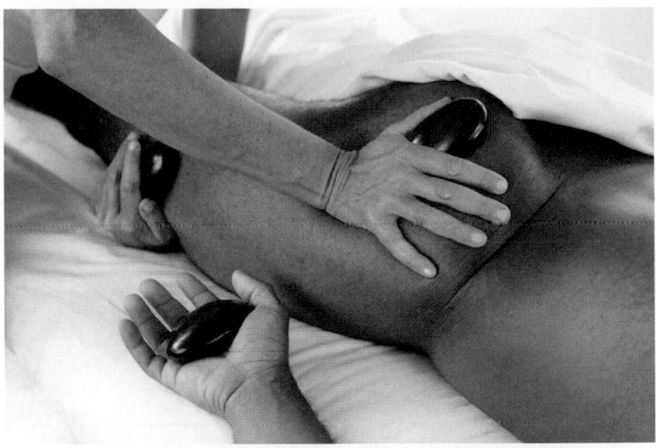

Figure 10-47 Three-Dimensional Leg Effleurage. Slide up the outside of the client's leg and onto the buttock with one hand and from the inside with the other hand to embrace the entire leg as you effleurage.

Pick up a new stone from the table.

Massage the client's **gluteus** muscles from the top with your stone-filled head-hand, while you work the **iliotibial band** and the **vastus lateralis** by reaching your stone-filled foot-hand from the inside of the client's thigh, then underneath and to the outside, as shown in Figure 10-47. You are now in position to transition seamlessly into shortened ham pump.

Shortened Ham Pump

Shortened ham pump is a stroke that works the hamstring muscles in their anatomically shortened position.

From three-dimensional leg effleurage, bring the client's foot up and sit down on the massage table, allowing the foot to rest upon your inner shoulder.

Lean forward, bringing the calf toward the buttocks and shortening the hamstring as you drop into its belly with the stones, as depicted in Figure 10-48. You can leave a stone behind the knee as you flex the foot forward, but be careful not to put the stone right against the popliteal area behind the knee or you could bruise it.

Continue to pump the calf forward as you drop into the hamstrings with depth, and then release the calf as you come out of the penetration, giving the hamstring a moment's rest.

While you penetrate the hamstrings in their anatomically shortened position, you can further enhance the penetration by manually shortening the muscle as well with the mother–father technique. After you have worked specifically with the stone, use its flat surface

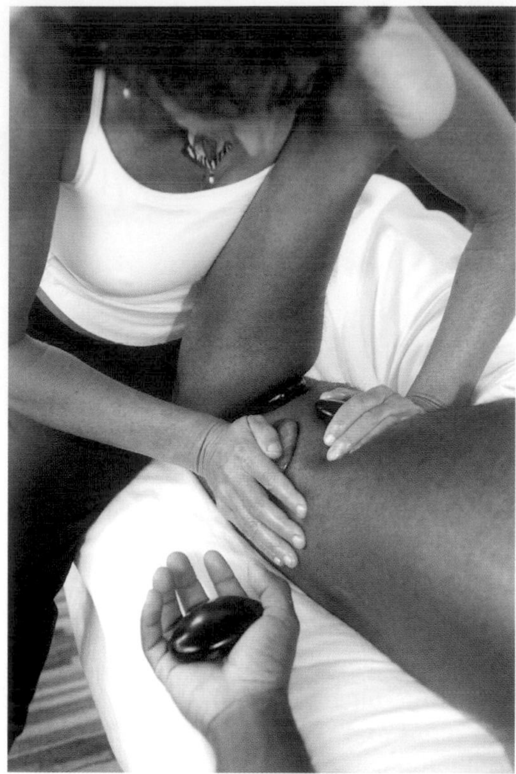

Figure 10-48 Shortened Ham Pump. With the client's foot on your shoulder, lean forward to shorten the client's hamstring as you drop into its belly with the stone. You can leave a stone behind the client's knee as you flex the foot forward.

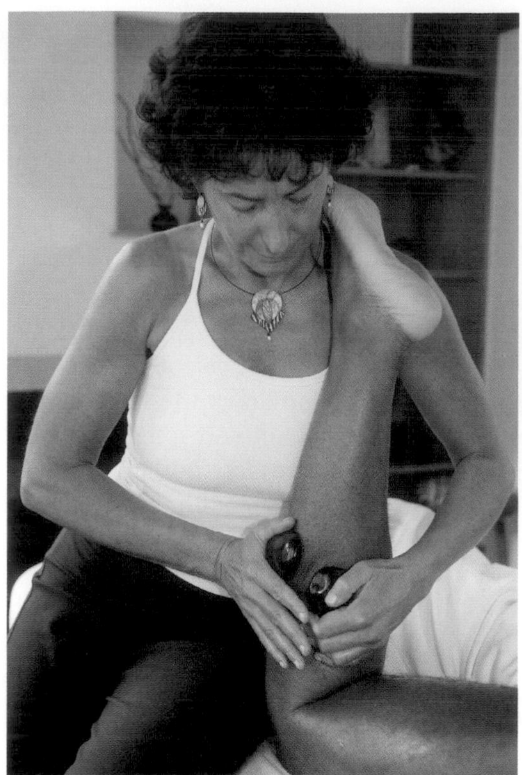

Figure 10-49 Calf Mush. Let client's foot rest on your shoulder as you massage the calf from both sides at once for a deep, cradling effect.

to make broad strokes over the hamstrings. You can also create resistance of the hamstring muscle by pushing the stone up toward the buttocks, while you pull the calf away from the buttocks toward you.

After you have completed working the hamstring, leave the calf in the upward position to move directly into the next stroke, calf mush.

Calf Mush

Calf mush is a stroke for working the calf from both sides at once. The following are just some of the ways you can work it. Feel free to improvise and include the mother–father technique to go deeper into the calf muscles without eliciting pain.

From shortened ham pump, the calf is already in the upright position resting on your shoulder. Work the calf broadly at first, with two stones, to warm up and loosen the **gastrocnemius** and **soleus** muscles, as shown in Figure 10-49.

Once the calf muscles are warmed up, massage the calf with more depth and specificity, using the stone as a tool.

Always end with broad mushy strokes to soothe the calf.

You are now in the perfect position to transition smoothly into reverse frog.

Reverse Frog

Reverse frog is a wonderful stroke for raising the leg off the table and working both sides of the thigh freely without obstruction.

Begin from the seated position of calf mush, with the calf still raised up.

Rotate the client's knee laterally with your inside arm, and gently press the client's calf medially with your outside arm. This moves the knee into the reverse frog position.

Allow the client's knee to rest on your thigh, raising the thigh slightly off the table and giving you access to both sides. Be careful not to lift the thigh too high with client's who suffer from low back pain or injury. Reach under the thigh with the stone-filled hand from your inner arm, while you place your stone-filled hand from your outer arm on the lateral side of the

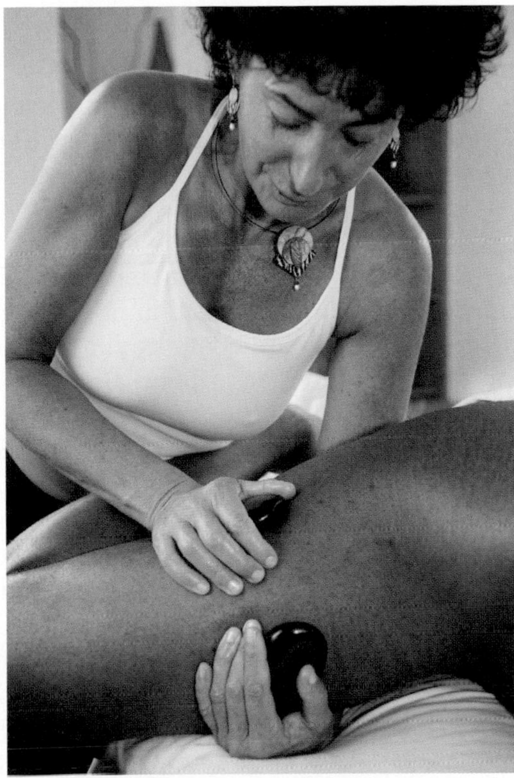

Figure 10-50 Reverse Frog. Rotate the client's knee laterally and rest the client's thigh on your thigh. Reach under the client's thigh and massage it three-dimensionally, from both sides at once.

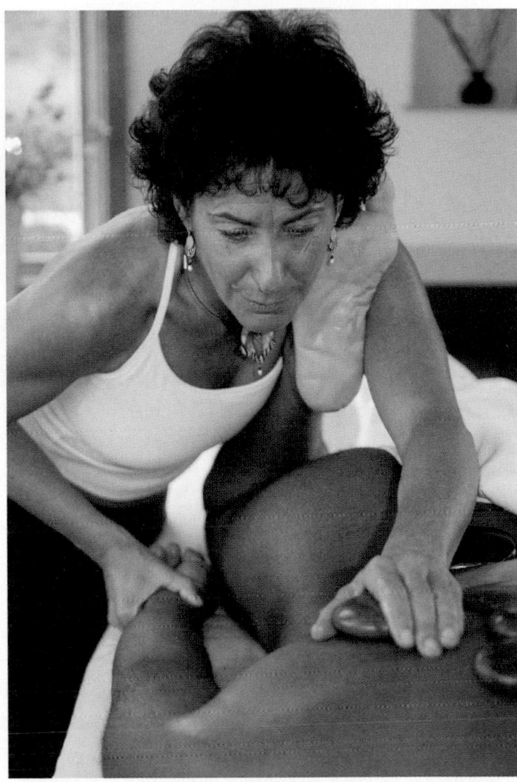

Figure 10-51 Calf Up-Arm Down. With the client's foot on your shoulder, lean forward with your body weight until the client's calf folds as far forward as it easily can. Continue to slide the stones up the back and down the arm. When you reach the hand, pull the hand down as you push the foot forward, creating a wonderful stretch.

thigh, as shown in Figure 10-50. From this position, you can easily massage the quads, hamstring, and iliotibial band. Place both of your hands on the lateral side of the client's thigh as you lean back and "paw" the outside of the buttock and thigh. Create your own variations of this tension-relieving stroke.

CLOSING STROKES

As with the opening strokes, there are many possibilities for closing a massage. I have included only two closing strokes here. Enjoy them and create some of your own as well.

Calf Up-Arm Down

The closing stroke I call calf up-arm down stretches the client's quadriceps and shoulder girdle muscles through an oppositional pull. Begin this stroke from calf mush, with the client's raised calf resting against your shoulder. Stand up, keeping the client's foot nestled against your shoulder.

Place your stone-filled inner hand on your client's low back.

Lean completely forward with your body weight until the client's calf folds as far forward as it can without injuring the client.

Slide your stone-filled hand up the client's back while you pull down the arm with your outside hand. Continue to pull down on the client's wrist as you lean forward into the calf, creating a wonderful stretch (Fig. 10-51).

Bubbling Spring/Palace of Weariness

The stroke bubbling spring/palace of weariness is named for the two acupuncture points that you stimulate at the end of the stroke. Begin by placing both of your stone-filled hands together, facing away from each other, on the client's buttocks, as shown in Figure 10-52.

Drop your weight into both stones and glide each hand away from the other. Continue gliding each of your hands in opposite directions, one down the client's arm, and the other down the client's leg.

Time your movements so that you reach the client's hand and foot at the same time.

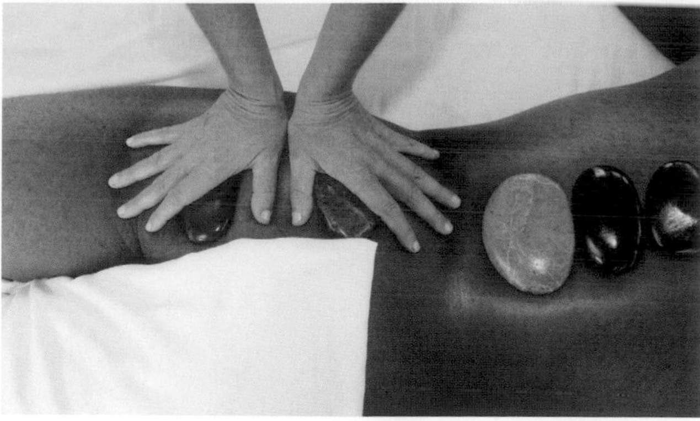

Figure 10-52 Opposing Hands. Place both stone-filled hands on the client's buttocks with fingers pointing in opposite directions. Then, slide one hand up the client's back and the other down the client's leg.

Complete the closing stroke by holding one stone on the client's foot at the acupuncture point called **bubbling spring** (ball of the foot) and one on the client's hand at the acupuncture point called **palace of weariness** (center of the palm of the hand), as pictured in Figure 10-53.

Sit in silence and breathe with your client.

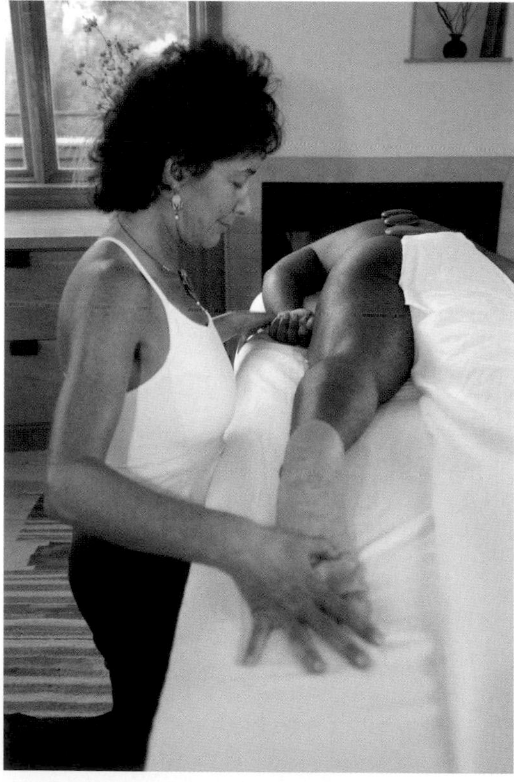

Figure 10-53 Bubbling Spring/Palace of Weariness. Complete the closing stroke by holding one stone on the client's foot at the bubbling spring acupuncture point and one on the client's hand at the palace of weariness acupuncture point.

SUMMARY

Grounded in the principles and basic stone techniques described earlier in this book, the three-dimensional strokes identified in this chapter will greatly enhance your hot stone massage. Practice each stroke without stones first and then, when comfortable, weave each of them into the hot stone massage.

The strokes included in this chapter are only some of the ones offered in the collection of Phenomenal Touch Massage. Many are complex and difficult to perform by their written description alone and thus require additional assistance from an experienced Phenomenal Touch Massage practitioner or through taking a three-dimensional hot stone training.

Strokes for the face include face flush, broad strokes around the entire face; infiniteye, specific small alternating circles around the eyes; and jaw melt, specific work in the masseter muscles.

Strokes for the neck include waterfall, a freeing backward drop and slide of the neck; neck drool, a slow gravitational fall of the head to the back and then to the side, as the neck is simultaneously lifted up; neck over, a specific penetration into the lateral neck muscles in their shortened position; and rock n' roll, which adds a rocking movement to the normal static neck stretches.

Strokes for the arm and shoulders include three-dimensional arm effleurage, an embracing stroke that goes up the arm, across the neck, beneath the shoulder, and back down both sides of the arm; altar-nater, an alternation of altars created by the stone beneath the shoulder; hand scrunch, which works both sides of the hands with stones; and lat pump, a penetration of the lat muscle in its shortened position.

Strokes for the torso include rag doll, a sideways rhythmical undulation of the spine; lumbar torque, a lift of the low back while pushing back on the armpit; undertow, a lift of the low back while pushing down on the opposite iliac crest; and belly waves, which embrace the belly and low back from the supine position, making wave-line motions between the two hands.

Strokes for the legs in the supine position include three-dimensional leg effleurage, a long embracing stroke that embraces both sides of the leg and extends up the back and down the arm; foot scrunch, which works both sides of the foot; leg over sequence, a crossing of the leg to the other side of the body; the frog, in which a bent knee that falls out laterally is torqued to the opposite side of the body, stretching the low back; and hip flip, a double-legged version of frog.

To turn your client over, begin with hip flip and then slowly bring the upper torso toward you, lift the opposite arm, flip the head over and then bring the legs to join. This series of movements is accompanied by many stretches and pauses to disguise that that the client is being turned over.

Strokes for the back include the fullback, a three-dimensional effleurage that extends onto the buttocks and belly and back up to the neck; forearm frenzy, a rhythmical alternation of forearms in the rhomboid area; chicken wing, a pectoralis stretch created by a fulcrum and lever; teres tango, a rhythmical penetration of the teres muscle in the shortened position; reverse belly wave, an embracing of the belly and low back from the prone position; and hip hop, a lift of the hip and push up the quadratus lumborum to create a lumbar torque and stretch.

Strokes for the legs in the prone position include three-dimensional leg effleurage, a long embracing stroke up both sides of the leg, then the back and down the arm; shortened ham pump, a penetration of the hamstring muscles in the shortened position; calf mush, an embracing of both sides of the calf in the upright position; and reverse frog, a bending of the knee outward while in the prone position, exposing the lateral aspect of the thigh.

Closing strokes include calf up-arm down, a pulling of the arm down as the calf is pushed up toward the back; and bubbling spring/palace of weariness, the holding of two acupuncture points at the same time, one in the ball of the foot and one in the center of the palm.

TIP

When doing the strokes, never abandon the principles that underlie each of them. Fancy strokes done without allegiance to the principles will result in a hollow disjointed experience for the client. Allow the strokes to unfold naturally from the foundations that helped form them. Refer to Appendix A, a full body guided hot stone massage, to bring all the pieces of this book together.

REVIEW QUESTIONS

TRUE/FALSE

1. Even though draping is important in all forms of massage, three-dimensional strokes require less attention to draping the sheet than regular massage does.

   Circle: True False

2. When doing the head stone cradle as an opening stroke, both your hands should be on top of the client's head.

   Circle: True False

3. In face flush, begin with the pointed edge of the stone.

   Circle: True False

4. Alternate the circles in infiniteye simultaneously but with a lag.

   Circle: True False

5. Jaw melt starts broad and then works specific points and then becomes broad again.

   Circle: True False

MULTIPLE CHOICE

6. The three-dimensional arm effleurage differs from a regular one in that it:
   a. Works both sides of the body at once
   b. Incorporates opposition
   c. Goes beyond the shoulder and neck
   d. Lifts the head up in space
   e. All of the above
7. Altar-nater does the following:
   a. Makes one altar under the shoulder
   b. Makes one altar under the leg
   c. Makes two altars that alternate under the low back
   d. Makes two altars that alternate under the shoulder
   e. All of the above
8. Hand scrunch is:
   a. Scrunching the hand backward with a stone
   b. Scrunching the hand forward with a stone
   c. A catchall name for all the ways to use stones on hand
   d. Scrunching the hand straight up with a stone on the fingertips
   e. None of the above
9. To perform the lat pump, you should:
   a. Pump the arm up and down, pressing on the lateral shoulder muscles

b. Pump the arm up and down, pressing on the latissimus muscle in its short pose
c. Pump the arm up and down, pressing on latissimus muscle in its long pose
d. Pump the arm up and down, pressing on the lateral rotators
e. None of the above

10. To perform the rag doll, you should:
    a. Push the shoulder forward at the same time as you push the hip forward
    b. Push the shoulder back at the same time as you push the hip back
    c. Let the hip fall back as you gently pull the shoulder forward, then reverse this
    d. All of the above are appropriate
    e. None of the above are appropriate

SHORT ANSWER

11. In lumbar torque, it is important to push down on the client's ___________ rather than his or her arm to avoid dislocating the shoulder.
12. Undertow is used to __________________ the client's hips.
13. In the large belly wave, it is best to have your _________ arm beneath the back so you can torque it against the client's hips.
14. In leg over, you need to make sure that you stay _____________ the client's leg as you cross it over and walk forward with it.
15. The frog should not be done on clients who have had recent _____________ injury or surgery.

Answers to Review Questions can be found in Appendix D.

APPENDIX A

Full-Body Three-Dimensional Hot Stone Massage Sequence

"Following this sequence helped me to bring together all of the separate pieces involved in giving a hot stone massage. It allowed me to get a sense of the flow so that I could eventually find my own rhythm."

Andy Oriel, Three-Dimensional Hot Stone Massage Practitioner, Boulder, Colorado

This guided massage sequence is one example of a three-dimensional hot stone massage that should take you approximately 90 minutes to perform. It does not include every move described in this book and is not "the way" to do hot stone massage. It is intended merely as a guide. Use it to gain a sense of all the components involved in giving a full-body hot stone massage. Then, once you have followed it a few times, make your own variations. Each massage you give should be a unique expression of your creative response to your client's needs.

Attempt to follow this sequence only after you have studied and practiced the principles and techniques in this book. Once you've done that, use this guided sequence to give you an overview of all that you have learned, including the set up, layout, stone management, and the order and flow of the strokes and techniques, which you can choose to incorporate as you wish.

For the sake of simplicity, throughout this guided massage, the client will be considered female; thus, the pronouns "she" and "her" will be used.

This guided massage uses eight stones in pile number one, eight stones in pile number two, and sixteen stones in pile number three. However, because stones vary in how long they hold their temperature, you may have to use more stones than I instruct to maintain proper warmth. Make adjustments and replenish your stone piles according to your particular situation if they do not coincide with mine.

It's important to remember that the four-pile stone system is a guideline, not a bible, for how to manage the stones. There is some variation as to when I return my stones to the skillet. Sometimes I return pile one to the skillet immediately after using it. Other times I use both pile one and two before returning the stones to the skillet. What's most important is what will support the best flow of the massage in that moment.

Throughout this guided massage, I do not make mention of when to dip your working stones into the cold water (for quick cooling) or the skillet (for quick reheating), as this is completely dependent on the temperatures of each specific stone you are using at the time. Dip your stones when you need to, based on their individual temperatures and the time frame in which you need to use them.

Throughout this guided massage, there is very little direction given as to which principles or techniques to use on each part of the body. Instead, its focus is on stone management and strokes. Feel free to incorporate any and all of the principles and techniques of stone use that you have learned in Chapters 8 and 9 any time you wish. This is really a matter of personal preference.

I hope you enjoy doing your very first three-dimensional hot stone massage. May the force be with you!

THE SET UP

Make sure you are completely prepared before your client arrives.

1. Turn the skillet to the highest setting approximately 20 minutes prior to client's arrival. Keep the lid on the skillet for the initial heating.
2. Double check to make sure that the thermostat device is pushed all the way into the skillet. Make sure the cord to the skillet is plugged into the wall socket or an appropriate extension cord. Turn off all unnecessary electrical appliances to avoid a short in the circuit.
3. Remove the lid from the cold stones bowl. Add ice to the water.
4. Once the stones have heated up, lower the temperature to the warm or low setting.
5. Remove the lid from the skillet. Be careful not to drip the condensed water on your hand. Place the lid out of the way.
6. Remove lids from the oil bowls and make sure the appropriate amount of oil is in each of them. If the room allows, set four oil bowls out: one on the stone table, one on a shelf on the other side of the massage table, and one on shelves at each end of the massage table.
7. Be sure that your stone table is covered in polyurethane (if it is wood) and that it has a thick towel over it to collect excess water from the stones.
8. Place the eye mask, foot straps, oven pockets, thin strip of material or pillowcase, spare towels, and sandbags where they are readily accessible. Make sure your slotted spoon and essential oils are close by.
9. Fill your spare pitcher with water.
10. Place your tiny stones in a small bowl so that they are readily available. Place your bowl of spare stones beneath the stone table.

Once all of this is in order, you are ready to begin to remove the stones from the skillet in order to make a layout on the massage table before the client arrives.

INITIAL LAYOUT AND STONE PILES

Begin with the super double spinal run layout. You will need 16 stones for this layout: one neck, two scapula, six spinal, one sacrum, two hand, two knee, and two foot stones. You will also want three stones for the top of the body: one heart, one solar plexus, and one large belly stone.

1. Remove the necessary stones from the skillet. Take the time to allow the water from the stones to run through the slots of the spoon before placing each of them on the towel-covered stone table. Keep in mind the size and shape of the stones you will want for the layouts and individual placements you are choosing and for the body parts you are planning to work first.
2. Dip the stones in cold water for a few seconds to cool them off slightly for the initial layout.
3. Shake off the excess water or dry the stones before you lay them on the table; otherwise, the sheet will get wet.
4. Lay out the stones on the table. Create the super double spinal run. The stones need to be fairly flat, and those that will be opposite each other along the spine should be of the same height. Leave approximately 1 inch between the two lines of stones for the spine. Place the neck stone so that there is enough room for the head.
5. Lie on the stones to see how they fit with your body and adjust them according to the approximate difference between your size and the client's (if you know it).
6. Once the stones are in place, cover them with a narrow strip of material in order to preserve their heat until the client arrives.
7. After the layout is ready, turn to the three stones you had picked out for the top of the body. Place those stones, along with two for the client's

hands, two for the feet, and two for the knees on the left side of the stone table for easy access.

8. Arrange all the stones that you did not use for the placement neatly on the stone table. These are the stones you will use to begin your pile system once the client arrives.
9. Make sure you have taken a sufficient number of small to medium-small stones out of the skillet, as you will be starting with the face.
10. Make sure the stones that remain in the skillet are all pushed to the right side.
11. Add some eucalyptus or lavender to the skillet to create a lovely aroma for when the client walks into the room.
12. Once the client arrives, show her the layout and how to lay on it (over the strip of material, unless the stones have cooled off too much, then, directly on top of the stones) and encourage her to adjust the location of the stones should she need to for comfort.
13. Once she has lain on the stones, wait a few moments and then check with her for approval on the temperature of the stones beneath her back, before placing stones on top of her body. If the stones are too hot, add another layer of material. If they are not hot enough, remove the piece of material.
14. Once approval of the stone layout and temperature has occurred, place the large belly stone, the solar plexus stone, and then the heart stone on top of her. The solar plexus and heart stone can double as working stones and be part of your pile two. The large belly stone is not considered part of your pile two, but instead a separate placement stone.
15. Place the two hand and two knee stones beneath her hands and knees.
16. Strap the two feet stones to the bottoms of her feet.

Now you are ready to make your piles. When you initially create piles, pile number two does not need to be placed on the client first, as she already has a placement on her. However, when all the piles are ready to be replenished, you would then follow the protocol of placing pile number two on the person before placing pile number one on the table.

17. Place pile one on the massage table with four stones on either side of her head. Add two tepid stones to your initial pile one to help introduce the heat gradually. Thus, the first pile one you make will contain ten stones, but the future ones will only contain eight.
18. Place pile two on top of her torso in between the layout stones (or include the smaller layout stones as part of your pile two).
19. Pile three is made up of the stones that remain on the stone table. Make sure there are approximately sixteen stones there. If not, take some hot ones from the skillet. Place them on the right end of pile three for easy temperature differentiation.
20. Push all the stones in the skillet to the right.

You are now ready to begin your massage!

OPENING STROKE

1. Standing to the side of the client, place one of your hands on the large belly stone and the other on the heart stone and breathe in silence for a few minutes, matching your client's breath.

THE HEAD AND NECK

1. Massage your client's head for a few minutes without stones.
2. When ready to massage the face, anoint your hands with face lotion. Slide your anointed hands over the stones in pile one and then make contact with the face.
3. Massage the face without stones for a few moments and then pick up two of the least hot stones from pile one. Enter on the face with fingertips first, edge of stone, and then full stone. Remember not to massage for too long with these stones, as a stone that has lost its heat is experienced as hard and boring.
4. As soon as these stones have lost their heat, place them down on the massage table and pick up two warmer stones from pile one and continue to massage the face doing the face flush.
5. Move into infiniteye using two new small stones from pile one. Alternate circles with the flat sides of the stones and then use the edges of the stones if deeper pressure is desired.
6. Continue into jaw melt, making slow circles around the temporomandibular joint with two somewhat pointed stones from pile one. Use the

ends of the stones to massage the belly of the masseter muscle. Slide up to the temples and do small slow circles over the temporal muscles.

7. Reach into the bowl of iced water with your hand; remove four cold stones and bring them to the head of the massage table.
8. Use one of your last two hot stones from pile one to introduce the cold stone. First, use the hot stone and then gently warn your client as you enter with the cold stone, alternating hot with cold.
9. When the hot stone has lost its heat, bring in a second cold stone to replace the hot one. Then, bring in the third cold stone so that you are now massaging with two new cold stones on the face.
10. When the cold stones have lost their coldness, put them down on the massage table. Now, pick up the last cold stone and continue working with it on the face. With your other hand, pick up the last hot stone from pile one and massage with it alternating between the hot and the cold.
11. End with the warm stone only.
12. Return the warm stones to the left side of the skillet and the cold stones to the bowl of ice water.
13. Retrieve five tiny stones from the small bowl. Place them in the slotted spoon and dip them in the hot water for approximately 5 seconds. Dry them and carefully place over the client's third eye, eyes, and cheeks, checking first to make sure their temperature is appropriate.
14. Place the eye mask over the face stones and strap it to the head.
15. Move the stones from on top of the client's torso (pile two) onto the massage table. This now becomes your new pile one.
16. Remove placement stones from beneath the neck and upper shoulders and return them to the left side of skillet.
17. Take eight stones from the left side of pile three (waiting in the wings) and place them on top of the client for your new pile two.
18. Push the eight remaining stones of pile number three to the left side of the stone table. Remove eight hot stones from the right side of the skillet (pile four) and add them to the right of pile three on the stone table. Push all remaining skillet stones to the right side.
19. First, lubricate your hands by dipping them into the oil bowl. Slide your oiled hands over the stones in piles one and two and then proceed to the neck.
20. Massage the neck without stones for a few minutes to make contact with the client and get a feel for what is going on in the neck.
21. Introduce two stones (from your new pile one) onto the neck with a hand-over-hand alternation.
22. Place these cooled off stones on the massage table and get one oblong warm stone from pile one to do waterfall. Make sure this stone is not too hot, as it will be held still against the neck.
23. Do waterfall with stone a few times. Then, place the stone on the massage table.
24. Move into neck drool with a new stone from pile one. Go slow with this move.
25. Perform approximately four neck drools.
26. Place the stone you were just using on the massage table. Remove the eye mask and tiny face placement stones. Place them in the slotted spoon and dip them in hot water for 10 seconds to clean them. Put them back in the little bowl.
27. Take a slightly pointed stone from pile one. Move right into neck over with this new stone. Do one side first, moving the stone altar to a new spot on the neck with each opening and closing of the neck.
28. Seamlessly switch hands and do neck over on the other side. Use a new stone for this side of the neck.
29. Put the cooled stone on the massage table. Pick up two new stones from pile one and go right into rock n' roll, alternating placing your stone-filled hands on the shoulders of the client.

Once you have completed rock n' roll, there should be no more warm stones in pile one.

30. Return pile one to the left side of skillet. Move pile two from the top of the client to the massage table. This is now your new pile one.

Before placing a new pile two on top of the client, you'll need to tend to the stone layout beneath the client because by now the client can no longer feel the heat through the fabric strip.

31. Standing on the side of the table closest to the skillet, remove large placement stone from the client's abdomen and place out of the way on the stone table (you will not be using this large stone again for a while, so don't take up room in the skillet for it just yet).
32. Gently roll the client's body toward you and remove the narrow strip of fabric from the spinal stone run. From this sideways position, massage the client's back for 30 seconds or so with two hot stones from your new pile one.
33. Slowly lower the client back down onto the exposed stones, making sure that they are not too hot.
34. Replace the hand placement stones, remove the knee placement stones, and replace the foot placement stones (without removing the straps) using four stones from the left side of pile three. Replace these stones to pile three on the right side of stone table.
35. Take stones from left side of pile three and replace pile two on the client's chest and belly.
36. Remove stones from right side of the skillet to replenish pile three. Push remaining skillet stones to the right side
37. Oil pile two and then return to the head to do a few stoneless rock n' rolls from a standing position.
38. Transition into three-dimensional arm effleurage on the arm that is furthest from the skillet. This will set you up for being on the proper side of the table for removing the placement stones from beneath the spine when it is time do so.

THE ARMS, SHOULDERS, AND TORSO

1. Use two stones from pile one to do a few three-dimensional arm effleurages.
2. Take two new stones from pile one and slide down the arm to the hand and do some hand scrunches with a stone on either side.
3. With two new stones from pile one, slide back up the arm while doing some heeling, circling, sandwiching, resistance, and point work.
4. By now you will have used up your pile one. Leave them on the table and take two stones off the client's torso from pile two to do one more three-dimensional arm effleurage.
5. Flow into the altar-nater with the same stones. As you continue alternating your altars, replace the stones in your hands with two new hot ones, taking your time with each stone altar that you make.
6. Lift the client's arm above her head, pick up a new stone from pile one and move right into lat pump. Continue to work the armpit area with another new stone from pile one.

There should be approximately two stones left on the client's torso.

7. Move the two remaining stones off the client's body to the far side of the massage table next to the hip and proceed directly into rag doll.
8. Reach across the table and lift the client's arm. Begin with step two of the rag doll sequence pulling the client's torso up and toward you, away from the skillet.
9. Do a few undulations on the client's torso and then push the placement stones away from you in the direction of the skillet, while staying in contact with and supporting her back with your upper arms.
10. Pick up the two hot stones you had previously placed by the client's hip and continue doing rag doll with the new stones.
11. Once you are finished with rag doll, move directly into lumbar torque and then undertow.

Now, you must replenish your stones.

12. Return all cooled stones (from both pile one and two) to the left side of the skillet.
13. Use the stones from the right side of pile three to replace pile two. Place pile two on the client's chest, but leave the belly without stones.
14. Use the stones from the left side of pile three to re-create a pile one. Place pile one next to the client's pelvis.
15. Replace the foot stones (without removing the straps) with stones from the left side of skillet. Use them on calf to diminish heat before placing on foot.
16. Get eight tiny stones from the little bowl, place them in the slotted spoon, and dip them in the hot water for approximately 5 to 10 seconds.

Dry them on the stone table and gently place them between the toes of both feet, making sure the temperature is appropriate for your client.

17. Replenish pile three and then push the remaining stones to the right side of the skillet. Add more water to the skillet and resume massage.
18. Oil the stones in both piles and then move back into undertow.
19. Use two new hot stones from pile one to do a few small belly waves.
20. Get two new stones from pile one and do a few large belly waves.
21. Seamlessly transition from large belly wave into three-dimensional leg effleurage.

THE LEGS—SUPINE

1. From belly wave, pick up two new hot stones from pile one.
2. Turn toward the client's feet and do a three-dimensional leg effleurage heading down the leg.
3. Once you reach the foot, turn toward the client's head and continue back up the body with a three-dimensional leg effleurage, letting both hands go all the way up her leg and beneath her lower back.
4. Pick up two more stones from pile one and work the whole leg from both sides at the same time with the stones. Then, using momentum, let your outside arm continue beneath the client's back to her shoulder, while the inside arm reaches under and creates a fulcrum on the thigh.
5. Using your outside arm, lift the client's shoulder slightly and leave your stone beneath it (make sure it is not hitting spine or scapula border).
6. Take your inside arm away from the thigh and bring it up to the client's shoulder to meet your other hand. Embrace the arm from both sides and slide the stone that is in your inside-hand down the arm, leaving it in the client's hand when you reach it.
7. Pick up two new hot stones from pile two, one for each hand, and massage both sides of her thigh.
8. Use two new stones from pile two to massage the calf. Work your way down the calf to the foot.
9. When you reach the foot, remove the foot stones, the toe stones, and the straps. Return the foot stones to the skillet. Dip the tiny toe stones in the hot water for a quick cleaning and return to them to the little bowl.
10. Use two new stones to do foot scrunches. Don't forget to use the mother–father technique to soften the pressure of the stone into the sole of the foot.
11. When finished with the foot, get two new stones from pile two to do a few more three-dimensional leg effleurages, using stones on either side of the leg.
12. Replenish your stone piles.

Normally, we would place pile two on the body first to keep the client warm while creating pile one on the massage table, but because of the nature of the massage strokes that follow, this time, rather than placing pile two on the client, leave it somewhere on the massage table separate from pile one so that you are aware of the temperature difference.

13. Place pile one by the hip of the leg you are working on.
14. Move into leg over.
15. Once you have done the three stretches, use all the stones from pile one (by the client's hip) to work the client's buttocks, low back, IT band, and shoulder.
16. Leave a stone beneath the client's low back as you move into the frog.
17. Return cool stones from pile one to the left side of skillet.
18. Using a stone from pile two perform the frog.
19. Move into hip flip, using a new stone. Remove the placement stone from beneath the client's low back before completing hip flip.
20. Pick up two stones from pile two and end this leg with a long three-dimensional effleurage.
21. Cover the leg with the sheet.
22. Remove the flowing placement stone from beneath the client's shoulder. Replace both hand and foot stones with stones from the left side of pile three. Replenish these stones to the right side of stone table.

Before proceeding to the next leg, you must replenish your stone piles.

23. If you wish, this time you can place pile two on the client's torso before you begin the other leg. Just make sure that there are no stones on top of

the client's body by the time you enter into leg over.

24. Place pile one on the massage table near the leg you are about to work.
25. Repeat the same moves on the second leg, using up both your stone piles; however, this time do not strap a new stone to the foot at the completion of massaging the leg, but instead remove the one that is still strapped onto the other foot.
26. Now, remove all stones that are left on the massage table and any flowing placements that are left beneath or on top of the client.

TURNING CLIENT OVER

1. Before the client is turned over, double check that all of the stones are removed from the massage table. They can hide in places you forgot about and can fall on your foot if you are not aware.
2. If you would prefer to have the client turn herself over, simply ask her to do so.
3. If, instead, you choose to turn your client over, start with hip flip and follow the instructions on how to turn a client over from the last chapter (Chapter 10).

Once the client is turned over, replenish all of your piles.

THE BACK

1. Begin by placing new hot stones onto the client's hands and feet (use straps on feet if necessary).
2. Place pile two on her buttocks and thighs.
3. Place pile one at the head of the table above the shoulders, by the outside of the arms, or between the arm and the side of the torso. Make sure the stones are not too close to the client's body. Let the client know where the stones are so she does not inadvertently move into them. If the client is very large and there is no space left on the massage table for pile one, place it on a table or shelf near you.
4. Replenish pile three.
5. Put the large placement stone back into the skillet for a future final back placement.
6. Add more water to the skillet, and move skillet stones to the right.
7. Stand at the head of the table. Oil your hands and then glide them over piles one and two before making contact with the back.
8. Do two fullbacks without stones.
9. Pick up two stones from pile one and enter your third fullback with finger-wrapped stones at the upper traps. Let the stones emerge from your hands and make full stone contact with the back.
10. Glide slowly and deeply with these stones down the back, over the buttocks, around the edges of the hips, under the belly, up along the sides, back up to the rhomboids, out the shoulders, and up the neck.
11. Using one stone from pile one, do some compression on the rhomboids.
12. Using one stone from pile one, do some mother–father along the spinalis.
13. Using another stone from pile one, do some edging along the multifidus.
14. Reach into the bowl of iced water and remove two cold stones. Bring them to the massage table. Take a hot stone from pile one and begin warming the area of the back where you will introduce the cold stone (ideally an area of inflammation or tension).
15. Warn the client as you enter with a cold stone. Alternate the hot stone with the cold stone. Replace the hot stone with a cold one and continue massaging with two cold stones. Replace the cold stones in their bowl of iced water.
16. Use the last two hot stones from pile one to do a few more fullbacks, ending by gliding down the arms and replacing the client's hand stones with these.
17. Enter into forearm frenzy without stones.
18. After a few strokes on the rhomboids with your forearms, seamlessly reach down the back and pick up two stones from pile two.
19. Enter the next four or five forearm frenzies first with stone-wrapped fingers and then with full contact of the stones.
20. Continue with these stones directly into chicken wing.
21. Perform both directions of the chicken wing stretch.

22. Grab a new stone from pile two and sit at the client's shoulder, facing her head.
23. Perform teres tango by placing your stoneless hand beneath the client's shoulder and use your stone-filled hand to penetrate the teres muscle.
24. Do teres tango for as long as you deem necessary.
25. Stand at the side of the table by the client's hip. Place two stones from pile two on the opposite side of the hip.
26. Begin reverse belly wave, by sliding your stoneless foot-hand underneath and across the belly. When your hand emerges out on the other side of the client's body, use your head-hand to put one of the pre-placed stones into it. Lift the other stone off the massage table with your empty hand and slide both stone-filled hands across either side of the torso until you reach the center. Make vertical waves with the belly and low back using both of your hands.
27. Slide your lower arm out and leave both of the used stones on the massage table before you pick up one new stone from pile two.
28. Move into hip hop. With a stone held only in your head-hand, paw hand over hand along the side of and slightly beneath the hip. Use the stone-hand to push up against the lower back when doing the "hop" part of the move. While still at the hip, undrape the leg you are going to work on next.
29. If you have a healing or warming balm that is in reach, rub some into any areas of the back that were extra tender or contracted.
30. Pick up the last two hot stones from pile two.
31. Facing the head, use your new stones to warm the areas where the healing balm was applied, and then make long and fast gliding strokes up and down the back flushing the entire area.
32. From the upper part of the back, let your hands slide down either arm allowing these stones to replace the existing ones in the client's hands.

You will now need to replenish your stone piles and make a back and belly placement.

33. Return all cold stones from the massage table to the left side of the skillet.
34. Using stones from the left side of pile three, make a single spinal run out layout along the entire spine. Depending on the temperature of the stones, you may need to place a thin strip of fabric beneath them.
35. Remove a large placement stone from the skillet, dry and place it in an oven pocket or wrap it in a towel. Standing at the client's hip, lean across to the other side of the client's back and lift her iliac crest high up off the table. As you lift the hip up with one hand, slide the large placement stone beneath her belly with the other. Slowly lower her down onto the placement stone making sure that the temperature is okay.
36. Place pile two on both sides of the client's low back, buttocks, and in the groin area.
37. Put pile one on either side of the client's leg that you are working on, careful not to place the stones too close to the client's body.
38. Remove stones from the right side of skillet to replenish pile three.
39. Push the remaining stones of pile four to the right side of the skillet.

THE LEGS—PRONE

1. Remove the placement stones and straps from both of the client's feet.
2. Oil your stone piles and then do a few three-dimensional leg effleurages without stones.
3. Pick up two stones from pile one and continue doing three-dimensional leg effleurages, changing stones when required. Use six stones total from pile one to complete the effleurages.
4. Move into calf mush, using the last set of stones from pile one.
5. Place all stones from the client's buttocks on the massage table for your new pile one.
6. Use two of these stones to do shorten ham pump.
7. Use four of these stones to do the many variations of reverse frog.
8. Use your last two stones to do one final three-dimensional leg effleurage moving directly into calf up-arm down, replacing the existing hand placement as you slide into the hand.
9. Cover this leg with the sheet.
10. Replenish your stones again before doing the other leg. However, this time you only need to leave four stones in pile three (on the stone table) for your closing stroke.

11. Work the second leg.
12. Once you have completed the second leg, ending with calf up-arm down, replace existing hand placement, and take all of the remaining cool stones from the massage table and put them back into the skillet.
13. Remove the single spinal run out from the back and return those stones to the skillet as well.
14. Remove the large placement stone from beneath the client's belly in the same way that you placed it. Return this stone to the skillet.

All of your stones should now be back in the skillet except for the last four you will use for your closing stroke.

15. Before you begin your closing stroke, turn the skillet to high, make sure the water covers the stones, add a few drops of the essential oil of your choice, and place the lid back on the skillet in order to boil and clean your stones.

CLOSING STROKE

1. Bring your four remaining stones from the stone table to the massage table, placing two stones on the outside of each leg.
2. Uncover the leg you worked on first as well as the same side of the back.
3. Take the two stones from that side and hold them on the client's buttock, with your fingers opposing each other.
4. Simultaneously slide each stone away from the other down the client's leg and up the back, then down the arm and lower leg, ending at the hand and foot at the same time.
5. Hold the stones over the bubbling spring point on the foot and palace of weariness point on the hand.
6. Match your client's breathing.
7. Take a few minutes in this position, giving both you and the client time to take in the entire experience, which is about to come to an end.
8. Leave the stones in place on the hand and foot. Cover this leg and go to the other side of the body.
9. Repeat this closing stroke leaving the two stones in place and cover that side of the body.
10. Sit by the head of your client with your hands on either side of her head and breathe with her in silence.
11. Slowly remove the last four stones from the client's hands and feet and return them to the (now boiling) water. Once again, replace the lid on the skillet.
12. Before you leave the room, turn your skillet off (unplug it to be absolutely safe). The water will continue boiling for a few more minutes after it is turned off, sanitizing the last four rocks you put in.

Congratulations! You have just completed your first three-dimensional hot stone massage. Take a bow!

APPENDIX B

Sources for Stone Kits and Essential Oils

Finding quality premade stone sets from stone companies can prove to be difficult. The majority of the stone sets sold are very limited in their colors, sizes, and shapes. Most of them are all gray or black with no color variation, and only one company pre-oils the stones. Thus, the photos of the stones sold are rarely indicative of the stones you receive in the mail. The photos show black glistening oiled stones, while the ones that are sent are dry, gray, and lusterless. Once oiled, the stones will pick up some luster; however, they are generally not as black, smooth, or flat as they appear to be in the advertisements. Most stone sets sold are more grainy, and larger than what is optimal to use in hot stone massage. This is why it is strongly recommended that you inquire in great detail about the stones before purchasing them. Ask for a few sample sizes of stones to be sent to you prior to ordering them so that you can see and feel the stone as well as get a sense of the size. It is also very important to find out ahead of time if the stone set is returnable so that you are not left with a set of stones that you do not like.

Out of the multitude of companies that sell stones, there are three companies that stand out. Only two of these companies include a variation in stone color. Thus, only these three stone companies will be included in this list; however, feel free to do research of your own as companies do change their stone sources and new companies may have come into existence since the publication of this book.

1. 3-D Hot Stone Massage
   Institute for Phenomenal Touch Massage
   Post Office Box 3084
   Eldorado Springs, Colorado 80025
   Phone: (303) 494-6204
   Email: massage@phenomenaltouch.com
   Web site: www.phenomenaltouch.com/hotstones/index.htm

3-D Hot Stone Massage is based within the Institute for Phenomenal Touch Massage and founded by Leslie Bruder. The stones sold by them are the ones photographed in this book, and a sample of their kits can be seen in Chapter 4, Figure 4-28. Their stones are naturally tumbled basalt and quartzite and include a gorgeous range in colors. They are hand-selected with careful attention to shape, category, and size from the banks of the Colorado River in Colorado and Utah and the beaches of the oceans in various locations in California and Mexico. They are pre-oiled to save you the step. They sell sets of 55 stones for a full body massage and sets of 35 stones for facials, manicures, and pedicures. Additionally, they offer complete sets that include a cooker and all accessories needed for performing hot stone massage. They also make and sell the stone wrappers discussed and photographed in this book. They can be sold either with a set of stones or separately.

3-D Hot Stone Massage is happy to customize stone sets for their customers. As each set is made to order, they will discuss hand size and the colors and types of stones preferred by their customers and adjust the kit accordingly. They also sell individual stones to supplement your own stone collection.

2. Desert Stone People
   Tomi and John Wertheim
   Tucson, Arizona
   Phone: (866) 616-7218 or (520) 616-7250
   Email: john@desertstonepeople.com
   Web site: www.desertstonepeople.com

Desert Stone People is a small company run by a lovely couple, Tomi and John Wertheim. Their stones come from the dry beaches of Arizona and Mexico. Their kits have a selection of different colors and shapes and are naturally tumbled. Their original stone set includes 56 stones made of basalt. They also sell sets of various shapes and sizes of both jade and marble stones. They sell individual stones as well as stone warmers and accessories. Visit their Web site for the latest prices of their various sets of stones.

3. Th Stone
   Tamarac, Florida
   Phone: (866) 680-5149
   Email: info@thstone.com
   Web site: www.thstone.com

Th Stone, founded by Sonia Alexandra and recently sold to Tom Wellman, sells naturally tumbled black volcanic stones and gray marine stones from the oceans of South America. They make a variety of stone sets. Their starter kit is versatile and includes 50 stones. The facial kits include 45 stones, and the pedicure/manicure kit includes 32 stones. Their stones come in separate bags for each category of stone. They also sell stone cookers and accessories. They arc a large company and yet maintain a high quality of standard for their stones, choosing beautiful, smooth, and nicely shaped stones that are very useful for a hot stone massage. Their stones are of high quality but lack in their variety of color and shape.

1. Young Living Essential Oils
   Independent Distributor: Nancy Cebula
   Boulder, Colorado
   Phone: (303) 499-1607
   Email: nancy@aromaticsandmassage.com
   Web site: www.aromaticsandmassage.com

Gary and Mary Young, founders of Young Living Essential Oils, are deeply committed to offering only the highest grade of essential oils available. Similar to food, cosmetics, and automobiles, there are many versions and qualities of essential oils. And while they all may look alike, there is a huge difference between low- and high-grade essential oils. The majority of essential oils that are bought over the counter are low-grade oils that may have strong aromas, but a very low therapeutic value.

The difference between a low-grade essential oil and a therapeutic-grade is thousands of petals! For instance, a 15 mL bottle off a low-grade rose essential oil may have been distilled from approximately 100 rose petals, whereas a therapeutic-grade rose essential oil would be distilled from 1,000 rose petals. One smells similar to a rose, and one is the essence of a rose. One has aromatic qualities, and the other can aid in healing disorders and conditions. Sourced from the world's finest and purest plants, Young Living's essential oils are not diluted with chemical and synthetic additives and are carefully prepared to maintain the integrity of the plants.

I only recommend using therapeutic-grade essential oils for hot stone massage. Anything less could not only diminish the experience for both the clients and the therapists but may also cause an adverse reaction to the oils. Young Living Oils are the world's premium essential oils and are perfect for using with hot stone massage.

Nancy Cebula is not only a representative for Young Living Oils, but she has also taken much time to study the individual therapeutic effects of each of the different oils. She can help inform you as to which oils would be best to use for each particular condition you want to treat. Her vast knowledge extends beyond that of the average representative, and she is happy to offer verbal or written information on the properties of the oils.

APPENDIX C

Training in Three-Dimensional Hot Stone Massage

Training in three-dimensional hot stone massage is offered in various locales; however, the instructors are also equipped to travel to your locale and teach at your house, spa, or school should you choose not to travel. Contact any of the following instructors to find out more about the training they offer. Please note that over time the phone numbers of these instructors may change, thus the email addresses may be more reliable to use.

1. The Institute for Phenomenal Touch Massage
   Eldorado Springs, Colorado
   Phone: (303) 494-6204
   Email: massage@phenomenaltouch.com
   Web site: www.phenomenaltouch.com/hotstones/index.htm
2. Mary Axelrod
   Fort Collins, Colorado
   Phone: (970) 204-1794
   Email: maryaxelrod@comcast.net
   Web site: www.callmary.net
3. Edye Rose
   Denver, Colorado
   Phone: (303) 916-0058
   Email: edye_rose@hotmail.com
4. Michelle Helms
   Bakersfield, Vermont
   Phone number available via email
   Email: michellehere4u@gmail.com
5. April Moon
   Spokane, Washington
   Phone: (509) 675-5399
   Email: april.moon21@gmail.com
6. Nolus Sunoon
   Denver, Colorado
   Phone: (303) 564-9205
   Email: nsunoon@hotmail.com
7. Cedar Johnson
   Santa Cruz, California
   Phone: (831) 234-3933
   Email: cedaronelove@gmail.com
8. Daniel Munoz
   Edwards, Colorado
   Phone: (970) 331-2244
   Email: mountainbare2002@yahoo.com
9. Andy Oriel
   Boulder, Colorado
   Phone: (720) 308-9355
   Email: hotriverstone@aol.com

10. Nora Keahon
    Boulder, Colorado
    Phone: (503) 536-5131
    Email: manifestnext2me@hotmail.com
    Web site: www.divineresonance.com
11. Jeffrey Chaplin
    Gardiner, Maine
    Phone: (207) 582-1600
    Email: jchaplin24@hotmail.com
    Web site: www.touchleaf.com
12. Jonathan Grassi
    Boulder, Colorado
    Phone: (303) 877- 7475
    Email: jmg94@cornell.edu
13. Paula Pearson
    Billings, Montana
    Work Phone: (406) 254-6399
    Cell Phone: (406) 860-2461
    Email: PAP0519@aol.com
14. Cary Ambraziunas
    Boulder, Colorado
    Phone: (303) 440-0390
    Email: carycreekside@gmail.com

APPENDIX D

Answers to Review Questions

CHAPTER 1

1. False 2. False 3. True 4. False 5. False 6. e 7. e 8. e 9. c 10. e 11. moxabustion 12. saunas 13. pointed tool stones 14. help children fall asleep 15. warm their hands or feet

CHAPTER 2

1. True 2. False 3. True 4. True 5. False 6. c 7. b 8. a 9. e 10. c 11. Hot Stone Massage Intake Form 12. Healing Crisis 13. hot 14. cold 15. moderate 16. e 17. d 18. b 19. c 20. a

CHAPTER 3

1. False 2. False 3. True 4. False 5. False 6. e 7. a 8. d 9. e 10. e 11. blow a circuit 12. turn off 13. ventilation 14. ice 15. towel, oven pocket, stone wrappers, and grain bag

CHAPTER 4

1. False 2. True 3. False 4. False 5. True 6. c 7. e 8. c 9. d 10. e 11. igneous, sedimentary, metamorphic 12. intrusive igneous, granite 13. extrusive igneous, basalt 14. sedimentary, limestone & sandstone 15. water, airtight plastic bag 16. b 17. c 18. e 19. a 20. d

CHAPTER 5

1. False 2. False 3. False 4. True 5. False 6. b 7. a 8. c 9. e 10. d 11. entrance 12. warn 13. alternate 14. ice 15. 15 16. b 17. d 18. a 19. c 20. e

CHAPTER 6

1. False 2. True 3. False 4. True 5. False 6. e 7. c 8. c 9. e 10. b 11. beginning / end 12. working / placement 13. quickly / slowly 14. spontaneous / cool off 15. themselves 16. d 17. c 18. e 19. b 20. a

CHAPTER 7

1. False 2. False 3. False 4. False 5. True
6. False 7. True 8. False 9. True
10. False 11. a 12. d 13. d 14. d 15. e
16. 6 to 8, 6 to 8, 12 to 16, 16 to 23 17. left
18. push stones to the right side of skillet
19. tend to the client then resume system
20. hands / stones

CHAPTER 8

1. False 2. True 3. False 4. False 5. False
6. False 7. True 8. False 9. True
10. False 11. c 12. b 13. c 14. c 15. e

16. movement of your own body 17. fulcrum / lever 18. momentum 19. space or an opening 20. weight / vertically / horizontally

CHAPTER 9

1. True 2. False 3. True 4. True 5. False 6. b 7. e 8. d 9. e 10. c 11. alternating 12. teetering 13. sneaking in 14. mother 15. clanking 16. b 17. c 18. a 19. e 20. d

CHAPTER 10

1. False 2. False 3. False 4. True 5. True 6. e 7. d 8. c 9. b 10. c 11. armpit 12. straighten 13. foot 14. behind 15. hip

APPENDIX E

Research Data on Stone Temperature

I did four different experiments. The first experiment, entitled "waiting stones," tested the length of time a stone held its heat when simply sitting on a table, waiting in the wings, with no human contact whatsoever. The room temperature was 65°F and there was a slight breeze coming in the window. Beginning with stones at a temperature of 165°F, readings were taken every 5 minutes for 20 minutes. The second experiment, entitled "placement stones," tested the length of time a stone held its heat when covered with a towel and placed on or beneath the body. Beginning with stones at a temperature of 170°F, readings were taken every 5 minutes for 20 minutes. The third experiment, entitled "working stones," tested the length of time a stone held its heat while being used to massage the body. Beginning with stones at a temperature of 130°F, the first reading was taken after the first 20 seconds and then readings were taken every 10 seconds thereafter for a total of 40 seconds. The fourth experiment, entitled "cold stones," tested the length of time a stone held its cold while being used to massage the body. For this experiment, I only used two stones for comparison, black basalt and white marble. Beginning with stones at a temperature of 35°F, readings were taken every 10 seconds for a period of 5 minutes.

The four stones that held the heat the longest overall from the four experiments were (in order of first to last) brown quartzite (large), white marble (medium and small), red quartzite (medium thick), and black basalt (large). The individual "winners" of each category were as follows. "Waiting stones": Brown quartzite (large) with a resultant temperature of 122°F after 20 minutes of waiting. "Placement stones": White marble (medium-thick) with a resultant temperature of 115°F after 20 minutes of placement. "Working stones": Red quartzite (medium-thick) with a resultant temperature of 118°F after 40 seconds of being massaged along the body. "Cold stones": White marble (medium-thick) took five times longer to go from a temperature of 35°F to 66°F than it took black basalt when massaged along the body. Jadestone (medium) and blue/green basalt (medium) were the stones next in order as far as heat retention. The rest of the stone types fell slightly below the abovementioned ones, with temperature ranges from 109°F down to 103°F in the duration time of the experiments. The varying temperature results of all stones included in the experiment ranged from 122°F to 103°F, which is an approximate difference of almost 20°F from the hottest to the coolest stone. The biggest difference in range of temperatures was found in the category of "waiting stones," which differed from 122°F down to 104°F, a total difference of 18°F. The resultant temperature range for the "placement stones" was 115°F to 103°F, a difference of only 12°F. And similarly, the resultant temperature range for the "working stones" was 118°F to 107°F, leaving a difference of 11°.

So, what is the significance of these data? Let us look at what the difference in temperatures actually means in real time for each category, beginning with "waiting stones." The large brown quartzite stone began with a temperature of 165°F and dropped to a temperature of 122°F, resulting in a total drop of 43°F in a period of 20 minutes. If, for the sake of convenience, we divide the time evenly, that would mean this stone lost its heat at a rate of approximately 2.15°F per minute. Given that there is a total range of 18°F of difference between the stones tested in the "waiting" category, this stone could possibly hold its heat approximately 9 minutes longer than the one that lost its heat the fastest. The significance of this finding is that the stones with the higher thermal emanation factors could add as much as 9 minutes more to their heat retention when waiting in the wings. Thus, it is safe to say that stones such as brown quartzite, white marble, red quartzite, and black basalt hold their heat (when waiting on a table with no body contact or movement) a reasonable amount of time longer than gray basalt, jadestone, and slate and even longer than a reasonable amount of time than blue/green basalt, green quartzite, and New England seastone.

Let's take a look at the category of "placement stones." Their resultant temperatures range from 115°F to as low as 103°F, creating a difference of 12°F. The white marble stone began at a temperature of 170°F and dropped to 115°F after 20 minutes of being placed on (or beneath) a body, creating a drop of 55°F. This means that this placement stone lost 2.75°F every minute. With a range of 12°F difference in the stones in this category, it would be safe to say that this stone held its heat for approximately 4.3 minutes longer than the one that lost its heat the fastest. Gaining 4 minutes for the duration of a placement stone is somewhat significant given that most placement stones lose their heat anywhere from 5 to 20 minutes depending on their size, thickness and the temperature at which they were placed. Thus, once again, the four leading stones still show good evidence for using them over others, as far as placement goes.

Let's now take a look at the category of "working stones." Their results range from temperatures of 118°F to 107°F, creating a total drop of 11°F. The three top stones, red quartzite, with a temperature of 118°F; white marble, with a temperature of 117°F; and brown quartzite, with a temperature of 116°F, all fell into a similar ranges. These stones began at a temperature of 130°F and ended with temperatures of approximately 117°F after being massaged over the body for a time period of 40 seconds. This means that these stones lost, on the average, 13°F in 40 seconds of use, which means a loss of about 1°F approximately every 3 seconds or 0.33°F every second (every degree of temperature gives this stone 3 seconds of use). Thus, with an 11°F range in the temperature loss of the stones in this category, these three stones could hold their heat for approximately 30 seconds longer than the stones that lost their heat the fastest. This is fairly significant in that this stone almost doubles the length of time it can be used for massage in comparison to the stones that lost their heat the fastest.

However, outside of the top three stones, marble, red quartzite, and brown quartzite, which were right around the same temperature, the rest of the stones all fell within a very close range to each other, so any of them would work as good as the other as a second choice, should a therapist choose to use them for their stones. And even though the top three stones do hold their heat longer, there are still valid reasons for using the stones that did not hold their heat as long. For instance, basalt is much more accessible, inexpensive, and smoother than quartzite, and jadestone is magnificent to behold and has special healing powers. And even though white marble seems to hold heat the longest, its smooth, round shape is not naturally found and must be shaped and tumbled artificially; thus, it is more expensive, less available, and has lost some of the energetic qualities found in a stone that has been naturally tumbled. The interesting thing for me about these data is that black basalt has been proclaimed to hold its heat the longest because it is black and originates in lava. But this is apparently not true. Its black color has nothing to do with heat retention, only heat absorption when it is out in the sun. In water, stones of all colors are heated to the same temperature and their retention seems to have more to do with their composition, size, and thickness rather than their color (which is especially proven in that white marble held heat longer than black basalt!).

As far as which stones are best to use for cold stone massage, white marble once again takes the door prize for its ability to retain cold. It took a marble stone, which started at a temperature of 35°F, 5 minutes to reach a temperature of 66°F, while it took a black basalt stone, also starting at 35°F, only 1 minute to reach the same temperature. This shows that white marble retains cold temperatures five times longer than does black basalt, releasing its cold very gradually in comparison to the basalt that releases its cold relatively quickly. Marble's gradual release of cold is very useful for treating injured areas of the body because therapists do not have to replace the cold stones every minute, but instead can keep working with it for up to 5 minutes at a time. Because of its unusual capacity to retain cold, white marble, however, may feel too cold for some clients who have a strong sensitivity and reaction to cold temperatures. For these clients, basalt may be less shocking and thus more useful. Marble is also approximately $25 a stone and must be purchased from a company that shapes it, in comparison to basalt, which can be purchased for $99 for 50 stones or found naturally on beaches or in rivers. Thus, each stone has redeeming qualities for being used with cold.

All of these data have served to gain insight into the stones that have the highest thermal emanation factor; however, it has also helped to make clear that stone choices cannot be based on heat retention alone. While it is advantageous to use stones that hold their heat the longest, other attributes such as cost, availability, texture, beauty, and their energetic state also need to be taken into consideration when choosing the best stones to use for giving a hot stone massage.

TABLES FOR RESEARCH DATA ON STONE TEMPERATURE

The following tables are based on the data derived from the four different experiments.

Table for Experiment #1 Waiting Stones

Room temperature = 65°F/heated 30 min. Temp taken in 5 min. intervals
Waiting stones
Heat lost from stones waiting (on table) to be used for massage

	Not in skillet	Not placed on body			
Time (min)	**Stone Type**	**Large**	**Medium-Thick**	**Medium-Thin**	**Small**
0	**Basalt**	165	165	165	165
5	black	152	140	139	144
10		136	130	129	125
15		128	121	119	110
20		**118**	111	106	105
0	**Basalt**	nda	165	nda	nda
5	gray		145		
10			130		
15			119		
20			**108**		
0	**Basalt**	nda	165	165	nda
5	blue/green		149	133	
10			131	119	
15			120	110	
20			**106**	**106**	
0	**Quartzite**	165	165	165	nda
5	red	141	147	140	
10		130	137	126	
15		120	126	116	
20		113	**119**	109	
0	**Quartzite**	nda	165	165	nda
5	green		143	138	
10			130	118	
15			116	109	
20			**105**	**105**	
0	**Quartzite**	165	165	165	165
5	brown	147	142	135	125
10		138	130	123	112
15		127	119	114	100
20		**122**	111	107	97

(continued)

Table for Experiment #1 Waiting Stones (*Continued*)

Room temperature = 65°F/heated 30 min. Temp taken in 5 min. intervals
Waiting stones
Heat lost from stones waiting (on table) to be used for massage
Not in skillet Not placed on body

Time (min)	Stone Type	Large	Medium-Thick	Medium-Thin	Small
0	**Slate**	165	nda	nda	nda
5		141			
10		134			
15		116			
20		**107**			
0	**New England Seastone**	nda	165	nda	nda
5			133		
10			122		
15			111		
20			**104**		
0	**Jadestone**	nda	165	165	nda
5	polished		137	127	
10			125	116	
15			112	105	
20			**107**	99	
0	**Marble**		165	165	165
5	polished		146	147	147
10			135	134	134
15			122	121	120
20			**120**	**119**	**119**

Table for Experiment #2 Placement Stones

Thermal Emanation factors for different types and sizes of stones
Temp. taken at intervals of 5 min/heated for 30 min/room temperature 65°F
Placement Stones
Heat lost from stones placed on body with no movement over the skin

Time (min)	Stone Type	Large	Medium-Thick	Medium-Thin	Small
0	**Basalt**	170	170	170	170
5	black	155	140	142	136
10		139	130	133	102
15		124	114	118	107
20		**106**	105	102	99
0	**Basalt**	nda	170	nda	nda
5	gray		147		
10			135		
15			120		
20			**103**		

Table for Experiment #2 Placement Stones (*Continued*)

Thermal Emanation factors for different types and sizes of stones
Temp. taken at intervals of 5 min/heated for 30 min/room temperature 65°F
Placement Stones
Heat lost from stones placed on body with no movement over the skin

Time (min)	Stone Type	Large	Medium-Thick	Medium-Thin	Small
0	**Basalt**	nda	170	170	nda
5	blue/green		144	142	
10			128	126	
15			112	110	
20			**105**	104	
0	**Quartzite**	170	170	170	
5	red	147	147	144	nda
10		134	134	128	
15		119	120	110	
20		108	**111**	102	
0	**Quartzite**	nda	170	170	nda
5	green		143	138	
10			128	124	
15			111	110	
20			**103**	**103**	
0	**Quartzite**	170	170	170	170
5	brown	147	144	144	133
10		135	129	131	116
15		123	114	115	105
20		**111**	105	106	100
0	**Slate**	170			
5		141	nda	nda	nda
10		125			
15		121			
20		**108**			
0	**New England Seastone**	nda	170	nda	nda
5			132		
10			124		
15			115		
20			**105**		
0	**Jadestone**	nda	170	170	nda
5	polished		143	136	
10			128	122	
15			119	114	
20			**107**	105	
0	**Marble**	nda	170	170	170
5	polished		159	156	154
10			133	132	128
15			129	126	123
20			**115**	**115**	**112**

Table for Experiment #3 Working Stones

Thermal Emanation factors for different types and sizes of stones
Temp taken after 20 sec and every 10 sec thereafter/
Working stones room temperature 65°F 30 min heat
Heat lost from stones as used in massage, moving over the skin

Time (min)	Stone Type	Large	Medium-Thick	Medium-Thin	Small
0	**Basalt**	130	130	130	130
20	black	119	118	116	116
30		115	114	110	110
40		**110**	103	105	105
0	**Basalt**	nda	nda	130	130
20	gray			118	115
30				114	113
40				**108**	107
0	**Basalt**	nda	130	130	nda
20	blue/green		123	118	
30			115	114	
40			**110**	108	
0	**Quartzite**	130	130	130	nda
20	red	120	122	112	
30		115	120	107	
40		110	**118**	105	
0	**Quartzite**	nda	130	130	nda
20	green		115	111	
30			112	106	
40			**107**	104	
0	**Quartzite**	130	130	130	130
20	brown	122	115	112	110
30		118	112	108	105
40		**116**	104	106	107
0	**Slate**	130	nda	nda	nda
20		120			
30		118			
40		**114**			
0	**New England Seastone**	nda	130	nda	nda
20			118		
30			115		
40			**109**		
0	**Jadestone**	nda	130	130	nda
20	polished		117	110	
30			113	106	
40			**110**	105	
0	**Marble**	nda	130	130	130
20	polished		127	125	119
30			121	119	113
40			**117**	115	108

Table for Experiment #4 Cold Stones		
Cold Stones Cold lost or Heat gained every 10 seconds **Time**	**Black Basalt**	**White Marble**
0	35	35
10 sec	57	45
20 sec	60	46
30 sec	62	47
40 sec	64	48
50 sec	65	49
1 min	**66**	50
1 min 10 sec		51
1 min 20 sec		51
1 min 30 sec		52
1 min 40 sec		51
1 min 50 sec		52
2 min		53
2 min 10 sec		54
2 min 20 sec		55
2 min 30 sec		56
2 min 40 sec		56
2 min 50 sec		57
3 min		57
3 min 10 sec		58
3 min 20 sec		59
3 min 30 sec		59
3 min 40 sec		59
3 min 50 sec		60
4 min		60
4 min 10 sec		61
4 min 20 sec		62
4 min 30 sec		63
4 min 40 sec		64
4 min 50 sec		65
5 min		**66**

Table for Data of End Results from the Four Experiments

Type of Stone	Waiting Stone	Placement Stone	Working Stone	Cold Stone
Marble (white) Medium-thick/medium	**120/119**	**115**	**117**	**66°F in 5 min**
Red Quartzite Medium-thick	**119**	**111**	**118**	
Brown Quartzite Large	**122**	**111**	**116**	
Black Basalt Large	**118**	106	**110**	66°F in 1 min
Gray Basalt Medium	108	103	108	
Jadestone Medium	107	107	**110**	
Slate Large-thin	107	108	109	
Blue/Green Basalt Medium	106	105	**110**	
Green Quartzite Medium	105	103	107	
New England Seastone	104	105	109	

APPENDIX F

Suggested Readings and References

SUGGESTED READINGS

The following books offer more information on various aspects of the anatomy, physiology, pathology, geology, energy of stones, gemstones, chakras, and alternative stone techniques. Again, these are just a handful of suggestions from the multitude of books on these topics. Don't limit yourself to these books for additional reading.

Alexandra S. *The Art of Stone Healing*. Boca Raton, FL: Sonia Alexandra Inc.; 2004.

American Geological Institute, Bates R, Jackson J. *Dictionary of Geological Terms*. Rev. ed. Garden City, NY: Anchor Press Doubleday; 1984.

Anagnostakos GJ, Tortora NP. *Principles of Anatomy and Physiology*. 10th ed. Hoboken, NJ: John Wiley & Sons Ltd; 2002.

Bates R, Jackson J. *The Glossary of Geology*. 2nd ed. Falls Church, VA: American Geological Institute; 1980.

Bentley E. *Head, Neck & Shoulders Massage: A Step-by-Step Guide*. New York: St. Martin's Griffin; 2000.

Blanche C. *The Book of Touch & Aroma: Sensual Ways with Massage and Aromatherapy*. Alexandria, VA: Time Life; 1999.

Dietrich R, Skinner B. *Rocks and Rock Minerals*. New York: John Wiley & Sons, Inc.; 2001.

Gardner J. *Color and Crystals: A Journey Through the Chakras*. Freedom, CA: The Crossing Press; 1988.

Greene L, Greene R. *Save Your Hands! Injury Prevention for Massage Therapists*, 1st ed. Coconut Creek, FL: Gilded Age Press; 2000.

Hess M, Mochizuki S. *Japanese Hot Stone Massage*. Boulder, CO: Kotobuki Publications LLC; 2002.

Higley C, Higley A. *Quick Reference Guide for Using Essential Oils*. 10th ed. Olathe, KS: Abundant Health; 2006.

Kunz GF. *The Curious Lore of Precious Stones*. New York: Dover Publications Inc.; 1913.

Lily S. *Healing with Crystals and Chakra Energies*. 2nd ed. New York: Barnes & Noble; 2004.

Mein CL. *Releasing Emotional Patterns with Essential Oils*. Rancho Santa Fe, CA: Vision Ware Press; 1998.

Premkumar K. *Pathology A to Z—A Handbook for Massage Therapists*. Calgary, Alberta, Canada: VanPub Books; 1999.

Scott-Moncrieff C. *Detox: Cleanse and Recharge Your Mind, Body and Soul*. London: Collins and Brown; 2001.

Thomas S. *Massage for Common Ailments*. London: Gaia Books Ltd.; 2006.

Thrash CL, Thrash A. *Home Remedies, Hydrotherapy, Massage, Charcoal and Other Simple Treatments*. Seale, AL: New Lifestyle Publishing; 1981.

Werner R. *A Massage Therapist's Guide to Pathology*. 4th ed. Baltimore: Lippincott Williams & Wilkins; 2008.

Zand J, Spreen A, LaValle J. *Smart Medicine for Healthier Living*. Garden City Park, NY: Avery Publishing Group; 1999.

REFERENCES

Chapter 1

No References

Chapter 2

1. Abbott GK. The Circulation-Hydrostatic Effects, Principles and Practice of Hydrotherapy for Students and Practitioners of Medicine, 1914. Available at: http://www.balneoklinika.com/ptbimf/hydro5.htm. Accessed August 8, 2008.
2. Kimball J. Organization of the nervous system. Available at: http://users.rcn.com/jkimball.ma.ultranet/BiologyPages/P/PNS.html. Accessed August 8, 2008.
3. Thrash A, Thrash C. *Home Remedies: Hydrotherapy, Massage, Charcoal and Other Simple Treatments*. Seale, AL: Thrash Publications; 1981:25, 140; reprint 2001.
4. Barnes T. Newsletter. Available at: http://www.Tanjabarnes.com/newsletter/Fall2001.html. Accessed August 8, 2008.
5. Cobb L. Herbal care for tired muscles. Available at: http://www.motherearthnews.com/Natural-Health/1982-11-01/Herbal-Care-for-Tired-Muscles.aspx. Accessed August 8, 2008.
6. Rouzier P. Heat therapy. University of Michigan Health System Web site. Available at: http://www.med.umich.edu/1libr/sma/sma_htherapy_sma.htm. Accessed August 8, 2008.
7. Klabunde R. *Cardiovascular Physiology Concepts*. Baltimore: Lippincott Williams & Wilkins; 2004.
8. Zand J, Spreen A, LaValle J. *Smart Medicine for Healthier Living*. Garden City Park, NY: Avery Publishing Group; 1999:341.
9. *Alternative Treatments for Aids;* 2001–2004. Life Research Universal. Acquired immunodeficiency syndrome. Available at: http://www.liferesearchuniversal.com/aids3.html. Accessed October, 2008.
10. Is HIV/AIDS contagious? WrongDiagnosis.com Web site. Available at: http://wrongdiagnosis.com/ h/hiv_aids/contagious.htm#contagiousness. Accessed August 8, 2008.
11. Mayo Foundation for Medical Education and Research. Arteriosclerosis/atherosclerosis. Available at: http://www.cnn.com/HEALTH/library/DS/00525.html. Accessed August 8, 2008.
12. Traditional Chinese medicine for arteriosclerosis. Available at: http://www.holistic-online.com/Remedies/Heart/arter_TCM.htm. Accessed August 8, 2008.
13. Medical College of Wisconsin. The Facts about Arthritis. Available at: http://healthlink.mcw. edu/article/960326819.html. Accessed August 8, 2008.
14. William C, Shiel WC, Jr., Schoenfield LJ. Ice or heat—"which should I apply?" Available at: http://www.medicinenet.com/script/main/art.asp?articlekey=18347. Accessed August 8, 2008.
15. Zand J, Spreen A, LaValle J. *Smart Medicine for Healthier Living*. Garden City Park, NY: Avery Publishing Group; 1999:121–122.
16. The Nemours Foundation. Can the Weather Affect My Asthma? Available at: http://kidshealth.org/kid/health_problems/allergy/weather_asthma.html. Accessed August 8, 2008.
17. Clot busting drugs. Your Total Health Web site. Available at: http://heart.healthcentersonline. com/bloodclot/clot-busters.cfm. Accessed August 8, 2008.
18. The Associated Press. Studies: more heat aids cancer therapies. Available at: http://uplink.space.com/showflat.php?Cat=&Board=humanbio&Number=347316&page=5&view=collapsed&sb=5&o=0&fpart.html. Accessed August 8, 2008.
19. American Cancer Society. Hyperthermia. Available at: http://www.cancer.org/ docroot/ETO/content/ETO_1_2x_Hyperthermia.asp. Accessed August 8, 2008.
20. Zand J, Spreen A, LaValle J. *Smart Medicine for Healthier Living*. Garden City Park, NY: Avery Publishing Group; 1999:240.
21. Bradley B. Hot weather concerns for pumpers. Available at: http://www.diabeteshealth.com/read,3003,4303.html. Accessed August 8, 2008.
22. Premkumar K. *Pathology A to Z—A Handbook for Massage Therapists*. Calgary, Alberta, Canada: VanPub Books; 1999:112.
23. Edema. e Notes Web site. Available at: http://health.enotes.com/medicine-encyclopedia/edema. Accessed August 8, 2008.
24. Zand J, Spreen A, LaValle J. *Smart Medicine for Healthier Living*. Garden City Park, NY: Avery Publishing Group; 1999:285.
25. Cohen MR, Gish R. *The Hepatitis C Help Book*. New York: St. Martin's Griffin; 2001:5–19.
26. Bricklin M. *The Practical Encyclopedia of Natural Healing*. Emmaus, PA: Rodale Press; 1983:306.
27. American Association for Clinical Chemistry. Kidney and urinary tract function, disorders, and diseases. Available at: http://www.labtestsonline.org/understanding/conditions/kidney-2.html. Accessed August 8, 2008.
28. Premkumar K. *Pathology A to Z—A Handbook for Massage Therapists*. Calgary, Alberta, Canada: VanPub Books; 1999:156–157.
29. Barnes A. The about MS section. Available at: www.netcomuk.co.uk/~abarnes/ms.html. Accessed August 8, 2008.
30. Premkumar K. *Pathology A to Z—A Handbook for Massage Therapists*. Calgary, Alberta, Canada: VanPub Books; 1999:229–230.
31. Stevens K. The proper use of heat and cold to manage pain. Available at: http://www.arthritisinsight.com/medical/pain/heat.html. Accessed August 8, 2008.
32. Neuropraxia. Available at: http://en.wikipedia.org/wiki/Neuropraxia. Accessed October 2008.
33. Parkinson's disease. FAQs.org Web site. Available at: http://www.faqs.org/health/Sick-V3/Parkinson-s-Disease.html. Accessed August 8, 2008.

34. Pownall M. Health news-Siestas may help to beat heat-waves. Available at: http://www.bupa.co.uk/health_information/html/health_news/190805copingwith-heat.html. Accessed August 8, 2008.
35. Medicines and Summertime Heat. Available at http://www.agingincanada.ca/medications_and_heat.htm. Accessed October 2008.
36. Pergament E, Schechtman AS, Rochanayon A. Hyperthermia and pregnancy. Available at: http://www.fetal-exposure.org/HYPERTH.html. Accessed August 8, 2008.
37. Raynaud's Disease: The Reason Behind Cold, White Fingers And Toes. Available at http://www.medicalnewstoday.com/articles/70780.php. Article date: May 13, 2007. Accessed October 2008.
38. The Effect of Limb Position on the Vasodilator Response to Cold in the Finger. John Dickson, Department of Physiology, The Queen's University of Belfast. Available at http://jp.physoc.org/cgi/reprint/135/1/93.pdf. Accessed October 2008.
39. Zand J, Spreen A, LaValle J. *Smart Medicine for Healthier Living*. Garden City Park, NY: Avery Publishing Group; 1999:500.
40. Mayo Foundation for Medical Education and Research. Scleroderma. Available at: http://edition.cnn.com/HEALTH/library/ DS/00362.html. Accessed August 8, 2008.
41. Premkumar K. *Pathology A to Z—A Handbook for Massage Therapists*. Calgary, Alberta, Canada: VanPub Books; 1999:6.
42. Chabot K. The art of stone therapy. *Massage Ther J* 2003;Fall:47.
43. Tendinitis. Available at: http://www.ajc.com/health/altmed/shared/health/alt medicine/ConsConditions/Tendinitiscc.html. Accessed August 8, 2008.
44. Facts about Temporomandibular Joint (TMJ) Dysfunction Syndrome and Related Headache, Neck Pain, Jaw and Face Pain. 2008 Head and Neck Pain Center. Available at http://www.headandneck.com/book/tmj.html. Accessed October 2008.

Chapter 3

No References

Chapter 4

1. Kunz GF. *The Curious Lore of Precious Stones*. New York: Dover Publications Inc.; 1913:Preface.
2. Breese R. Personal communication. March 30, 2007.
3. Dietrich R, Skinner B. *Rocks and Rock Minerals*. New York: John Wiley & Sons, Inc.; 2001:4.
4. Raup O. Personal communication. June 21, 2007.
5. Bates R, Jackson J. *The Glossary of Geology*. 2nd ed. Falls Church, VA: American Geological Institute; 1980:513.
6. Chesterman C. *The Audubon Society Field Guide to North American Rocks and Minerals*. New York: Alfred A. Knopf; 1978:715.
7. Liddicoat RT Jr.. *Handbook of Gem Identification*. 9th ed. Los Angeles: The Gemological Institute of America; 1993:247–248.
8. Levine JS. The Repair, Replacement & Maintenance of Historic Slate Roofs: Where Does Slate Come From. Available at: http://www.slateroof.com/tech4.htm. Accessed August 7, 2008.
9. Crichton C. *Healing Stone Massage*. Director: Sean Riehl; 2001.
10. American Geological Institute, Bates R, Jackson J. *Dictionary of Geological Terms*. Rev. ed. Garden City, NY: Anchor Press Doubleday; 1984:103.
11. Chabot K. The Breath within the Stone. Available at: http://www.massagetherapy.com/articles/index.php/article_id/56. Accessed Aug 7, 2008.

Chapter 5

No References

Chapter 6

No References

Chapter 7

No References

Chapter 8

No References

Chapter 9

No References

Chapter 10

No References

Glossary

A

Active hyperemia—Physiologic response in which blood rushes to an area recovering from an application of cold.

Acute—Having a sudden onset and involving intense pain and other symptoms that typically resolve promptly with appropriate medical intervention. Contrast *Chronic*.

Alternating—A technique that involves alternating the stone-held hands beneath any part of the body.

Aromatherapy—The use of essential oils to promote health and well-being. The fragrances and oils can be applied to the body or introduced into the air through a variety of heating methods.

Ayurveda—A 2,000-year-old system of medicine practiced in India that is based on a holistic approach, which focuses on establishing and maintaining balance of the life energies within us, rather than on individual symptoms. The Sanskrit definition of *ayu* is life, while *veda* means knowledge.

B

Balm—An ointment, cream, or other skin product that relieves muscular pain and inflammation through dissemination of heat.

Basalt—A dark-colored extrusive igneous rock with small fine-grained crystals that forms as a result of rapid cooling on the earth's surface.

Bubbling spring—The acupuncture point kidney 1, located at the ball of both feet. Holding this spot at the end of a massage is very calming and grounding.

C

Carpal tunnel syndrome—A type of entrapment neuropathy in which the median nerve, which runs through a narrow tunnel formed by ligament and carpal bones at the base of the hand, is compressed by inflammation of the nearby tendons and surrounding tendon sheath. This inflammation is typically caused by chronic repetitive stress, such as from working with the wrist in a bent position.

Chi—A form of energy that the ancient Chinese believed flowed through the body via channels called *meridians*. Traditional Chinese medicine explains that the blockage of chi causes both mental and physical diseases.

Chronic—Having a gradual onset and characterized by signs and symptoms that are difficult to interpret, persist for a long time, and generally cannot be prevented by medical interventions. Contrast *Acute*.

Circling—A technique that involves the vertical dropping of weight through the heel of the hand to make circles with the stone.

Clanking—A technique where the edges of placement stones are struck against one another.

Compression—A calming technique that utilizes the weight of an additional stone or sand/grain bag laid on top of the placement stones. Compression can be increased by adding the weight of the hands.

Concave tool stone—A stone with a concave or indented surface that accommodates the contours of a bony protuberance.

Counterirritant—Substance applied topically to produce a slight irritation or inflammation in order to relieve pain or deeper inflammation.

Criss-crossing—A technique that is similar to gliding but done in crossing patterns.

Cryotherapy—Clinical application of cold to treat an ailment, relieve pain, and/or improve the client's general state of well-being.

Crystal—A regular polyhedral form bounded by plane surfaces that are formed by a repeating internal arrangement of atoms. Crystals are found within mineral stones.

Curved tool stone—A stone with a curve, either on its side or tip, that is useful for working the various shapes and contours of the body.

D

Deltoid—A thick triangular muscle covering the shoulder joint used to raise the arm from the side. It originates on the lateral third of the clavicle, acromion, and spine of scapula and inserts in the middle of the lateral surface of the humerus.

Derivation—Physiologic process by which heat draws blood to the surface of the body.

Draping—A technique that allows the client's body weight to drape or fall over the stone.

E

Edging—A technique that opens a muscle by using the edge of a stone to push or "scrape" the muscle fibers into submission.

Elephant walking—Is similar to compression but done with alternating hands that move up and down the body slowly like an elephant's feet walking.

Embracing—A technique for encompassing and massaging both sides of the client's body simultaneously.

Energetic vibration—Using stones to create a vibration that sends energy deep into the body by means of tapping, clanking, or rubbing together.

Erector spinae—The largest muscle mass of the back. It lies near the vertebral column and runs along the length of the spine. It is divided into three longitudinal columns, the iliocostalis, longissimus, and spinalis muscles, and assists in extension, lateral flexion, and rotation of the spine.

Extrusive—A type of igneous rock that is formed as magma erupts from a volcano and pours as lava onto the earth's surface, where it cools rapidly.

F

Flowing placement—Use of warm working stones for placement on the body during the flow of a massage.

Flushing—A technique that uses light, sweeping strokes with a large flat stone to soothe and "clean out" an area that has just received deep specific work.

Foot-hand or arm—The therapist's hand or arm that is closest to the client's foot when facing the side of the table.

Four-pile system—A system of stone management created by the author to reduce the amount of interruption necessary during a hot stone massage.

Friction—A technique similar to rubbing, but instead of rubbing stones against each other, they are rubbed back and forth against the client's skin.

Fulcrum—The point at which a lever's force is transmitted to a weight.

G

Gastrocnemius—The largest and most prominent muscle of the calf whose action is to extend the foot and bend the knee. It originates on the lateral condyle of femur and highest of three facets on lateral condyle (above knee joint) and it inserts into the calcaneus at the same place as the soleus muscle joining tendons to make up the *achilles'* tendon.

Geo-thermotherapy—Use of stones to deliver heat to the body to treat an ailment, relieve pain, and/or improve the client's general state of well-being.

Gliding—A technique that involves sliding a hot oiled stone along the muscle in a long sweeping motion.

Gluteus—A broad and thick fleshy mass made up of three gluteal muscles (gluteus maximus, minimus, and medius) and otherwise known as the buttocks.

Granite—An intrusive igneous rock generally light in color, high in silica, and composed of coarsely grained large crystals that result from slow cooling in the earth's interior.

H

Hamstrings—The three tendons that insert behind the knee and connect to the muscles located in the back of the thigh, referred to as the *semitendinosus*, *semimembranosus*, and the *biceps femoris*.

Head-hand or head-arm—The therapist's hand or arm that is closest to the client's head when facing the side of the table.

Heeling—A technique that utilizes the heel of the hand to increase the depth or specificity of gliding.

Hogu—A large intestine acupuncture point located in the middle of the meaty part of the webbing of the thumb. This spot is known to relieve headaches when worked. It is often very painful to work.

Hot stone massage—The incorporation of heated (and cooled) stones into a session of traditional massage or other bodywork.

Humerus—A long bone in the arm that runs from the shoulder to the elbow, anatomically sitting between the scapula and the radius and ulna.

I

Igneous rock—Type of rock that arises from the cooling and solidification of molten matter from the earth's interior.

Iliac crest— The long curved upper border or crest of the wing of the ilium, or the upper part of the bony pelvis. It is thinner at the center than at the extremities.

Iliotibial band—A thick, wide fascial layer that runs from the iliac crest of the pelvis to the knee joint. It is often referred to as the *IT Band*.

Infrared temperature gun (also called an *optical pyrometer*)—A tool that measures temperature by aiming its infrared laser beam at an object.

Infraspinatus—A thick triangular muscle that originates from the infraspinous fossa of the scapula and inserts laterally to the greater tubercle of the humerus. It is a lateral rotator of the glenohumeral joint and an adductor of the arm.

Inside hand or arm—The therapist's hand or arm that is closest to the client when facing the client's head or feet.

Intrusive—A type of igneous rock that is formed within the earth's interior from magma trapped in pockets within a magma reservoir and cooled slowly.

J

Jadestone (or **jade**)—An extremely tough, fine-grained metamorphic stone consisting of jadeite or nephrite.

L

Laminar groove—The groove that runs along either side of the entire spinal column made of paraspinal tissue. It is the dip that exists between the transverse process and the erector spinae mass.

Latissimus dorsi—A pair of fan-shaped muscles across the middle and low back that attach to the arms and the spine and work to adduct, extend, and medially rotate the arm. They are often referred to as the *lats*.

Lava—Molten rock that has erupted from an active volcano.

Lever—A rigid object, such as a metal bar or long bone, fixed to a stationary fulcrum and used to lift a weight.

Lift and drag—A technique that involves lifting a stone against the underside of the body so that it drags rather than glides along the muscle.

Limestone—A sedimentary rock composed chiefly of the mineral calcium carbonate derived from the remains of marine animals.

M

Magma—A naturally occurring molten rock material generated within the earth and capable of intrusion and extrusion from which igneous rocks are derived.

Marble—A rock formed by the metamorphic recrystallization of limestone or dolomite.

Masseter—A thick, somewhat quadrilateral muscle, consisting of two portions, superficial and deep, both originating from aspects of the zygomatic arch and inserting into aspects of the mandible. It aids in chewing or masticating.

Metamorphic rock—Type of rock that is formed through the transformation and change of preexisting rocks due to heat, pressure, or changes in chemical environment.

Mineral—A naturally formed element or compound having a specific and definite range in chemical composition and a characteristic crystal form.

Molten—Melted state of rock.

Mother-father technique—Massage technique used to shorten muscle fibers in an area of the body that cannot be anatomically moved into its short position. The "father" hand uses the thumb or a stone to penetrate the muscle while the "mother" hand pushes the tissue towards the father hand. The term originated with massage therapist Grant Freeman of Crestone, Colorado.

N

Nerve conduction velocity—The speed of conduction of impulses through a nerve.

New England seastone—A conglomerate metamorphic granitic stone consisting mostly of mineral composites such as granite, feldspar, magnetite, dark- and light-colored quartz, and ore.

O

Occipital ridge—The region at the back of the head where the base of the skull meets the spine.

Occlusion—Clinically induced temporary blockage of the blood supply, trapping toxins next to the skin.

Opposition—The movement of opposite ends of a muscle or body part further away from each other, which lengthens and (when released) softens the tissue.

Outside hand or arm—The therapist's hand or arm that is furthest from the client when facing the client's head or feet.

P

Palace of weariness—The acupuncture point pericardium 8, located in the center of the palm of both hands. Holding this spot at the end of a massage is very calming and grounding.

Paws digging—A technique for softening tissues using stones in a motion similar to that of a dog digging in the sand with its two front paws.

Pectoralis—Two muscles, one major and one minor, located on the lateral edges of the upper chest just medial of the shoulders. They originate from the sternum, clavicle, and ribs and insert on the bicipital groove of the humerus and anterior lip of the deltoid tuberosity as well as the coracoid process of scapula. They serve to flex, adduct, and medially rotate arms, as well as elevate ribs and aid in inspiration.

Phenomenal Touch Massage—Massage modality created by the author from which the three-dimensional principles and moves (used in this book) are derived. Phenomenal Touch is a trademarked name.

Pin and stir—A technique that involves pinning the tip of a stone in place on the belly of a muscle and moving the limb in a range of motion around the pinned stone.

Placement stones—Stones that are used for static placement on the body.

Pointed tool stone—A stone with a pointed tip that is used for working trigger points and very specific areas of tension.

Q

Quadratus lumborum—A muscle that is irregularly quadrilateral in shape, broader below than above. It originates from the iliolumbar ligament at the iliac crest and inserts into the lower border of the last rib for about half its length and into the transverse processes of the upper four lumbar vertebrae.

Quadriceps—The large four-part extensor muscle at the front of the thigh often referred to as the *quads*. The four parts of this large muscle mass are named rectus femoris, vastus lateralis, vastus medialis, and vastus intermedius.

Quartzite—A metamorphic rock that is formed from the sedimentary rock sandstone (or chert) that has been heated and recrystallized during metamorphic processes.

R

Reactive hyperemia—Physiologic response to the removal of an occlusion in which blood rushes to the site.

Resistance—Tension created when a muscle opposes pressure. This tires and thereby relaxes the muscle.

Retrostasis—Physiologic process in which cold draws blood away from the surface and to the interior of the body.

Rhomboid(s)—Two muscles, comprised of a major and minor, that originate on the spines of the seventh cervical and upper thoracic vertebrae and supraspinous ligaments and insert into lower half of the posteromedial border of scapula. Their purpose is to retract scapula and rotate it to the rest position of the glenoid cavity.

Rock—Any naturally formed aggregate or mass of mineral matter making up an appreciable part of the earth's crust.

Rolling—A simple technique accomplished by rolling a round stone back and forth or up and down the body.

Rotator cuff—A set of muscles and tendons that secures the arm to the shoulder joint and permits rotation of the arm. It is comprised of four muscles—supraspinatus, infraspinatus, teres minor, and subscapularis.

Rubbing—A technique that is accomplished by vigorously rubbing the sides of two stones against each other.

S

Sandstone—A classic sedimentary rock that is formed from the cementing together of sand-sized grains. Quartz is the most abundant mineral in sandstone.

Sandwiching— A technique that involves covering a body part with a stone on either side.

Sedimentary rock—A stratified soft rock that is formed by the consolidation of transported sediments derived from the physical and chemical breakdown of pre-existing rocks or from chemical precipitation from solution.

Semiprecious gemstones—An arbitrary designation of a gemstone of lesser value than a diamond, ruby, or emerald. Some examples are jasper, jade, and turquoise.

Slate—A metamorphic rock that is formed from the consolidation of shale, a sedimentary rock composed of fine silts, clays, volcanic dusts, or other very fine-sized grains of rock.

Snaking the spine— A technique that uses the point of a stone to carve an S-curve down the spine.

Sneaking under—A technique that involves bringing a stone beneath the body in a smooth and subtle fashion.

Soleus—A broad flat muscle in the calf of the leg that lies under the gastrocnemius muscle and plantar flexes foot. It originates on the soleal line and posterior border of tibia and posterior shaft of fibula and inserts in the calcaneus at the same place as the gastrocnemius muscle.

Squeeze, twist, and slide—A technique that involves squeezing a stone up from beneath a body part and then rapidly twisting and sliding it the rest of the way.

Static placement—Use of individual stones or layouts of several stones underneath or on the client's body before or during the massage. These stones are used solely for placement and not for massage.

Stone entrance—The way in which a stone is brought into the massage and first makes contact with the skin.

Stone flipping—A technique used with a very hot stone to prevent burning or discomfort for both the client and the therapist.

Stone table—The table on which the stones, skillet, and accessories are placed.

Stone wrapper—Elastic Velcro strap used to hold stones in place.

T

Tapping—A technique whereby very specific vibration is sent vertically into the body by tapping one stone directly down onto a placement stone.

Teetering—A technique that utilizes draping on a very specific part of the body.

Temporal—A muscle that originates in the temporal fossa and fascia and inserts in the coronoid process of the mandible. Its location is normally referred to as the temples and its purpose is to close the jaw.

Temporomandibular joint—The joint between the head of the mandible (lower jaw bone) and the tubercle of the temporal bone, otherwise known as TMJ.

Teres minor—Is a narrow, elongated muscle of the rotator cuff that originates from the axillary border of the scapula and inserts into the lowest impression on the greater tubercle of the humerus. Its purpose is to stabilize the shoulder joint and medially rotate and adduct the arm.

Thermal emanation factor—The measured length and rate of time in which a stone gives off heat.

Thermo-cryotherapy—Clinical application of alternating heat and cold to treat an ailment, relieve pain, and/or improve the client's general state of well-being.

Thermotherapy—Clinical applications of heat to treat an ailment, relieve pain, and/or improve the client's general state of well-being.

Three-dimensional hot stone massage—An approach to hot stone massage in which the therapist effortlessly moves the client's body in space in order to massage both sides simultaneously with stones.

Tonify—To enhance or restore balance and to strengthen various parts of the body, including blood and all organs.

Tool stones—Concave, arched, or pointed stones used to massage the body in a specific manner.

Trapezius—A muscle commonly known as the *trap(s)*, extending from occipital bone and nuchal plane to the clavicle. Its purpose is to draw the scapula backward and rotate it to raise the shoulder.

Trigger point—A small, isolated tight spot in the muscle tissue that is tender to touch and causes referred pain to another area distant from itself.

U

Undulation—A wavelike rippling motion created by moving the client's body in a gravitational dance.

V

Vascular gymnastics (also *vascular whip* or *circulatory whip*)—Physiologic response to the rapid and constant alternation of applications of heat and cold in which vessels repeatedly dilate and constrict.

Vastus lateralis—A muscle that originates from the posterior ridge of the femur as far as the greater trochanter and inserts into the tibia in order to extend the leg.

W

Working stones—Stones that are actively used to massage the client.

Z

Zygomatic arch—A paired bone of the human skull that articulates with the maxilla, temporal bone, sphenoid bone, and frontal bone. It forms a part of the orbit and is commonly referred to as the cheekbone.

Index

Page numbers followed by f indicate figure; those followed by t indicate table.